Laboratory-acquired Infections

History, incidence, causes and prevention

Fourth edition

C. H. Collins
MBE, DSc, FRCPath, FIBiol

Senior Visiting Research Fellow, Department of Microbiology, Imperial College School of Medicine at the National Heart and Lung Institute, London, UK

and

D. A. Kennedy
MA, PhD, CBiol, MIBiol, FIBMS, FIOSH

Visiting Fellow, Cranfield Biomedical Centre, Cranfield University, Bedfordshire, UK

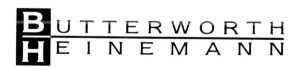

OXFORD   AUCKLAND   BOSTON   JOHANNESBURG   MELBOURNE   NEW DELHI

Butterworth-Heinemann
Linacre House, Jordan Hill, Oxford OX2 8DP
225 Wildwood Avenue, Woburn, MA 01801-2041
A division of Reed Educational and Professional Publishing Ltd

A member of the Reed Elsevier plc group

First published 1983
Second edition 1988
Third edition 1993
Fourth edition 1999

British Library Cataloguing in Publication Data
A catalogue record for this book in available from the British Library

Library of Congress Cataloguing in Publication Data
A catalogue record for this book is available from the Library of Congress

ISBN 0 7506 4023 5

Typeset by Keytec Typesetting Ltd, Bridport, Dorset, UK
Printed and bound in Great Britain by MPG Books Ltd, Bodmin, Cornwall

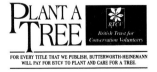

FOR EVERY TITLE THAT WE PUBLISH, BUTTERWORTH-HEINEMANN
WILL PAY FOR BTCV TO PLANT AND CARE FOR A TREE.

Contents

Preface to the fourth edition

Since 1983, when the first edition of this book was published, about 150 new cases of laboratory-acquired infections have been reported, and not a few earlier ones have come to light. The number of unreported cases will never be known and those we do hear about may well represent only the tip of an iceberg. During the same period there have been many official (and a fair number of private) reports expressing concern and offering advice about safety in microbiology. A number of authoritative guidance documents and regulations have been promulgated, designed to protect the worker from infection.

We have considered the failure to stem the flow of these infections and suggest that the following are contributory factors: (1) lack of instruction in safe procedures for handling infected material; (2) the removal of trained and experienced workers from the laboratory to managerial posts elsewhere; (3) the emergence of new and the resurgence of old diseases which have caught some people unaware; (4) poorly designed and ill-equipped laboratories; (5) lack of protection of workers; and (6) an inadequate system of inspection of premises where pathogens are handled.

In this edition, as well as updating accounts of infections, we have tried to address these shortcomings and have included sections on precautions in work with new agents and procedures, as well as risk assessments.

Once again, we are indebted to our colleagues for help and advice, and for tracing references. To those named in earlier editions, we must add Dr A. Arai (Japan), Professor R. Clark (Cranfield University), Professor S. Honjo (Japan), Professor S. Shibata (Japan) and Dr R. Slade (London).

C. H. Collins   D. A. Kennedy
Hadlow   Kingston upon Thames

Preface to the first edition

Public concern about the hazards, real, potential and imaginary, of work with pathogenic microbes was aroused recently by the smallpox incidents in London and Birmingham, and by fears of epidemics arising from the importation of viruses such as those of Lassa fever and of the products of recombinant DNA research.

Laboratory-associated infections are not new phenomena, however, as this book is intended to illustrate. My personal interest in them and their prevention was aroused in the late 1950s when the risks of inhaling aerosols from liquid cultures of tubercle bacilli became apparent and an enlightened employer, the Public Health Laboratory Service (PHLS) Board, supplied its workers with the first effective commercially produced biological safety cabinets which had been designed by its own scientists. Further interest was stimulated when Dr G. Briggs Phillips visited the London (County Hall) laboratory during his world-wide study (1959–1960) of safety in microbiological laboratories. Dr Phillips' report led me to collect information from published material and individuals and institutions. It resulted in the firm conviction that good laboratory practice is the key to laboratory safety and this was the theme behind the various editions of the book *Microbiological Methods* (1974–1979) and the PHLS Monograph *Prevention of Laboratory Acquired Infection* (1974–1976).

Continued interest brought participation in official inquiries and reports, such as those of Godber (Category A pathogens), Maycock (hepatitis), Howie (Category B and C pathogens) and the Safety Measures in Microbiology programme of the World Health Organization.

The information presented here has been garnered from many publications and in conversations with many scientists during meetings, official and casual, and visits to 103 laboratories in the UK and six other countries. The book is mainly concerned with infections caused by those agents which do not excite public or political concern. No particular reference is made to recombinant DNA research as this is no longer an emotive subject: there is no evidence to suggest that the methods used in microbiological laboratories to contain pathogens are not equally adequate for such research and its industrial applications.

Personal opinions expressed in this book on the causes and prevention of laboratory-associated infections are my own and do not reflect those of my employers or of any other official body. I am, however, deeply grateful to the PHLS Board and to past and present Directors of the Service and of the London (County Hall and Dulwich) laboratories for time and facilities to continue these studies alongside my official duties. I am particularly indebted to the following scientists who have given me specific information and advice which could not reasonably be acknowledged in the references: Dr T. Bektemirov (USSR); Mr W. Bruce (UK); Dr M. A. Buttolph (UK); Dr D. Coates (UK); Surgeon Commander H. M. Darlow (UK); Dr J Forney (USA); MR W. J. Gunthorpe (UK); Mr G. Harper (UK); Sir James Howie (UK); the late Dr R. J. C. Harris (UK); Professor M. L. Koch (FRG); Dr S. W. B. Newsom (UK); Mr V. R. Oviatt (WHO); Dr K. M. Pavri (India); Captain W. V. Powell (USA); Dr J. Richardson (USA); Dr J. Songer (USA); Dr M. Scruton (UK); Dr A. E. Wright (UK).

C. H. Collins
Hadlow

Chapter 1

Laboratory-acquired infections

In spite of an ever-increasing number of official and other publications, guidelines and codes of practice there is still an annual increment of reports, in print and anecdotal, of laboratory workers who have become infected with microorganisms with which they work. Since the 1890s more than 5000 cases of laboratory-acquired infections have been reported and at least 200 of these caused the death of the worker. The annual numbers of reported infections remained steady at something less than 100 until 1990, but are now declining. Figure 1.1, adapted from Williams (1981) and extended, shows the numbers of publications, and the numbers of reports of laboratory-acquired infections

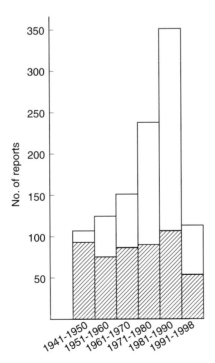

Figure 1.1 The numbers of publications about laboratory-acquired infections in the last six decades. The hatched areas show the number that reported actual infections

between 1941 and 1998, culled from our own literature searches and the
Laboratory Safety Listings of the Canadian Laboratory Centre for Disease
Control.

There can be little doubt, however, that such laboratory-acquired infections
are still under-reported. There are three possible reasons for this:

1. In many countries there is no statutory requirement for such notification.
Nor is there any machinery for collecting such data. (In the UK, however, there
is a legal requirement to report laboratory-acquired infections under the *Reporting of Injuries, Diseases and Dangerous Occurrences Regulations 1994*,
although the information collected is regarded as confidential and therefore not
in the public domain.)

2. Some laboratory directors and managers back away from admitting that
infections have occurred among their staff for fear of reprisals or opprobrium.

3. Pressure of space in scientific and medical journals discourages editors
from publishing such reports unless they refer to new, rare or unusual infections.

Unfortunately, some of these infections have been transmitted from those
workers to members of their families and to others outside the laboratory. Yet
again, biological agents, as they are now known, have 'escaped' from laboratories and infected members of the public and contaminated the environment.
Although the deliberate release of genetically-modified microorganisms into the
environment is generally well regulated (Chapter 19) there is still the public
perception that if they *are* accidentally or deliberately released into the environment further genetic recombination between them and the 'natural' microbial
flora may result in new biological agents having the ability to cause disease.

What is a laboratory-acquired infection?

It is not always easy to define a laboratory-acquired infection or to conclude
with certainty that one has occurred.

If a person is working with a microorganism which is not present in the
community in which he or she lives and he or she becomes ill with a disease
caused by that organism, there can be no doubt that he or she became infected in
the course of his or her work. If another individual, who does not handle that
microorganism but works in the same room, another part of the building or is
merely a visitor, becomes ill and the organism is recovered from his or her body
he or she also qualifies as a case of laboratory-acquired infection. The criterion
in these cases is proximity to an organism that is not present at that time in the
community: the disease is unlikely to have been contracted elsewhere.

Problems arise when a laboratory worker's illness is caused by an organism
that is present in the laboratory and *also* in the community. There is always the
possibility that he or she will acquire such an infection during the 16 hours of
the day when not at work. Evidence that an infection with such organisms is
acquired in the laboratory is usually circumstantial. There may have been an
accident that released the organisms into the room. Apart from traditional
bacteriological and serological typing of the organism from the worker which
may suggest that it is a current laboratory strain, it is now possible, by restriction
fragment length polymorphism (RFLP) analysis, to confirm in some cases that
the strains are identical. This has been done recently in cases of laboratory-
acquired tuberculosis (Peerbohms *et al.*, 1995). There may also be clinical

evidence suggesting, for example, that the individual received an unusually large dose of the infecting organism or that it entered his body by an unusual route. Epidemiological investigations, made during outbreaks or epidemics, may indicate a laboratory rather than a natural infection because of discrepancies in incubation times or activities that do not fit into the general patterns. Subclinical infections cannot be quantified unless there are reasons, such as accidents or known exposures, for serological testing when seroconversion is evidence of infection.

It is especially difficult to assess the likelihood that diseases such as tuberculosis (which have long and uncertain incubation periods) and those where the presentation is atypical (because the route of infection is not that occurring in the community) are contracted in the laboratory. Again, the evidence may be circumstantial: the individual may have worked with the organism for a long period. A single case could be of doubtful origin, but two or more in the same laboratory in a short period would be regarded with much more suspicion.

Laboratory-associated infections

It may also be difficult to decide whether an infection that arises from contact with a microorganism outside the laboratory can be defined as laboratory acquired. Sulkin and Pike (1951) included infections such as relapsing fever resulting from the collection, during field work, of ticks for laboratory examinations but excluded infection acquired during contact with patients in hospitals. They excluded a case of chicken pox in a laboratory technician which resulted from contact with a patient in hospital. It is not clear if the technician was performing some laboratory exercise on the patient. Today, if she were collecting blood from such a patient she might be included in the statistics of laboratory-acquired infections on the grounds that she was engaged in laboratory work at the time, although this was not specifically directed at chicken pox, unlike that of the tick collectors, who were probably looking for spirochaetes. If the chicken pox patient carried hepatitis virus, and the technician contracted hepatitis after pricking herself with the hypodermic needle she certainly would be recorded as having a laboratory-acquired infection. Again, one would exclude an infection acquired by a physician during the examination of a patient unless he or she was obtaining material for laboratory tests or conducting an autopsy.

The problem, therefore, is in making a distinction between laboratory-acquired and laboratory-associated infections. Sulkin and Pike (1951) attempted to classify the infections reported to them as definite, probable or possible with respect to their origin in the laboratory. The classification was based on the opinion of the person who reported the case or incident, or, if this was not given, on the circumstances and nature of the infection. They considered that a laboratory-acquired infection was one that resulted from laboratory work, whether it occurred in a laboratory worker, or in another person who happened to be exposed as a result of work with infectious agents. It is important that they used the words *resulted from*, rather than *during* laboratory work. This takes care of the woman with chicken pox, the tick collectors and the doctors. It can also include people who do not work in the laboratory building but to whom the infection is transmitted by one who does, and those who become infected as a result of the escape of agents handled therein, e.g. the smallpox cases in England (Report, 1974; DH, 1980a) and the Sverdlovsk anthrax incident in 1979 (see Meselson *et al.*, 1994). It would be difficult to find a better definition today.

Autopsy-associated infections

A number of the infections mentioned in this chapter were acquired by pathologists, technicians and assistants during autopsies. It may be argued that they are not 'laboratory acquired', but in the first four decades of this century pathology had not separated into distinct disciplines and the staff moved freely between laboratories and mortuaries. Today, autopsy work is restricted to histopathologists, forensic pathologists and their staff, but it still cannot be divorced from clinical laboratory activities.

Shifts and trends in laboratory-acquired infections

Although the total number of infections has fallen in the past few years, there appears to have been a shift away from those associated with the inhalation of infected airborne particles, loosely termed aerosols, towards those where mucocutaneous and percutaneous exposure has been incriminated. One reason for this may well have been the mandatory, instead of voluntary, use of microbiological safety cabinets (Kiley, 1992), e.g. in the European Union as a result of the general adoption of the Biological Agents Directive (EC, 1990).

Table 1.1 compares the most commonly reported laboratory-acquired infections in four surveys (Harrington and Shannon, 1976; Pike, 1978; Miller *et al.*, 1987; and Grist and Emslie, 1985, 1987, 1989, 1991). Although not strictly comparable, as some are global and others are for England and Wales only, they show a shift away from brucellosis and Q fever. It is of interest that laboratory-acquired shigellosis was much more of a problem in the UK than elsewhere.

TABLE 1.1 The most commonly reported laboratory-acquired infections, 1975–91

Harrington and Shannon, 1976[a]	Pike, 1978[b]	Miller, 1987[c]	Grist and Emslie, 1981–91[d]
Brucellosis	Brucellosis	Brucellosis	Shigellosis
Tuberculosis	Q fever	Tuberculosis	Tuberculosis
Q fever	Hepatitis	Psittacosis	Hepatitis
Hepatitis	Typhoid	Leptospirosis	Salmonellosis
Tularaemia	Tularaemia	Dermatomycoses	
Typhus	Tuberculosis	Newcastle disease	
Typhoid	Dermatomycoses	Salmonellosis	
Psittacosis	Venezuelan equine		
Fungal infections	encephalitis		
Shigellosis	Psittacosis		
	Coccidiomycosis		

[a] UK clinical laboratories.
[b] Global.
[c] US Animal Diseases Center.
[d] UK clinical laboratories.

Tuberculosis remains high in the lists, as may be expected in view of the resurgence of the disease (WHO, 1996). Numbers for laboratory-acquired hepatitis have declined also, possibly as a result of the AIDS epidemic, which has led laboratory workers, regardless of the new regulations, to handle blood with greater care—although this epidemic has itself resulted in a number of laboratory-acquired infections.

Some laboratory-acquired infections are now history. For example, since 1991 (when material for the third edition of this book was assembled) no new reports have been found of tularaemia, plague, leptospirosis, cholera and typhoid fever, nor of the many rarer viral infections. Others, however, like the poor, are always with us and some have not been previously reported (Table 1.2)

Fortunately, the emergence of 'new' microbial diseases, and the resurgence of some thought to be in decline, if not well under control, have resulted in comparatively smaller numbers of some laboratory-acquired infections (Table 1.3). Infections from newly identified agents are still a risk, however (Kruse *et al.*, 1991), e.g. the recent report of a laboratory infections with Sábia virus, *Escherichia coli* O157 and hantaviruses (see below).

TABLE 1.2 The changing pattern of laboratory-acquired infections since 1991

New reports not found	Continuing infections	'New' infections
Cholera	Brucellosis	*E. coli* O157
Leptospirosis	Cryptosporidiosis	Helicobacteriosis
Plague	Hantavirus	*Haemophilus ducreyi*
Rat-bite fever	Hepatitis B	Parvovirus B19
Tularaemia	Lymphocytic choriomeningitis	Schistosomiasis
Typhoid	HIV	Sabia virus
	Meningococcal disease	
	Murine typhus	
	Q fever	
	Salmonellosis	
	Shigellosis	
	Sporotrichosis	
	Tuberculosis	

TABLE 1.3 Emergent and resurgent microbial agents, 1976–96, that have been associated with or have a potential for laboratory-acquired infections

Vibrio cholerae	S. America, India, Asia
Cryptosporidium spp.	Europe, USA
Dengue fever virus	Australia, C. and S. America
Corynebacterium diphtheriae	Russia
Escherichia coli O157	Europe, S. Africa, USA
Hantaviruses	Europe, Mexico, USA, S.E. Asia
Hepatitis C virus	Worldwide
Neisseria meningitidis	Worldwide
Sabia haemorrhagic fever virus	Brazil
Tuberculosis	Worldwide
Yellow fever (sylvan)	Kenya

Data from CDC (1994).

Surveys and accounts of infections

There are two kinds of reviews and surveys of laboratory-acquired infections: those that report a wide range of infections and those that deal with diseases caused by specific organisms or groups of related or similar organisms often occurring as institutional and common-source outbreaks.

Some doubts are often cast on the usefulness of both kinds because they are retrospective, some even relating to events that occurred 20, or even 40, years ago. As indicated above, some of the microorganisms that were important agents of infection among laboratory workers in the 1950s to 1970s are no longer a problem. Some, that report point-source incidents where a number of people have been infected, are unique: they are unlikely to be repeated.

Nevertheless, these reports will be useful in making risk assessments in institutions that handle microorganisms. The general surveys will be considered first.

General surveys

The most extensive, and historically the most important, of these surveys was initiated by Sulkin and Pike (1951) who sent questionnaires to about 5000 laboratories in the USA, including those belonging to state and local health departments, hospitals, medical and veterinary schools, teaching institutions, commercial biological laboratories and government departments. An attempt was also made to obtain estimates of the numbers of people at risk, but through no fault of the investigators this was not very successful. The total number of infections, including those culled from the literature, was 1342, of which 1275 had occurred since 1930. Sulkin and Pike maintained files on laboratory infections and, in 1964, reported that the total number had risen to 2348 cases with 107 deaths (Sulkin, 1964).

The next paper in this series was by Pike et al. (1965) who widened the investigation to include countries outside the USA and accumulated 641 additional reports of infections. Significant changes were observed in the ratio of bacterial to virus infections. The former had predominated in the two decades 1930–50, with 57% bacterial and 20% viral infections. Between 1950 and 1965 the percentage of bacterial infections fell to 30% and virus infections had risen to account for 39%; 11 of the 13 additional deaths were due to viruses. There appeared to be a reduction in the incidence of reported infections, which had reached a peak in the USA about 1950 and this was attributed to an increased awareness of the risks of infection and to better protective measures. Although tularaemia was now the commonest infection, only three (research) laboratories were involved. Brucellosis and leptospirosis followed in the bacterial league tables. Tuberculosis was thought to be under-reported, because of the well-known problem of establishing that it was acquired in the laboratory. All the tuberculosis cases in this report were extrapulmonary; these were easier to relate to laboratory activities. Among the virus infections, hepatitis fell to second place after encephalitis and yellow fever disappeared, probably because of immunization practices. Attention was drawn to the hazards of attenuated organisms and old laboratory strains, several of which had caused infections. These included *Salmonella typhi*, *Brucella abortus* Str 19, *Bacillus anthracis* and chlamydia.

Ten years elapsed, and Dr Sulkin died before the next report (Pike, 1976) was published. In this one a total of 3921 infections was reported, with 164 deaths (4.1%). The number of different kinds of microorganisms involved had risen to 164; 37 of these were bacteria, 90 viruses (some recently identified), three chlamydia, nine fungi and 16 parasites. Bacterial infections now numbered 1669 (42.6%) with 69 deaths (4.1%); viral infections, 1049 (26.7%) with 54 (5.1%) deaths; rickettsial infections, 573 (14.6%) with 23 (5.6%) deaths; chlamydial infections, 128 (3.3%) with 10 (7.8%) deaths; fungal infections, 353 (9.0%) with five (1.4%) deaths; parasitic infections, 115 (2.9%) with two (1.7%) deaths, and unspecified infections, 34 (0.9%) with two (2.9%) deaths. It is worth noting that the number of bacterial infections was some 600 more than that of virus infections. The death rates were not very different, 4.1% for bacterial and 5.1% for viral diseases. The death rate for rickettsial infections was 4.0%. The 'top ten' had changed too, although brucellosis was still at the top of the table with 423 infections (10.8%), followed by Q fever 278 (7.1%); typhoid 256 (6.5%); hepatitis 234 (8.3%); tularaemia 225 (5.7%); tuberculosis 176 (4.5%); dermato-mycoses 161 (4.1%); Venezuelan equine encephalitis (VEE) 141 (3.6%); psittacosis 116 (3%); and coccidiomycosis 93 (2.4%).

Pike reiterated the earlier observations of himself and his colleagues that the numbers of any infections are likely to be inflated by institutional outbreaks: for example, 45 of the brucella infections resulted from a common exposure; tularaemia occurred only in the few laboratories that handled it; 13 of the erysipeloid infections occurred in one institution and one laboratory reported 23 cases of cutaneous anthrax. About half the cases of Venezuelan equine encepha-litis were reported by four laboratories and in one of these a single accident was responsible for 24 cases; 53 of the 67 Kyasanur Forest virus infections occurred in one laboratory and 31 of the 40 cases of vesicular stomatitis occurred in one other. Each of several laboratories reported more than 15 infections with the agent of Q fever.

Pike (1978) reviewed past and present hazards of working with infectious agents and observed that since his 1976 summary 158 more cases, with four deaths had been reported, bringing the total to 4079 and 168 deaths. The 'top ten' remained much the same except that hepatitis was promoted over typhoid fever. The last of Pike's reviews (1979) was concerned largely with institutional and common source infections (which are considered later) and with individual infections.

The surveys conducted by Dr Pike and his colleagues were not the only ones that were published in this period. Cook (1961) had already published an account of 26 laboratory-acquired infections (and two allergic reactions) that had occurred in the Texas State Health Department laboratories between 1934 and 1958. Seven of these were due to bacteria, eight to viruses, 10 to rickettsias and three to parasites.

Oya (1975) reported that there had been 33 bacterial or fungal, 22 viral and 14 rickettsial infections in the Japanese National Institute of Health laboratories in a period of 25 years. In another report from Japan Shimojo (1975) reported 61 incidents of viral infections among 35 laboratories, in some of some which more than 10 people were involved. Influenza virus was the most common, occurring in the preparation of vaccine as well as in diagnostic work, although Australia antigen (hepatitis B) and rickettsias also figured. These may have been included in Pike's figures, but they are not referenced in any of his papers. There do not appear to be any later reports from Japan. It is also not clear if any of the

423 cases of laboratory-acquired infections that occurred at one US institution (Wedum, 1978) were included by Pike.

Since Pike's last report (1979) there have been five further surveys, all in the USA. An 8-year survey conducted by Jacobson *et al.* (1985) of laboratory-acquired infections in Utah showed an annual incidence of 3 per 1000 workers. Hepatitis was the most frequent infection, with shigellosis and tuberculosis trailing. The numbers of cases were small, making interpretation difficult.

Miller *et al.* (1987) carried out a 25-year survey of laboratory-acquired human infections at the National Animal Center. Of 128 exposures 103 resulted from known accidents; the remaining 25 were identified only after clinical or serological evidence had accrued. Brucellas were the most commonly reported followed by chlamydia and mycobacteria.

Vesley and Hartman (1988) assessed infection incidence in 54 state and territorial public health laboratories and 165 hospital clinical laboratories in Minnesota. The infection rates were 1.43 for the former and 3.5 per 1000 full-time equivalents for the latter.

Sewell (1995) built on the earlier American reports, adding a number of new cases or reports of infections with agents mentioned earlier and also some that had not previously been incriminated (parvovirus B19, hantaviruses, cryptosporidia).

Harding and Lieberman (1995) reviewed 58 publications with the following findings: 65 bacterial infections, predominantly with *Salmonella typhi*, *Brucella melitensis* and chlamydia; 119 viral infections, mostly miscellaneous, with arboviruses and hantaviruses, 162 rickettsial infections, 153 of which were caused by *Coxiella burnetii*; 13 with protozoa and three with fungi. Of particular interest was evidence of seroconversion, in the absence of symptoms, with an Ebola-related filovirus, parvovirus B19, ECHO and orf viruses.

No comparable surveys have been carried out in Europe, but two morbidity surveys (i.e. all infections among laboratory workers, whether occupational or not) among workers in the UK have yielded useful information. The first of these was by Harrington and Shannon (1976) who sent questionnaires to 24 000 medical laboratory workers in England, Wales and Scotland asking if, during 1971 (England and Wales) or 1973 (Scotland), they had developed tuberculosis, hepatitis, shigellosis or brucellosis. Other information about age, sex, laboratory duties, etc. was also requested. Replies were received from more than 90% of laboratory staff. Pulmonary tuberculosis was reported in 21, hepatitis in 38, shigellosis in 45 and brucellosis in one.

A few years later a series of investigations into the morbidity rates in clinical laboratory workers was started in the UK on behalf of the Association of Clinical Pathologists and (later) the Institute of Medical Laboratory Sciences (now the Institute of Biomedical Science) by Grist (1975, 1976, 1978, 1980, 1981a,b, 1983) and Grist and Emslie (1985, 1987, 1989, 1991). The first four of these were concerned only with hepatitis and the last five included other infections. Not all of the infections reported were clearly laboratory acquired. Those that could be attributable during the years 1979–89 are listed in Table 1.4. It is interesting to note that shigellosis, which does not figure very highly in the American reports, tops this list (23 cases), with hepatitis B second (18). Unfortunately, this useful investigation seems to have been discontinued.

The Subcommittee on Arbovirus Laboratory Infections (SALS, 1980) listed

TABLE 1.4 Attributable infections in the UK, 1979–89

Shigellosis	23	Zoster	2
Hepatitis B	18	Malaria	1
Tuberculosis	8	Erysipelas	1
Salmonellosis	8	Glandular fever	1
'Bowel infections'	3	Herpes	1
Streptococcal	3	Vibriosis	1
Brucellosis	2	Staphylococcal	1

From Grist (1981a, 1983); Grist and Emslie (1985, 1989, 1991).

TABLE 1.5 Laboratory infections with arboviruses*

Apeu	2	Mayoro	5
Bebaru	1	Modoc	1
Bhanja	6	Mucambo	10
Bluetongue	1	Muructucu	1
Bunyanwera	4	O'nyong-nyong	1
Caraparu	5	Oriboco	1
Catu	5	Oropouche	7
Chikungunya	39	Orungo	13
Colorado tick	16	Ossa	1
Dugbe	2	Piry	13
Germiston	6	Pichende	17
Hypr	37	Powassan	2
Issyk-kul	1	Spondweni	4
Japanese encephalitis	22	Semliki Forest	3
Keystone	1	Tacaribe	2
Koutango	1	Wesselbrun	13
Kunjin	5	West Nile	18
Machupo	1	Ziki	4
Marituba	1		

Data from the Subcommittee on Arbovirus Laboratory Safety of the American Committee on Arthropod-borne Diseases (SALS, 1980)

infections with those agents. Those for which no individual publications (see below) were found are summarized in Table 1.5.

Recorded cases: published reports

Reports of infections with specific organisms are scattered through medical and scientific literature published over the last 90 or so years. Although we have attempted to document as many as possible there are probably more cases than those listed below, but enough are cited to illustrate their importance. There may, of course, be some overlapping as more than one group of workers sometimes publish accounts of the same outbreak or incident, and authors tend to review one another's work. The agents causing infections have been classified as bacterial, viral, rickettsial and chlamydial, fungal and protozoal and within each group are presented in alphabetical order rather than in order of numerical incidence.

The numbers of cases of infections by various agents cited will facilitate the assessment of risk in laboratories that handle them. An agent summary is included, following the example of Richmond and McKinney (CDC/NIH, 1993), as are some comments on some recent cases. The mode of laboratory-acquired infection is given (ingestion, inhalation, through the skin (cutaneous, muco- or percutaneous (see Chapter 2)) or vector), as is the availability of a vaccine. The circumstances surrounding some of the infections are outlined in Chapter 2.

This information is also included in a bibliography of occupationally-acquired infections available on the Internet (http:/www.boku.ac.at/iam/efb/lai.htm) by courtesy of the Institut für Angewandte Mikrobiologie, Universitat für Boden-kultur, Vienna and the Safety in Biotechnology Working Party of the European Federation of Biotechnology.

Principal bacterial agents

BACILLUS ANTHRACIS

Agent summary:
Aerobic Gram-positive spore-bearing bacillus. Worldwide. Anthrax, pulmonary or cutaneous. Zoonosis: cattle, sheep, wild animals. Laboratory infection: inhalation, cutaneous. Vaccine (only for those at risk).

Infections have been reported by Popov (1914), Lubarsch (1931), Shanahan *et al.* (1947), Soltys (1948) and Krug and Glen (1953). Pike's (1976) tables include 45 cases with five deaths. Ellingson *et al.* (1946) reported 25 cases of cutaneous anthrax among armed forces personnel in one institution. In 1979 there was an escape of anthrax from an establishment in the former USSR (Sverdlovsk). There were 96 cases of anthrax among the local population, 76 of which were gastrointestinal and 17 cutaneous, with 64 deaths (reviewed by Meselson *et al.*, 1994).

BORDETELLA PERTUSSIS

Agent summary:
Aerobic Gram-negative non-sporing bacillus. Worldwide. Whooping cough (pertussis). Laboratory infection: inhalation. Vaccine.

Cook (1961) reported an infection in a worker who had aerated liquid cultures for vaccine preparation. McKinney *et al.* (1985) described a possible infection in a person who worked in a building where research was being done on pertussis vaccine. The organism was recovered from this patient but not from several others who may have been infected.

BORRELIA RECURRENTIS; B. DUTTONI

Agent summary:
Spirochaete. Arthropod vectors. European (*B. recurrentis*) and African (*B. duttoni*) relapsing fever. Laboratory infection: per/mucocutaneous (blood), vector.

Infections were reported by Alexandroff (1927), Iwanowa (1928), Namikawa (1929) and Grunke (1933). Pike (1976) lists 45 cases with two deaths.

BRUCELLA SPP.

Agent summary:
Aerobic (some capnophilic) Gram-negative non-sporing bacilli. Worldwide. Undulant and Mediterranean fevers. Zoonosis: cattle, goats, etc. *B. abortus*, *B. melitensis*, *B. suis*. Laboratory infection: inhalation, muco/percutaneous. Animal vaccine only.

Brucellosis has the distinction of being the most frequently-acquired laboratory infection in the past (Pike, 1978) and infections still occur. According to Dalrymple-Champneys (1960) 'anyone working for any considerable time with cultures of brucella is likely to become infected'.

A comprehensive survey of the incidence of laboratory infections with brucellas made in the 1950s gave a total of 1334 cases (US Treasury, 1950). This report concluded that handling large volumes of cultures, with consequent aerosol release, was a more important factor than poor technique.

The first report found was that of Birt and Lamb (1899), and thereafter reports and reviews of laboratory infections were made by Nicolle (1906), McCulloch *et al.* (1907), Arloing *et al.* (1910), Burnet (1925), Huddleson (1926), Hardy *et al.* (1927), Gilbert and Coleman (1928), Moss and Castenada (1928), Amoss (1931), Humphreys and Guest (1932), Burke-Gaffney (1934), Meyer and Geiger (1935), Tung and Zia (1936), Newitt *et al.* (1939), Huddleson and Munger (1940), Green (1941), Meyer and Eddie (1941), Meyer (1943), Hernandez-Morales (1946), Evans (1947), Spink (1946, 1956), Howe *et al.* (1947), Joiris (1950), Cowan (1951), Biscay and Carbonelle (1951), Green (1951), Merger (1957), Trever *et al.* (1959), O'Brien (1962), Joffe and Diamond (1966), Anon (1969), Smith *et al.* (1980), Gopaul *et al.* (1986), Olle-Goig and Canelar-Soler (1987), Vesley and Chagla (1989), Al-Aska and Chagla (1989), Georghiou and Young (1991), Staszkiewicz *et al.* (1991) and CDSC (1991).

Evidence that laboratory-acquired brucellosis is still a problem is indicated by three more recent reports: Staszkiewicz *et al.* (1991) reported eight cases where work was done on the open bench; Reuben *et al.* (1991) described two cases, one in a laboratory worker who then transmitted the infection to his wife. Batchelor *et al.* (1992) reported three cases resulting from misidentification; Luzzi *et al.* (1993) reported further cases.

Gruner (1994) identified five cases; Martin-Mazuuelos *et al.* (1994) four cases (safety cabinet not used); and Grammont-Cupillard *et al.* (1996) three cases as a result of sniffing cultures; the last report found was by Zervos *et al.* (1997).

The vaccine strain S19 used to immunize cattle has also caused infections, mostly, of course, among veterinary staff: Gilman (1944), Anon (1945), Spink and Thompson (1953), Bardenwerper (1952), Spink (1957), Sadusk *et al.* (1957), Revich *et al.* (1961), McCulloch (1963), Pivnick *et al.* (1966), and Montes *et al.* (1986).

Pike's (1978) worldwide survey revealed 426 brucella infections this century, but Harrington and Shannon (1976) uncovered only one case in the UK in 1971. Miller *et al.* (1987) reported 24 cases in a 25-year review of veterinary laboratory staff. No cases were reported to Grist during 1979–81 (Grist, 1979, 1983) but one laboratory worker was infected with *Brucella melitensis* in 1982 (Grist and Emslie, 1985).

BURKHOLDERI (PSEUDOMONAS) MALLEI

Agent summary:
Aerobic, Gram-negative, non-sporing bacilli. Glanders, systemic disease in humans. Zoonosis: equines. Laboratory infection: inhalation, mucocutaneous.

Anecdotal evidence suggests a high rate of infection among those who handle cultures. The first report of human infection with the glanders bacillus was by Stewart (1904); this was followed by the accounts of Robbins (1906), Bernstein and Carling (1909), Gaiger (1913) and von Brunn (1919). There then seems to have been a gap of several years until the report of Hunter (1936) and another gap before that of six cases by Howe and Miller (1947). The last recorded case seems to be that of Redfearn and Palleroni (1975).

BURKHOLDERI (PSEUDOMONAS) PSEUDOMALLEI

Agent summary:
Aerobic, Gram-negative, non-sporing bacilli. Melioidosis. Far East. Zoonosis, rodents. Laboratory infection: mucocutaneous.

Cases were reported by Cravitz and Miller (1950), Fournier (1960), Nigg (1962), Green and Tuffnell (1974) and Schlecht *et al.* (1981). Ashdown (1992) reported serological evidence of subclinical infection in three workers in one laboratory. Pike's (1976) tables show 20 cases with seven deaths.

CAMPYLOBACTER SPP.

Agent summary:
C. pylori, C. jejuni. Aerobic curved bacilli. Worldwide. Gastroenteritis. Laboratory infection: ingestion.

Oates and Hodgkin (1981) reported an incident but there were earlier reports (Ward, 1948; Jennis and Mazo, 1971) in which the organism was described as *Vibrio fetus.* Penner *et al.* (1983) investigated a laboratory-acquired case of *C. jejuni* enteritis.

CLOSTRIDIUM TETANI

Agent summary:
Anaerobic Gram-positive spore-bearing bacillus. Worldwide. Tetanus. Laboratory infection: mucocutaneous. Vaccine (toxoid).

There was a very early report of a tetanus infection by Nicholas (1893) and two more by Scheidt (1939) and Kucharski *et al.* (1960). Pike (1976) gives 11 cases, six with the organisms and five with tetanus (toxin).

CORYNEBACTERIUM DIPHTHERIAE

Agent summary:
Aerobic Gram-positive non-sporing bacillus. Diphtheria; primary infection usually localized in the upper respiratory tract. Laboratory infection: usually cutaneous. Vaccine (toxoid).

Although diphtheria attracted the attention of many early bacteriologists only one laboratory infection was reported (Riesman, 1898), until well into the twentieth century, when several accounts appear (Mallory, 1913; Baldwin *et al.*,

1923; Hammerschmidt, 1924; Taylor, 1927; Spray, 1927; Wicht, 1969). Most of these were cutaneous infections but Chin (1998) reported a throat infection arising from a quality assurance specimen. Pike (1976) reports 33 cases but no deaths.

ERYSIPELOTHRIX RHUSIOPATHIAE

Agent summary:
Aerobic Gram-positive bacillus. Erysipeloid. Worldwide. Zoonosis: animals, fish (usually). Laboratory infection: cutaneous.

Infections with erysipelothrix have been recorded by Gross (1940), Price and Bennett (1951), Sneath *et al.* (1961) and Ajmal (1969). Pike (1976) records 43 cases.

ESCHERICHIA COLI

Agent summary:
Aerobic Gram-negative bacillus. Some serotypes are agents of gastroenteritis. Laboratory infection: ingestion.

A urinary tract infection was associated with a laboratory strain (Parry *et al.*, 1981). Burnens *et al.* (1993), Gopal *et al.* (1996) and Phillips and Old (1997) all reported laboratory-acquired infections with verotoxin-producing strains (O157) and Booth and Rowe (1993) reported a possible case.

FRANCISELLA TULARENSIS

Agent summary:
Aerobic Gram-negative non-sporing bacillus. North America, Scandinavia. Tularaemia. Zoonosis: rodents, other small mammals, ticks. Laboratory infection: cutaneous, inhalation. Vaccine (restricted).

In spite of its limited distribution, and the relatively small numbers of laboratories that have handled it, *F. tularensis* has acquired an evil reputation for infecting laboratory workers. Very few have escaped infection: Newsom (1976a) remarked that 'Sir John Ledingham is said to be the only bacteriologist in England to have worked on francisellas and to have escaped infection'. Certainly all the original investigators were infected (Lake and Francis, 1922). Laboratory infections have been reported and discussed by McCoy and Chapman (1912), Wherry and Lamb (1914), Ledingham and Frazer (1924), Francis (1922; 1925; 1936; 1937), Dieter (1926), Parker and Spencer (1926), Simpson (1929), Weilbacher and Moss (1938), Johnson (1944), Cooper (1948), Green and Eigelsbach (1950), Kadull *et al.* (1950), Carr and Kadull (1957), Charkes (1959), van Metre and Kadull (1959), Overholt *et al.* (1961) and Ringertz and Dahlstrand (1968). Pike's tables (1978) show 225 infections with two deaths.

HAEMOPHILUS DUCREYI

Agent summary:
Aerobic Gram-negative non-sporing bacillus. Meningitis, conjunctivitis, secondary pulmonary, etc. infections.

Only one report was found: Trees *et al.* (1992).

HAEMOPHILUS INFLUENZAE

Agent summary:
Aerobic Gram-negative non-sporing bacillus. Meningitis, conjunctivitis, secondary pulmonary, etc. infections. Laboratory infection: inhalation.

Two cases have been revealed by a literature search (Walker, 1928) and an eye infection (Jacobson *et al.*, 1985). Pike (1976) noted four cases.

HELICOBACTER PYLORI

Agent summary:
Aerobic, Gram-negative, non-sporing curved bacillus. Associated with gastric disorders. Laboratory infection: ingestion but may be inhalation.

One case was reported by Matysiak-Budnik *et al.* (1995).

LEPTOSPIRA SPP.

Agent summary:
Spirochaetes. Several species and serotypes. Leptospirosis (may develop into Weil's disease). Zoonosis: rats, cattle, dogs (urines). Laboratory infection: muco/percutaneous.

Rodents and dogs, which are common laboratory animals, are the natural reservoir of pathogenic leptospires so laboratory infections are not unexpected. There were early reports by Goebel (1916), Martin and Pettit (1916), followed later by that of Uhlenhuth and Grossman (1926). There was then a steady stream of reports of infections by the different species by Uhlenhuth and Zimmermann (1933; 1934); Korthof (1937); Blumenberg (1937); Welcker (1938); Farrell (1939); Stiles and Sawyer (1942); Schuffner and Bolhander (1942); Borst *et al.* (1948); *Lancet* (1949); Barciszewski and Domanski (1951); Mochaman and Schmutzler (1956); Broome and Norris (1957); Stoenner and MacLean (1958); Kleinschmidt and Christ (1959); Goley *et al.* (1960); Bertok *et al.* (1960); Kappeler *et al.* (1961); Brand and Kathein (1962); Kathe and Mochaman (1962); Sarasin *et al.* (1963); Barkin *et al.* (1974). The most recent is by Gilkes *et al.* (1988). Pike's (1976) survey lists 67 cases with 10 deaths; Miller *et al.* (1987) list four cases.

LISTERIA SPP.

Agent summary:
Aerobic, Gram-positive non-sporing bacilli. Listeriosis. Animals, soil, fodder. Laboratory infection: ingestion.

Although no reports of overt infection were found, Ortell (1975) noted the excretion of listerias by laboratory workers.

MYCOBACTERIUM TUBERCULOSIS AND *M. BOVIS*

Agent summary:
Aerobic, acid-fast, non-sporing bacilli. Tuberculosis: pulmonary and extrapulmonary. Laboratory infection: inhalation, percutaneous. Vaccine (BCG).

As indicated above it is not easy to define laboratory-acquired tuberculosis.

The incidence of pulmonary disease in the general population, its mode of spread, the opportunities for exposure to infection outside the laboratory and the long incubation period make it difficult to determine the source of infection. Anecdotal evidence of laboratory infections is plentiful, but published reports are not.

The high incidence of the disease in medical students compared with that in other students attracted the attention of Hedwall (1940), Myers (1941), Myers *et al.* (1941) and Morris (1946). The difference between the groups was attributed to the periods spent by the medical students in postmortem rooms and pathology laboratories. There are reports and discussions on pulmonary infections by Gruber (1949), *JAMA* (1950), Koch (1951), Canetti *et al.* (1951), Gale (1957), Ebring (1969) and Saint-Paul *et al.* (1972). In the case described by Canetti *et al.* the organisms were resistant to streptomycin; that of Ebring involved super-infection by isoniazid-resistant bacilli. Tuberculosis has also been associated with tissue processing. Workers exposed during the freezing for cryostat sectioning have converted to positive Mantoux tests (Anon., 1980; CDC, 1981b; Duray *et al.*, 1981).

In more recent years infections have been reported by Müller (1988a, 1988b) who found a higher rate in laboratories using Class II safety cabinets than in those that used Class I cabinets or none. Peerbohms *et al.* (1995) reported two infections, one of which is important because restriction fragment length analysis showed that the infecting strain was identical to those from a patient handled by the worker on the day of an accident. Ridzon *et al.* (1997) reported an infection in an HIV-positive phlebotomist who had been exposed to drug-resistant *M. tuberculosis*.

Non-pulmonary infections have also been reported: Alderson (1931) gives an account of disease following a knife wound in a postmortem room; 'Prosector's wart' acquired through injury during autopsies was described by Wilks and Poland (1862), later by Minkowitz (1969) and Allen *et al.*, 1979. Infections arising from pricks and cuts are also described by Stokes (1925), O'Leary and Harrison (1941), Borgen (1953), Webber (1956) and Sahn and Pierson (1974). Sakula (1977) told of a laboratory worker who developed a serious localized chronic tuberculoid granuloma after accidentally inoculating himself with Freund's complete adjuvant containing heat-killed tubercle bacilli. A case of endometrial tuberculosis acquired by a health worker in a clinical laboratory was documented by Shireman (1992).

Chatigny (1961) considered that most of the infections described by Smith (1953) and associated with autopsies were acquired in this way. Tegestrom (1942) reported an infection arising from a splash in the eye; Miller *et al.* (1987) reported four cases. Lundgren *et al.* (1987) reported infections acquired during autopsies and Anon (1995) reported a further five cases.

Infections have also occurred in the laboratory with BCG vaccine material (Hollstrom and Hard, 1953; Engbaek *et al.*, 1977).

For some assessment of the problem one must turn to surveys rather than case histories. In the report by Sulkin and Pike (1951) 153 cases are noted, but Long (1951) pointed out that only 25 of these were definitely associated with laboratory work. Mikol *et al.* (1952) found that the incidence of tuberculosis among technicians in a tuberculosis hospital was nine times that of the community and Merger (1957) writing from Ontario found that the incidence among laboratory staff there was 26 times that among the general population. The numbers involved in these two reports are quite small and the figures may be viewed with some suspicion. Nevertheless, in the UK, Reid (1957) found 98 cases of what he considered to be proved laboratory-acquired tuberculosis among a total of 153 such cases (55 were unproved) and concluded that the various categories of laboratory workers were from two to nine times as likely to contract tuberculosis as matched controls in other occupations. Saint-Paul *et al.* (1972) found a similar incidence among French laboratory technicians. Carbonelle *et al.* (1975) surveyed 23 laboratories and identified 20 accidents among technicians engaged in tuberculosis work. They concluded that in France there were more cases of laboratory-acquired tuberculosis than in other states.

Harrington and Shannon (1976) questioned 21 000 medical laboratory workers in the UK and found 21 new cases of tuberculosis: a five times greater risk than the general population. Pike's (1978) list includes 194 cases with four deaths. Grist (1981, 1983) and Grist and Emslie (1985) reported 33 cases of tuberculosis among laboratory workers and postmortem-room staff between 1979 and 1983, 19 of which were possibly attributable to laboratory exposure. Grist and Emslie (1987) reported another three cases of suspected occupational origin, that occurred during 1984–5, but none in their later surveys.

In a survey carried out by Kao *et al.* (1997) in the USA, 13 of 49 laboratories reported that, between 1990 and 1994, 21 laboratory employees were tuberculin-skin test converters and that seven of these were documented as laboratory-acquired infections.

Regrettably, tubercle bacilli have been used by individuals with suicidal tendencies. There are at least four reports of self-inoculation: Lemiere and Ameuilly (1938), Jones *et al.* (1949), Chien and Wiggins (1954) and Mikhail and Tattersall (1954).

The prevention of laboratory-acquired tuberculosis is discussed in Chapter 13.

MYCOBACTERIUM LEPRAE

Agent summary:
Aerobic, acid-fast, non-sporing, non-cultivable bacilli. Humans. Leprosy. Vaccine trials are in progress.

Marchoux (1934) described one case and this may be the one listed by Pike (1976).

MYCOBACTERIUM MARINUM

Agent summary:
Aerobic, acid-fast, rapid grower. Fresh and salt water, fish. Opportunistic human pathogen—cutaneous lesions.

Chappler *et al.* (1977) reported an infection arising from a needle-stick injury with a culture.

MYCOPLASMA CAVIAE

Agent summary:
Aerobic bacteria not having a cell wall. Pathogenicity uncertain.

Hill (1971) reported an infection following a needle-stick injury.

NEISSERIA GONORRHOEAE

Agent summary:
Aerobic/microaerophilic, Gram-negative diplococci. Humans. Gonorrhoea. Laboratory infection: contact, usually cutaneous or conjunctival.

A cutaneous infection was reported by Sears (1947) and cases of gonococcal conjunctivitis by Diene *et al.* (1976), Bruins and Tight (1977), McCarthy (1978) and Hackney *et al.* (1985).

NEISSERIA MENINGITIDIS

Agent summary:
Aerobic/microaerophlic, Gram-negative diplococci. Meningitis. Laboratory infection: inhalation, conjunctival. Vaccine (some types only).

Hunter (1936) described a fatal infection that occurred in 1918 and *JAMA* (1936) a fatal infection where the eye was the portal of entry. Another was reported by Bhatti *et al.* (1982). More cases have been reported since then (CDC, 1991—two cases; DH, 1993a—three cases; Anon., 1994). Pike (1976) lists eight cases.

PASTEURELLA SPP.

Agent summary:
Aerobic, Gram-positive non-sporing bacilli. Infections of wounds (animal bites and scratches), respiratory tract infection, meningitis. Zoonosis: dogs, cattle, poultry. Laboratory infection: inhalation, mucocutaneous.

Pasteurella infections have been recorded by Boisvert and Fousek (1941), Robinson (1944) and Bergogne-Berezin *et al.* (1972). Pike (1976) notes two cases.

SALMONELLA SPP. (OTHER THAN *S. TYPHI*)

Agent summary:
Aerobic, Gram-negative, non-sporing bacilli. Many species/serotypes. Paratyphoid fevers and food poisoning (salmonellosis). Laboratory infection: ingestion. Vaccine.

Laboratory-acquired salmonella infections other than typhoid fever are not widely reported, possibly because of the usually mild nature of the disease. Some cases that have been reported have been unusual in some respect, such as those of Bruner (1946) involving *S. abortus equi*; Perch (1947), *S. senegal*, and Baumberg and Freeman (1971) where the infecting strain of *S. typhimurium* was thought to have become avirulent. Blaser and Lofgren (1981) reported an infection with *S. agona*, and Steckelberg *et al.* (1988) another with *S. typhimurium*. Pike's tables (1976) show 48 cases. Two cases of suspected occupational origin occurred in the UK in 1984 (Grist and Emslie, 1987) and three in 1986–7 (Grist and Emslie, 1989). Miller *et al.* (1987) list two cases. Wormald (1950) reported two salmonella infections in postmortem-room staff after autopsies on known cases of salmonellosis.

SALMONELLA TYPHI

Agent summary:
Aerobic, Gram-negative, non-sporing bacilli. Typhoid fever. Water- and food-borne. Laboratory infection: ingestion. Vaccine (monovalent).

Among the enteric pathogens typhoid fever is probably the most serious disease. The first known laboratory infection occurred in 1893 (Kisskalt, 1915). Later Kisskalt (1929) reviewed other cases and further reports were published by Achard (1929), von Gara (1931), Draese (1939), Haedicke (1947), Schaefer (1950), Albrecht (1957), Olson *et al.* (1961), Kunz and Ewing (1965), Cook (1961), and Nikodemusz (1975). In 1976 a laboratory porter succumbed to an infection (*Times*, 1977). The latest incident was reported by Hoerl (1988). Among the surveys Pike's tables (1978) show 258 cases up to 1974 with 20 deaths. The UK surveys reported single cases in 1985, 1987 and 1991 Grist and Emslie, 1987, 1989, 1991).

All these cases were presumably associated with the examination of clinical specimens, but Blaser and Feldman (1980) reported the acquisition of typhoid from proficiency-testing specimens and indicted laboratories themselves as reservoirs of infection; they found that, of 24 cases, 21 were associated with proficiency-testing specimens. Earlier the Centers for Disease Control (CDC, 1979a) identified six such cases. Holmes *et al.* (1980) also reported such cases. Stock laboratory strains have also been involved. Olson *et al.* (1961) described an infection with a strain that had been isolated 41 years earlier and the CDC (1979a) noted that 11 cases that were associated with laboratory stock strains. Blaser and Lofgren (1981) reported that a symptomless laboratory worker who handled a stock strain but did not develop the disease, nevertheless transmitted it to two members of his family.

SERRATIA MARCESCENS

Agent summary:
Aerobic, Gram-negative, non-sporing coccobacilli. Upper respiratory tract. Formerly used in aerobiology investigations. Laboratory infection: inhalation.

S. marcescens, formerly used as a marker in aerobiology has caused a number of infections: those reported by Paine (1946), Reitman *et al.* (1955), and probably included in the five listed by Pike.

SHIGELLA SPP.

Agent summary:
Aerobic, Gram-negative non-sporing bacilli. Bacillary dysentery: *S. sonnei*, *S. flexneri*, *S. dysenteriae*. May be zoonotic (monkeys). Laboratory infection: ingestion.

Laboratory-acquired bacillary dysentery is said to be relatively common among laboratory workers (Wilson and Miles 1975). Reports of cases are few, however, and include those of Hirschbruck and Thiem (1918), Lippincott (1925), Kobayaski (1931), Woolpert *et al.* (1939), Rewell (1949) and Sutton and Shanahan (1954). Cook (1961) listed two infections with *S. alkalescens*, one with *S. boydii* and a double shigella/salmonella infection. In spite of this Pike's tables (1976) show 58 cases (but no deaths) and Harrington and Shannon (1976) found 45 cases among technicians in the UK since 1971. Grist (1981, 1983) and Grist and Emslie (1985) reported 15 cases, all 'attributable' or 'occupational' between 1979 and 1983. Seven of these were due to *S. sonnei*, six to *S. flexneri* and two to *S. boydii*. Ghosh (1982) and Dadswell (1983) each reported a laboratory infection with *S. flexneri* but these may also have been reported to Grist. Jacobson *et al*. (1985) reported three cases, two of *S. flexneri* (one from proficiency test material), one *S. sonnei* and one '*Shigella* sp.'. Four *S. flexneri* infections were reported to Grist and Emslie (1989) and in 1991 their survey included one *S. flexneri* and three *S. boydii* infections.

STREPTOBACILLUS MONILIFORMIS

Agent summary:
Aerobic, Gram-negative, non-sporing bacillus. Rat-bite fever and Haverhill fever. Zoonosis: rodents.
    Laboratory infections, mostly resulting from rat bites, have been reported by Clearkin (1928), Allbritten *et al*. (1940), Brown and Nunemaker (1942), Borgen and Gustad (1948), Hamburger and Knowles (1953), Glenhill (1967), Cole *et al*. (1969), CDC (1974a) and Hayes *et al*. (1950).

STREPTOCOCCUS SPP.

Agent summary:
Aerobic, Gram-positive, non-sporing cocci in chains. Scarlet fever, septicaemias. Laboratory infections: inhalation, mucocutaneous.
    There seem to be surprisingly few published reports of streptococcal infections, in spite of the 78 in Pike's survey. Five reports tracked down are pre-penicillin: Freidman (1928), Moltke and Poulsen (1929), Bormann (1930), Habobou-Sala (1932) and Flowers and Hall (1962). Another, more recent and probably acquired from experimental intranasally-infected mice, was noted by Kurl (1981). Streptococcal infections in the mortuary are discussed by Hawkey *et al*. (1980).

TREPONEMA PALLIDUM

Agent summary:
Spirochaete. Worldwide. Syphilis. Laboratory infection: percutaneous.
    No reports of recent infections were found, the latest being in 1976. Infections were reported by Metchnikoff and Roux (1905, 1906), Buschke (1913), Graetz and Delbanco (1914); Levaditi and Marie (1919), Gahylle (1924), Shaw (1941), Wakerlin (1932), Greenbaum (1937), Chacko (1966) and Fitgerald *et al*. (1976). In those of Wakerlin, Shaw and Chacko the rabbit-adapted strain was responsible.

VIBRIO CHOLERAE

Agent summary:
Aerobic, Gram-negative, non-sporing curved bacilli. Mostly tropical and subtropical areas. Asiatic cholera and cholera-like intestinal diseases. Water- and food-borne. Laboratory infection: ingestion. Vaccine.

Among recognized pathogens the cholera vibrio was probably the first to be incriminated in laboratory-acquired infections. Koch (1886) reports that a student in Berlin who handled a culture contracted the disease at a time when no other cases had been reported in that country. Other examples of laboratory infections with this organism were reported in the next few years (Reinicke, 1894; Zlatgoroff, 1909). Since these early days laboratory workers seem to have been able to protect themselves against infection, although there has been a resurgence of the disease in the last few years. Pike's (1976) tables show 12 cases.

VIBRIO PARAHAEMOLYTICUS

Agent summary:
Aerobic, Gram-negative, non-sporing curved bacilli. Gastroenteritis. Seafood. Food-borne. Laboratory infection: ingestion.

Sanyal *et al.* (1973) reported an infection. Pike (1976) reported two non-cholera vibrio infections.

YERSINIA PESTIS

Agent summary:
Aerobic, Gram-positive, non-sporing bacillus. Middle, and Far East, India. Plague (bubonic, pneumonic, septicaemic). Zoonosis: rats, fleas. Laboratory infection: inhalation, mucocutaneous. Vaccine (restricted use).

Plague is an emotive subject and it is not surprising that it has attracted laboratory investigations and as a result has yielded a crop of infections. The first report seems to have been by Wu *et al.* (1923) followed by that of Wu (1926), Hsu (1943), Anon. (1944), *Public Health Reports* (1944), Munter (1945), Lewin *et al.* (1948), Huang *et al.* (1948), Meyer (1950), Link (1951, 1955), Eskey and Haas (1962), Kartman *et al.* (1962), Smirnov (1963) and two from defence establishments, Burmeister *et al.* (1962) and *Lancet* (1962). Pike's tables show only 10 infections (which does not agree with these published reports). Four of these infections were fatal.

Chlamydia, Coxiella and *Rickettsia*

CHLAMYDIA PSITTACI

Agent summary:
Gram-negative, obligate intracellular parasites with some properties in common with bacteria. Causes (1) psittacosis/ornithosis, (2) ovine enzootic abortion. Zoonoses. Laboratory infection: inhalation.

Although natural infections of humans from birds are uncommon, laboratory infections unfortunately are not. There are reports by McCoy (1930; 1934), Hamel (1931), Schmid (1931), Neufeld and Leventhal (1932), Fortner and Pfaffenberg (1934, 1935), Fortner (1936), Rosebury *et al.* (1947), Green (1950), Barwell *et al.* (1955), Cook (1961), Sawyer *et al.* (1968), Schacter *et al.* (1968). Pike's (1978) total was 116 cases, 89% of which occurred before 1955.

CHLAMYDIA TRACHOMATIS

Agent summary:
Gram-negative, obligate intracellular parasites with some properties in common with bacteria. Trachoma, conjunctivitis, urethritis, etc. Laboratory infection: mucocutaneous (airborne).

Trachoma is a comparatively recent addition to the lists. The first reported laboratory infection was by Smith (1958), followed by those of Magruder *et al.* (1963) and DH (1974).

COXIELLA BURNETII

Agent summary:
Gram-negative, obligate intracellular parasites with some properties in common with bacteria. Q fever. Zoonosis: sheep, cattle, ticks. Laboratory infection: inhalation (infected dust), mucocutaneous.

In Pike's (1978) records Q fever was the second most frequently reported laboratory-acquired infection with a total of 280 cases since the first account in 1938, by Dyer. Rapid spread of the disease in the community especially among members of the armed forces led to intensive laboratory investigations especially after the Second World War. Most of the laboratories involved reported more than one case which is evidence of the high infectivity of the agent. Reports of infections have been made by Burnet and Freeman (1939), Smith *et al.* (1939), Hornibrook and Nelson (1940), Robbins and Rustigian (1946), the Commission on Acute Respiratory Diseases (1946), Huebner (1947), Spicknall *et al.* (1947), Lennette *et al.* (1948), Oliphant *et al.* (1949), Kikuth and Bock (1949), Nauck and Weyer (1949), Meiklejohn and Lennette (1950), Lippelt (1951), Stokes (1953), Stoker (1957), Johnson and Kadull (1966), Curet and Faust (1972), Kosina and Kolouch (1975), CDC (1979b), Dritz *et al.* (1979), Bayer (1982), Hall *et al.* (1982), Graham *et al.* (1988) and Hamadeh *et al.* (1992). A case reported by Oliphant and Parker (1948) occurred in a laundry worker (laboratory clothing?) and one by Beeman (1950) was a household contact of a laboratory worker.

Curet and Faust (1972) found that 15 of 29 workers had antibodies to *C. burnetii* and eight had clinical symptoms. Hall *et al.* (1982) found antibodies in 28 of 91 people who handled gravid sheep in a research unit; 14 showed symptoms of infection.

RICKETTSIA MOOSERI

Agent summary:
Gram-negative, obligate intracellular parasites with some properties in common with bacteria. Murine typhus. Zoonosis: rats, fleas. Laboratory infection: mucocutaneous, inhalation. Vaccine.

Six reports were found, one quite recent: Nicolle (1935), Van den Ende *et al.* (1943), Antoine *et al.* (1965), CDC (1978), Berlanca *et al.* (1978), Woo (1991), Norazah *et al.* 1995.

RICKETTSIA ORIENTALIS

Agent summary:
Gram-negative, obligate intracellular parasites with some properties in common with bacteria. Scrub typhus (tsutsugamushi fever). Zoonosis: mongooses, bird, mites. Laboratory infection: mucocutaneous, inhalation. Vaccine (restricted).

Reports of infections include those of Ogata *et al.* (1931), Buckland *et al.* (1945), Van den ende *et al.* (1946), Tullis *et al.* (1947). Pike (1976) reported 35 cases with eight deaths. No recent reports were found.

RICKETTSIA PROWAZEKI

Agent summary:
Gram-negative, obligate intracellular parasites with some properties in common with bacteria. Epidemic typhus. Louse-borne. Laboratory infection: mucocutaneous, inhalation. Vaccine (restricted use).

All reports pre-date 1968: Okamoto and Masayama (1937), Gear and Becker (1938), Gold and Fitzpatrick (1942), Loffler and Mooser (1942), Larsen and Lebel (1943), Tokarevich (1944), Silva and Kopscionska (1945), Cook (1961) and Wright *et al.* (1968).

RICKETTSIA RICKETTSII

Agent summary:
Gram-negative, obligate intracellular parasites with some properties in common with bacteria. Rocky Mountain spotted fever. Zoonosis: dogs, rodents, rabbits, ticks. Laboratory infection: mucocutaneous, inhalation. Vaccine.

Reports of infections have been made by Wolbach (1919), Badger *et al.* (1931), Parker (1938), Campbell and Ketchum (1940), Johnson and Kadull (1967), Calia *et al.* (1970), Sexton *et al.* (1975), Oster *et al.* (1977), CDC (1977a). Pike (1976) noted 63 cases with 11 deaths (17%).

NB. Ricketts died in 1910 and Prowazek died in 1915, both of laboratory-acquired typhus. Several of the above reports originated from establishments producing various typhus vaccines. The number of laboratory infections has declined since successful vaccines were developed.

Viruses

References cited here are limited to published reports of individual infections. For any not listed (e.g. arbovirus infections) see SALS (1980) and Table 1.5 above.

ADENOVIRUS

Agent summary:
Adenoviridae. Worldwide. Upper respiratory tract, meningitis, infantile gastro-enteritis. Laboratory infection: inhalation.

Two reports were found: Jawets *et al.* (1959) and Nasz *et al.* (1963), both with type 8 virus.

BHANJA VIRUS

Agent summary:
Bunyaviridae. Fever, muscle and joint pain, headaches. Laboratory infection: mode not known.

Only one report was found: Callisher and Goodpasture (1975) in a worker who titrated the virus in mice. SALS (1980) gives six infections.

CHIKUNGUNYA VIRUS

Agent summary:
Togaviridae (Alphavirus). Africa. Chikungunya haemorrhagic fever. Zoonosis: monkeys, mosquitoes. Laboratory infection: percutaneous.

Again, only two reports: Ramachandra *et al.* (1964), Shish and Baron (1965). SALS (1980) reported 39 cases.

COXSACKIE VIRUSES

Agent summary:
Picornaviridae. Worldwide. Aseptic meningitis. Humans. Laboratory infection: mucocutaneous.

There are reports by Shaw *et al.* (1950) and Dietzman *et al.* (1973).

CRIMEA CONGO HAEMORRHAGIC FEVER VIRUS

Agent summary:
Bunyaviridae (Nairovirus). Africa, Iraq, Eastern Europe. Haemorrhagic fever. Zoonosis: cattle, small mammals, tick-borne. Laboratory infection: percutaneous.

We found only one report: Karimov (1975) but SALS (1980) mentions eight cases (one fatal).

DENGUE VIRUS

Agent summary:
Togaviridae (Flavivirus). Haemorrhagic fever. Asia, India, Caribbean. Zoonosis: monkey, mosquitoes. Laboratory infection: percutaneous.

There are reports by Melnick *et al.* (1948) and Okunyo (1982). SALS (1980) lists 11 cases.

EASTERN EQUINE ENCEPHALITIS VIRUS

Agent summary:
Togaviridae (Alphavirus). Encephalitis, etc. Central and S. America. Zoonosis: birds, mosquitoes. Laboratory infection: percutaneous.

Olitsky and Morgan (1939), Fothergill *et al.* (1938) and Gold and Hampil (1942) report infections and SALS (1980) lists four.

EBOLA VIRUS

Agent summary:
Filoviridae. Ebola haemorrhagic fever. Zaire, Sudan. Zoonosis (?) monkeys (?),
Laboratory infection: percutaneous.
    Only one report was found: Emond *et al.* (1977).

GANJAM VIRUS

Agent summary:
Bunyaviridae. Nairobi sheep disease. Africa. Zoonosis: sheep, mosquitoes.
Laboratory infection; muco/percutaneous (blood).
    There appears to be only two reports: Dandewate *et al.* (1969) and Rao
(1981).

HANTAVIRUSES

Agent summary:
Arenaviridae. S.E. Asia, N. America, Europe. Emerging disease. Hantaan fever,
Korean haemorrhagic fever, Hantavirus fever with renal syndrome, hantavirus
fever with pulmonary syndrome. Zoonosis: rodents, mites. Laboratory infection:
inhalation.
    Infections were reported by Kulagin *et al.* (1962), Umenai *et al.* (1979), Lee
and Johnson (1982), Desmyter *et al.* (1983), Durin *et al.* (1984), Lloyd and
Jones (1986), Tsai (1987), Wong *et al.* (1988), Pether *et al.* (1993) and CDC
(1994).

HEPATITIS B VIRUS

Agent summary:
Hepadnaviridae. Serum hepatitis. Worldwide. Humans. Laboratory infection:
muco/and percutaneous. Vaccine (recombinant).
    Studies have indicated (Grist, 1987) that the rates of hepatitis B infections
were several times greater among laboratory staff than in the community in
certain geographical areas. It has been one of the most frequently reported
laboratory-acquired infection and in clinical laboratories it is still the most
feared, possibly because it is the only one that is more likely to infect chemists
and haematologists than microbiologists. Although there are at least seven
hepatitis viruses, A, B, C, D, E, F and G, hepatitis B has been responsible for
most of the known laboratory-acquired infections.
    Donovan (1974) cites what may have been the first case of laboratory-
acquired hepatitis, in 1929. This was followed by the report of Findlay *et al.*
(1931). Further cases among laboratory workers were reported by Sheehan
(1944), Liebowitz *et al.* (1949), Kuh and Ward (1950), Trumbell and Greiner
(1951), Hillis (1961), McCollum (1962), Byrne (1966), Ruddy *et al.* (1967),
Sutnick *et al.* (1971), Bone *et al.* (1971), Anido (1973), Kew (1973), Westwood
et al. (1973), Lo Grippo and Hayashi (1973), Skinhoj (1974, 1980), Pattison *et
al.* (1974), Krassnitsky *et al.* (1974), Saslow and Iammarino (1974), Seder *et al.*
(1975), Thomson and Inwood (1976), Levy *et al.* (1977), Shimojo (1975), Lauer
et al. (1977), Marimuthu (1980), Callender *et al.* (1982), Gerberding *et al.*

(1985), Polakoff (1986), Douvin (1990). Later incidents are recorded in surveys as they appear to be too common for individual accounts—although no cases of laboratory-acquired hepatitis B were reported for 1996 (Heptonstall, personal communication).

Harrington and Shannon (1976) identified 35 cases that occurred in laboratories in England and Wales during 1971, an overall attack rate of 170 per 100 000 person years. In a series of surveys carried out in British laboratories over several years Grist (1975, 1976, 1978, 1980, 1981b, 1981c, 1983) and Grist and Emslie (1985, 1987, 1989, 1991) declined from double to single figures. In a laboratory population averaging about 27 000 the numbers were 17 in 1971–2; 14 in 1973–4; three in 1975–6; six in 1977–8; none in 1979; three in 1980; six (three occupational) in 1981; six (four occupational) in 1982; seven (four occupational) in 1983; eight (six occupational) in 1984–5; one in 1986–7; and none in 1988–9. Skinhoj and Soeby (1981) identified 22 laboratory technicians in Denmark who had viral hepatitis during the years 1974–8, a significantly higher rate than, for example, among nurses. Compared with the population as a whole a fivefold increase was found for laboratory workers. Jacobson et al. (1985) reported that the incidence of clinical hepatitis B in their laboratory surveys was 10 times higher than that in the general US population.

Common source and institutional outbreaks seem to have occurred more often in hospital departments outside pathology, e.g. in dialysis units, but work with primates accounted for three incidents involving a total of 48 individuals.

Because of its importance in clinical laboratories hepatitis is also considered in Chapter 12.

HERPESVIRUS SIMIAE (B VIRUS)

Agent summary:
Herpesviridae. Encephalomyelitis. Africa. Zoonosis: monkeys, especially macaques), Laboratory infection: percutaneous.

Although this herpes disease is common in Old World monkeys it is fortunately rare in humans (possibly because of cross-immunity against human herpes virus). There have been over 30 cases with 17 deaths since 1934, when the virus was isolated post mortem from Dr W. Brebner (hence the initial) by Sabin and Wright (1934). Infection has followed bites and laboratory accidents. The 20 cases have been well documented by Sabin (1949), Pierce et al. (1958), Nagler and Klotz (1958), Breen et al. (1958), Hummeler et al. (1959), Davidson and Hummeler (1961), Love and Jungherr (1962), Hartley (1966; 1968), Hennessen (1968), Fierer et al. (1973), Brynat et al. (1975), CDC (1987a), Holmes et al. (1990).

HUMAN IMMUNODEFICIENCY VIRUS

Agent summary:
Retroviridae. Worldwide. Humans. Associated with AIDS. Laboratory infection: muco/percutaneous.

Although there have been at least 223 confirmed and posssible cases of occupational transmission of HIV (Heptonstall *et al*. 1995), the numbers of laboratory workers involved are low: 17 documented and 17 possible in clinical laboratory staff and three documented and two possible in non-clinical laboratory workers.

Reports of individual cases, including seroconversions, include those of CDC (1988a,b), Palca (1987), Weiss *et al*. (1985), Haley *et al*. (1989), CDC (1992b), Lot and Abiteboul (1993), Tokars *et al*. (1993), Pincus *et al*. (1994) and Fitch *et al*. (1995).

INFLUENZA VIRUS

Agent summary:
Orthomyxoviridae. Influenza. Worldwide. There are vaccines for current strains. Laboratory infection: inhalation.

Although Pike (1976) mentions 15 cases, there appear to be only few references: Smith and Stuart-Harris (1936) and Cook (1961)

JUNIN VIRUS

Agent summary:
Arenaviridae. Junin and Argentine haemorrhagic fevers. South America. Zoonosis: rodents (?), ticks. Laboratory infection: percutaneous, inhalation (?).

Rugiero *et al*. (1962) reported laboratory infections; Weissenbacher *et al*. (1978) noted inapparent infections among laboratory workers. SALS (1980) records 21 cases (one death).

KYANSANUR FOREST DISEASE VIRUS

Agent summary:
Togaviridae. Encephalitis, etc. India. Zoonosis: monkeys, rodents, ticks. Laboratory infection: percutaneous, inhalation.

Although this is high in Pike's (1976) league tables, with 67 cases, only a few laboratories seem to have been involved. All the infections reported up to 1955 occurred in only two places. Since then reports have been published by Work *et al*. (1957) and Morse *et al*. (1962). Hanson *et al*. (1967) reported 53 cases in one laboratory, and Banerjee *et al*. (1979) 87 cases in another. SALS (1980) reports 133.

LASSA VIRUS

Agent summary:
Arenaviridae. Haemorrhagic fever. Africa. Zoonosis: Mastomys rats. Laboratory infection: percutaneous, inhalation (?).

Although a rare disease this has a high mortality rate and in the 1970s it generated a great deal of fear in the UK. SALS (1980) reports only two laboratory-acquired infections, those of Leifer *et al*. (1970) and Frame *et al*. (1970).

LOUPING ILL VIRUS

Agent summary:
Flaviviridae. CNS involvement. Worldwide. Zoonosis: sheep, ticks. Laboratory infection: percutaneous, inhalation (during intranasal inoculations).

The earliest reports seem to have been those of Rivers and Schwenker (1934), followed by those of Wiebel (1937), Davison *et al.* (1948), Cooper *et al.* (1964), Webb *et al.* (1968), Reid *et al.* (1972). SALS (1980) lists 22 cases.

LYMPHOCYTIC CHORIOMENINGITIS VIRUS

Agent summary:
Arenaviridae. Aseptic meningitis. Worldwide. Zoonosis: mice, food. Laboratory infection: mucocutaneous, inhalation.

Infections have been reported by Lepine and Sautter (1938), Milzer and Levinson (1942), Farmer and Janeway (1942), Smadel *et al.* (1942), Hayes and Hartman (1943), Schied *et al.* (1956), Lewis *et al.* (1965), Baum *et al.* (1966), Hotchin *et al.* (1974), Hinman *et al.* (1975), Gregg (1975), Bowen *et al.* (1975) and Biggar *et al.* (1977). Pike (1978) noted that 49 of a total of 76 infections known to him had occurred since 1955. Dykewicz *et al.* (1992) reported a laboratory outbreak associated with nude mice. SALS (1980) records 15 cases.

MARBURG VIRUS

Agent summary:
Filoviridae. Haemorrhagic fever. Africa. Zoonosis: vervet monkeys. Laboratory infection: muco/percutaneous.

This disease is named after the place where it was first reported. Laboratory infections arose from contact and accidents with blood and tissue from vervet monkeys from Uganda. The incidents were spectacular, are well documented, and are reviewed by Hull (1973). Reports include those of Smith *et al.* (1967), *Lancet* (1967, 1971), Martini and Schmidt (1968) (secondary, spermatogenic), Stille *et al.* (1968), Kissling *et al.* (1970) and Bechtelsheimer *et al.* (1970). Pike (1976) numbers 31 cases with nine deaths, but SALS (1980) reports 25 cases with nine deaths.

NEWCASTLE DISEASE VIRUS

Agent summary:
Paramyxoviridae. Conjunctivitis in laboratory workers. Worldwide. Zoonosis: chickens. Laboratory infection: mucocutaneous.

Laboratory-acquired infections with this avian disease have been reported by Burnet (1943), Yatom (1946), Shimkim (1946), Anderson (1946), Freyman and Bang (1948), Hunter *et al.* (1951), Gustafson and Moses (1951), Divo and Lugo 1952), and Bortsov *et al.* (1976), Mustaffa-Babjee *et al.* (1976). Morgan (1987) reported one case of conjunctivitis and Miller *et al.* (1987) reported two more infections.

OMSK HAEMORRHAGIC FEVER VIRUS

Agent summary:
Togaviridae (Flavivirus). Haemorrhagic fever. Siberia. Zoonosis: rodents, ticks. Laboratory infection: muco/percutaneous.
   There are reports by Jelinkova-Skalova (1974) and Nikodemusz (1975). SALS (1980) records five cases.

PARVOVIRUS B19

Agent summary:
Parvoviridae. Arthropody, facial rash. Worldwide. Laboratory infection: muco-cutaneous.
   Cohen *et al.* (1988) reported nine probable cases and there is another report by Shiraishi *et al.* (1991).

PICHENDE VIRUS

Agent summary:
Arenaviridae, not considered to cause disease in humans but Buchmeier *et al.* (1974) found antibodies in six of 13 people who worked with the virus and reported one infection from a needle-stick injury.

POLIOVIRUS

Agent summary:
Picornaviridae. Poliomyelitis. Worldwide. Laboratory infection: ingestion.
   Laboratory infections have been reported by Sabin and Ward (1941), Wenner and Paul (1974) and Beller (1949). Pike's (1976) list gives 13 cases.

RABIES VIRUS

Agent summary:
Rhabdoviridiae. Rabies. Worldwide. Zoonosis: canines, bats, others. Laboratory infection: mucocutaneous. Vaccine.
   Infections were reported by: Winkler *et al.* (1973), Varela-Diaz *et al.* (1974), Conomy *et al.* (1977), Tillotson *et al.* (1977) and CDC (1977b). Cook (1961) three cases of bat rabies.

RIFT VALLEY VIRUS

Agent summary:
Bunyaviridae. Haemorrhagic fever. East and South Africa. Zoonosis: sheep, cattle, mosquitoes. Laboratory infection: percutaneous, inhalation.
   According to Newsom (1976) this arbovirus seems to have caused infections in every laboratory where it has been studied. The natural disease occurs in sheep in Africa (Kenya). Infections have been reported by Findlay (1932), Kitchen (1934), Schwentker and Rivers (1934), Francis and Magill (1935), Sabin and Blumberg (1947). Smithburn *et al.* (1949), Stern (1958), Shimojo

(1975), Murphy and Easterfay (1961). Pike (1976) records 28 infections and SALS (1980) 47 (one death).

RUSSIAN SPRING-SUMMER ENCEPHALITIS VIRUS

Agent summary:
Flaviviridae. Encephalitis. Siberia. Zoonosis: rodents, ticks. Laboratory infection: percutaneous, inhalation.

Infections are reported by Haymaker *et al.* (1955) and Jervis and Higgins (1973). SALS mentions eight cases.

SABIA VIRUS

Agent summary:
Arenaviridae. Tacaribe complex. Haemorrhagic fever. Brazil. Rodents. Laboratory infection: (?).

This is a 'new' virus (Lisieux *et al.*, 1994) reported from Brazil and an infection was acquired by a laboratory worker in the US the following year (Barry *et al.*, 1995). See also Ryder *et al.* (1995) and Gandsman (1997).

ST LOUIS ENCEPHALITIS VIRUS

Agent summary:
Flaviridae. Central and South America. Fever, aseptic meningitis. Zoonosis: birds, mosquitoes. Laboratory infection: percutaneous.

Only one report was found: von Magnus (1950).

SIMIAN IMMUNODEFICIENCY VIRUS

Agent summary:
Retroviridae. African green monkeys and macaques. Laboratory infection: muco/percutaneous.

There was serological (but not clinical) evidence of transmission to humans (CDC, 1992; ACDP, 1997a) and Khabbaz *et al.* (1994) reported evidence of infection in a laboratory worker who was receiving corticosteroids.

VACCINIA VIRUS

Agent summary:
Poxviridae. Vaccine. Laboratory infection: mucocutaneous.

Jones *et al.* (1986) and Openshaw *et al.* (1991) reported accidental infections of laboratory workers with recombinant vaccinia virus.

VARIOLA VIRUS

Smallpox has now been eradicated and laboratory-acquired infections are therefore of historical interest only. Benn (1963) reported on a pathologist who contracted the disease and died after conducting an autopsy on a smallpox victim. In the London incident, in 1973 (three cases, two deaths), the index case was a visitor to the laboratory and the fatal cases were contacts (Report, 1974). In the Birmingham (UK) incident, in 1978, the victim worked in the same building as the smallpox laboratory (DH, 1980a). Pike (1976) lumps variola with vaccinia and notes 18 cases but no deaths.

VENEZUELAN EQUINE ENCEPHALITIS

Agent summary:
Togaviridae. Encephalitis. Central and South America. Zoonosis: rodents, birds, mosquitoes. Laboratory infection: percutaneous.

Infections with viruses of Venezuelan, eastern and western equine encephalitis are usually associated with egg culture techniques and suckling mice but the much quoted Moscow outbreak (Slepushkin, 1959) was airborne, from broken containers of freeze-dried material. Other infections have been reported by Casals *et al.* (1943), Lennette and Koprowski (1943), Koprowski and Cox (1947), Olitsky and Casals (1952), Alekseeva *et al.* (1959), Schublaadze *et al.* (1959), Kuehne *et al.* (1962). SALS (1980) records 150.

VESICULAR STOMATITIS VIRUS

Agent summary:
Rhabdoviridae. Influenza-like fever. Worldwide. Zoonosis: mammals (cattle). Laboratory infection: inhalation, mucocutaneous.

Cases have been reported by Hanson *et al.* (1950), Fellows *et al.* (1957), Patterson *et al.* (1958), Hanson and Brandley (1957) and Johnson *et al.* (1966). Pike's (1976) tally was 40 cases, 31 of which occurred in one institution (Patterson *et al.*, 1958). SALS (1980) records 46.

WESSELBRON VIRUS

Agent summary:
Flaviviridae. Fever, hepatitis. Laboratory infection—route not known
    Only two reports were found: Bres (1965), Justines and Shope (1969).

WESTERN EQUINE ENCEPHALITIS VIRUS

Agent summary:
Togaviridae (Alphavirus). Encephalitis. Central and South America. Zoonosis: birds. mosquitoes. Laboratory infection: percutaneous.

There are reports by Fothergill *et al.* (1939) and Helwig (1940). SALS (1980) records seven cases with two deaths.

YABA AND TANAVIRUS

Agent summary:
Poxviridae. Host, non-human primates; oncogenic (monkey tumour). Laboratory infection: mucocutaneous.

According to Pike (1976) there have been 24 cases, all in the USA of infection with these African viruses, but the only reference to laboratory infection readily found was that of Grace and Mirand (1963).

Agent summary:
Flaviviridae. Yellow fever. Tropical Africa, South and Central America. Zoonosis: monkeys, mosquitoes. Laboratory infection: percutaneous. Vaccine.

Laboratory-acquired infections were reported by Berry and Kitchin (1931) and Lowe and Fairly (1931) but Pike (1978) mentions a total of 40. SALS (1980) gives 38 with eight deaths.

Fungi

BLASTOMYCES DERMATITIDIS

Agent summary:
Dimorphic fungus. Soil. North America, but occurs elsewhere. North American blastomycosis; cutaneous; pulmonary/disseminated disease. Laboratory infection: muco/percutaneous, inhalation.

The number of infections recorded is small and they appear to be well documented. The first was reported by Evans (1903), followed by that of Morris (1913). No more reports were found until those of Schwarz and Baum (1951), Ramsey and Carter (1952), Wilson *et al.* (1955), Smith *et al.* (1955), Harrel and Curtis (1959), Baum and Schwarz (1959), Denton *et al.* (1967), Palmer and McFadden (1968), Obenour (1969), Baum and Lerner (1970), Landay and Schwarz (1971), Onstad (1971), Larsh and Schwarz (1977). Pike's (1976) tally, however, was 11 with two deaths.

COCCIDIOIDES IMMITIS

Agent summary:
Dimorphic fungus. Soil. North America. Pulmonary disease. Laboratory infection: inhalation.

In a review of laboratory-acquired mycoses Hanel and Kruse (1967) concluded that *Coccidioides* caused most fungal infections. Fiese (1958) considered that 'The only occupations more hazardous than agriculture and allied pursuits are those that involve the handling of coccidioides in the laboratory'. This is probably because of the ease with which the arthrospores are dispersed when cultures are opened.

The list of reports of infections is long: Guy and Jacob (1927), Tomlinson and Bancroft (1928; 1934), van Cleve (1936), Dickson (1937), Dickson and Gifford (1938), Smith (1943), Bush (1943), Willett and Weiss (1945), Smith and Harrell (1948), Nabarro (1948), Looney and Stein (1950), Trimble and Doucette (1956), Fiese (1958), Chatigny (1961), Smith *et al.* (1961), Kruse (1962), Overholt and Hornick (1964), Johnson *et al.* (1964), Klutsch *et al.* (1965), Fischer and Kane (1973), Wegman and Plempel (1974), Drouhet *et al.* (1974) and Carroll *et al.* (1977). The geographical distribution of coccidioidomycosis is important: most cases occur in the south west of the USA. Only one of the above (Nabarro, 1948) occurred in the UK. Pike (1976) records 93 infections, but in their earlier report Hanel and Kruse (1967) had collected 108; they included subclinical infections, based on skin tests which would not have been counted by Pike.

CRYPTOCOCCUS NEOFORMANS

Agent summary:
True yeast. Worldwide, bird (pigeon) faeces. Meningitis, pulmonary disease. Laboratory infection: inhalation.

Cryptococci, but not HIV, were transmitted from an AIDS patient to another person by needle-stick (Glaser and Gordon, 1985).

HISTOPLASMA CAPSULATUM

Agent summary:
Dimorphic fungus. Pulmonary histoplasmosis. Soil, bird and mammal faeces. Laboratory infection: inhalation.

The first laboratory infection was reported by Furcolow *et al.* as recently as 1952. Other reports were made by Nilzen and Paldrock (1953), Dickie and Murphy (1955), Willis and Furcolow (1956), Spicknall *et al.* (1956), Furcolow (1961, 1965), Hartung and Salfelder (1962), Vanselow *et al.* (1962), Murray and Howard (1964), Tesh and Schneidau (1966), Chick *et al.* (1972). Again this is a geographically restricted infection, but there were 17 infections (all in expatriates) in the UK according to Newsom (1976a). Pike (1976) recorded 71 infections but Hanel and Kruse (1967) collected 81. The difference is probably due to the inclusion of clinically inapparent cases by the earlier authors. Furcolow *et al.* (1952) suggested, on the basis of skin test results, that there were more subclinical than overt infections.

SPOROTHRIX SCHENKII

Agent summary:
Dimorphic fungus. Pyogenic granulomatous disease. Europe and USA. Wood and plant material. Laboratory infection: muco/percutaneous.

Only a few laboratory-acquired infections associated with *Sporothrix schenkii* have been reported and they are spread over a long period (1909–77). The first was by Fava (1909) followed by Jeanselme and Chevalier (1910, 1911), Fielitz (1910), Wilder and McCullough (1914), Meyer (1915), Jeanselme *et al.* (1928), Norden (1951), Thompson and Kaplan (1977) and Ishizaki *et al.* (1979). Pike (1976) records only 12 cases.

TRICHOPHYTON SPP.

Agent summary:
Filamentous fungi, several species. Worldwide, humans, animals. Tinea (ringworm) of nails, hair, skin. Laboratory infection: cutaneous.

Trichophyton mentagrophytes would seem to be the fungus most frequently associated with laboratory infections. Accounts of dermatophyte infections are given by Rowsell *et al.* (1954), Meyer (1957), Dolan *et al.* (1958), Kaffka and Rieth (1958), Mantkelow and Russell (1960), Mackenzie (1961), Sonck (1961),

Alteras (1965), Hanel and Kruse (1967), Kamelam and Thambia (1979). Miller *et al.* (1987) found two cases. Pike's (1976) total was 161 cases.

Endoparasites

CRYPTOSPORIDIUM

Agent summary:
Free-living protozoan. Worldwide. Water, calves. Intestinal infections (especially in immunocompromised subjects). Laboratory infection: ingestion.
   A laboratory infection was reported by Blagburn and Current (1983).

GIARDIA

Agent summary:
Protozoan, usually water borne. Diarrhoea, abdominal discomfort. Laboratory infections: ingestion, aerosol(?).
   One case was reported by Cook (1961) in a worker who handled large numbers of stools. Transmission was thought to be airborne.

LEISHMANIA SPP.

Agent summary:
Flagellate protozoan (Trypanosomidae). Tropical and subtropical areas. Humans and dogs. (1) *L. donovani*: Kala Azar, visceral leishmaniasis; (2) *L. tropica*: Oriental sore; (local names); (3) *L. braziliensis*: naso-pharyngeal (American) leishmaniasis. Vector, sandflies (*Phlebotomus* spp. Laboratory infection: muco/percutaneous.
   Cases were reported by Chung (1931) and Terry *et al.* (1950), Sampaio *et al.* (1983), Freedman *et al.* (1987), Evans and Pearson 1988), Herwaldt and Juranaek (1993), Knobloch and Demar (1997).

PLASMODIUM SPP.

Agent summary:
Protozoa with complex life cycles. Tropical and subtropical, areas. Humans, other mammals, birds. Some animal species transmissable to humans. Vectors and definitive hosts are anopheline mosquitoes. Laboratory infection: percutaneous (vector).
   Laboratory-acquired infections by human strains have been reported by Holm (1924), Stuppy (1936), Burne (1970), Garnham *et al.* (1962), Cannon *et al.* (1972), Petithory and Lebeau (1977), Bouvret and Fouquet (1978), Bending and Maurice (1980), Jensen *et al.* (1981), Varma (1982) and Williams *et al.* (1983), Herwaldt and Juranek (1993b).
   Plasmodium cynomolgi was the agent in the cases decribed by Eyles *et al.* (1960), Schmidt *et al.* (1961), Most (1973) and Cross *et al.* (1973). Pike's (1976) total of 18 cases included eight such infections, indicating that mosquitoes infected with this parasite offer as much hazard as those infected with the usual human pathogens.

SCHISTOSOMA SPP.

Agent summary:
Trematoda. Africa, Middle East, South America. Infective stage—metacercaria; Laboratory infection: cutaneous.
Only one report was found: Van Gompel *et al.* (1933).

TOXOPLASMA GONDII

Agent summary:
Protozoan. Worldwide, humans and animals. CNS involvement in children, visceral in adults. Laboratory infection: ingestion.
This seems to be the most commonly-acquired parasitic disease in the laboratory, although it does not have a very long history (the first case was reported in 1956). Neu (1967), reporting on toxoplasmosis transmitted at autopsy, considered that 'Most of our knowledge of acquired toxoplasmosis is based on infections in laboratory workers'. Laboratory infections seem to have been associated with accidental inoculations and autopsies. Reports include those of Strom (1950–1), Magnusson (1951), Sexton *et al.* (1953), Beverley *et al.* (1955), van Soestbergen (1957), Rawal (1959)(summary of 18 cases), Radacovici *et al.* (1962), Ludlam and Beattie (1963), Neu (1967), Feldman (1968), Remington and Gentry (1970), Field *et al.* (1972), Zimmerman (1976),Wright (1985), Hermentin 1989), Parker and Holliman (1992), Herwaldt and Juranek (1993b). Pike (1976) collected 28 reports.

TRYPANOSOMA SPP.

Agent summary:
Flagellated protozoan. Tropical areas. *T. brucei gambiense*, *T. brucei rhodesiense*: African sleeping sickness, transmitted by tsetse fly (*Glossina*); reservoirs, cattle. *T. cruzi*: American trypansomiasis, Chagas' disease, transmitted by reduviid bugs (faeces contamination of bug bites); reservoirs, various mammals. Laboratory infection: mucocutaneous (blood, bug faeces), possibly inhalation.
Cases of laboratory-acquired Chagas' disease (*T. cruzi*) were reported by Herr and Brumpt (1939), Aronson (1962), Pizzi *et al.* (1963), Hanson *et al.* (1974), CDC (1980), Hofflin *et al.* (1987). Robertson *et al.* (1980) reported an infection *T. brucei rhodesiense* which occurred in the UK. Brenner (1987) reported an infection with *T. cruzi*, Herbert *et al.* (1980) one with *T. brucei*. Emeribe (1988) reported one with *T. gambiense*. In Pike's (1976) list there were 17 cases.

Places and people involved

The diversity of the agents that have been responsible for diseases among laboratory workers suggests that infections occurred in widely differing kinds of laboratories. Some of the organisms are handled only in research establishments, while others are encountered daily in diagnostic and clinical laboratories.
As with the numbers of infections, up-to-date information about the laboratories where infections occurred, and the status of the people who became infected are not available because of the absence of governmental,

and even private, surveys. We therefore can only use material dating from 1952 to 1991.

In their surveys Sulkin and Pike recorded the types of laboratories in which infections occurred as research, diagnostic, manufacture of biological products, teaching and unspecified. Table 1.6, from Pike's (1976) figures, shows that over half of the 3921 infections which they had identified in the first three-quarters of this century affected workers in research laboratories. This is not really surprising, as the research worker is usually in close daily contact with relatively large amounts of single agents or with groups of associated microorganisms. Many infections have occurred during work on hitherto unknown or newly-discovered bacteria or viruses, whose potential for infecting laboratory workers could not have been assessed. Many of these infections had a common source, i.e. a number of workers became infected as a result of a single accident or procedure.

The low numbers for institutions concerned with 'biological products' reflects the high standards of safety in the pharmaceutical industries which use pathogenic organisms to manufacture vaccines and antisera. The only incident to be reported was the escape, in 1979, of anthrax from an institution in the former USSR (Meselson, 1994; see also p.10) in which 96 people in the neighbourhood became infected.

In spite of fears expressed in the 1970s and 1980s about the use of genetically-modified microorganisms, no infections have been reported from the biotechnology industry, although there has been one report of a laboratory-acquired infection with a vaccinia virus expressing nucleoprotein (Jones *et al.*, 1986) and another with recombinant smallpox vaccine (Openshaw *et al.*, 1991).

Infections in diagnostic laboratories accounted for only 17.3% of Pike's (1976) total. Although a wide variety of microorganisms are handled in clinical laboratories the quantities cultured are less than in research institutes and exposure is intermittent. Nevertheless, a wider population is at risk. Table 1.7, adapted from the single-year surveys, in the UK, of Harrington and Shannon (1976) and of Grist (1981, 1983) and Grist and Emslie (1985, 1987, 1989, 1991) shows that infections are not confined to microbiologists. Other workers, who handle but do not culture clinical specimens, may become infected. Haematology and clinical chemistry staff examine many more blood specimens than those in microbiology and morbid anatomy departments. It is interesting to note at this point that during the 11 years (1979–89) of the Grist surveys the numbers of infections reported have decreased substantially.

TABLE 1.6 Types of laboratories where infections have occurred

	Number	%
Research	2307	58.8
Diagnostic	677	17.3
Biological products	134	3.4
Teaching	106	2.7
Unspecified	698	17.8
Total	3291	

From Pike (1976).

TABLE 1.7 Infections occurring in different departments of clinical laboratories in the UK[a]

	Year	Micro-biology	Haema-tology	Clinical chemistry	Morbid anatomy[b]	Others[c]	Not stated	Ancillary workers[d]	Totals
Harrington and Shannon (1976)	1971	29	13	8	14	28	1	11	104
Grist (1976)[f]	1979	9	3	0	1	–	1	1	15
Grist (1983)	1980–1	19	5	5	16	0	0	3	48
Grist and Emslie (1985)	1982–3	10	6	4	4	0	0	5	29
Grist and Emslie (1987)	1984–5	14	4	1	1	0	–	8	28
Grist and Emslie (1989)	1986–7	10	2	0	0	0	–	3	15
Grist and Emslie (1991)	1988–9	13	1	0	0	0	–	3	17

[a] Average number at risk 2500.
[b] Includes blood transfusion staff.
[c] Porters, domestic, clerical staff.
[d] 1971 in England and Wales; 1973 in Scotland.
[f] Includes some infections acquired by contact with other workers or with agent outside the laboratory (chicken pox, 4; tuberculosis, 1; salmonella, 1; hepatitis A, 1).

What is particularly disturbing, though, is the distribution of infections between 'trained' and 'untrained' staff. It is reasonable to follow the example of Sulkin and Pike (1951) and to include in the first group graduates, state registered medical laboratory scientific officers (MLSOs) and technicians, and in the second, junior and student MLSOs and technicians not yet qualified for registration, laboratory aides, domestic and clerical staff. Table 1.8 shows the percentages of trained and untrained workers who became infected according to four surveys. In that of Pike and Sulkin (1952), which was concerned with infections in the USA, 22% were untrained. Reid (1957) found that 64% of laboratory workers in the UK who contracted tuberculosis were also untrained. Wedum (1964) reported that of 369 workers who became infected, 82% were trained and 18% untrained. In Harrington and Shannon's (1976) survey, 37% of UK laboratory workers who became ill with hepatitis, tuberculosis or shigellosis were untrained.

Further distinctions may be made among untrained workers, depending on whether they support trained staff in the laboratories or are engaged in clerical or maintenance activities. Pike and Sulkin (1952) found 10% of their infections

TABLE 1.8 Proportion of trained to untrained[a] workers who became infected

	No. of infections	% Trained staff	% Untrained staff
Pike and Sulkin (1952)	1286	78	22
Reid (1957)[b]	96	36	64
Wedum (1964)	3698	21	8
Pike (1976)[c]	3921	65	35
Harrington and Shannon (1976)[d]	104	63	37

Adapted from the above authors.
[a] Trained: medical and scientific staff. Untrained: juniors, students, ancillary, domestic and clerical staff.
[b] Tuberculosis only, in the UK.
[c] All infections, 1900–74, worldwide.
[d] Tuberculosis, hepatitis and tuberculosis, 1971 (England and Wales); 1973 (Scotland).

in the first group and 7% in the second. Reid (1957) found 55% and 8% for tuberculosis only, while Harrington and Shannon (1976) reported 26% and 7% for tuberculosis and hepatitis. They did not separate trained from junior technicians in their shigellosis figures. Grist and Grist and Emslie did not distinguish between trained and junior MLSOs in any of their surveys. It is interesting, however, that three separate surveys yield figures suggesting that 7–8% of laboratory-acquired infections are likely to occur in clerical and maintenance staff.

While too much reliance should not be placed on comparisons of these figures, and even on the figures themselves, considering the ways in which they have been collected and their scatter in place and time, they illustrate that laboratory-acquired infections are not confined to any one kind of laboratory or group of people. They do suggest that the incidence of infection among untrained and ancillary workers is rather high. They are also likely to assist in the assessment of risk and the development of reasonable and appropriate precautionary measures and training programmes. It is particularly important that trainee (i.e. preregistration) and junior staff are included in any surveys. In UK clinical laboratories they are the people who do most of the bench work.

Malignant disease

Certain viruses are known to be associated with tumours in animals and may be transmitted horizontally. Although there seems to be no evidence of such transmission to humans, there is a report by Gross (1971) about two cases of malignancy following accidental injection of material aspirated from patients with cancer. Gugel and Sanders (1986) reported that a laboratory worker accidentally punctured her hand with a needle that had been used to draw up a suspension of a human colonic adenocarcinoma cell line. A nodule subsequently developed at the site of inoculation; histological examination revealed adenocarcinoma.

In 1986 there were seven cases of cancer among workers in a French laboratory where viruses and DNA were handled. This seemed to indicate a higher incidence than that in the general population. In 1991 Rutty and Doshi reported three workers in a UK laboratory who developed brain tumours over a 10-year period. Harrington and Oakes (1986) had already noted a higher incidence of cerebral tumours among British pathologists compared with a control group.

Chapter 2

Exposure, sources and routes of infection

It is not unreasonable to expect that any person who works with pathogenic microorganisms will be more likely than other members of the community to become infected. Evidence has already been presented that some organisms cause more infections than others and that the incidence of infections varies according to the nature of the work and the status of the worker. Attention must now be paid to the ways in which laboratory workers are exposed and may become infected.

Exposure

In simple terms an infection occurs when microorganisms that are capable of causing disease enter the body by a particular route, and in sufficient numbers to overcome that body's natural defences. For details of what is called the mechanism of infection the reader is referred to Mims (1982) and other textbooks on medical microbiology and immunology.

Sources and reservoirs of infection

All clinical laboratory workers are exposed to various infections while they are at work. The surveys of Grist and Emslie (1981, 1985, 1987, 1989), however, indicate that those engaged in microbiology are most at risk and that medical laboratory scientific officers and technicians are the most vulnerable. Recently, however, those who handle large numbers of blood specimens, e.g. in haematology and clinical chemistry laboratories consider themselves to be equally, or even more at risk. It is also apparent from the various surveys cited that 'exposure' or 'working with the agent' is more likely to result in infection than overt accidents.

Infectious materials, including large numbers of blood samples and cultures of microorganisms, accumulate in clinical and microbiological laboratories and, as it is necessary to transfer them from one container to another and to manipulate them in various ways, the potential hazards are considerable. There are several ways in which laboratory infections can be initiated. Some of these are obvious to the individual concerned: he knows that he has had a personal accident. In others it is known that organisms have been released

38

into the laboratory but there is no immediate evidence that anyone has been infected.

Accidents

Accidents involving infectious materials, and not always attributable to human error, occur in the best regulated laboratories. Even skilled workers are not immune. Tables 2.1, 2.2 and 2.3 give examples of the ways in which laboratory workers may become infected (Pike, 1976; Miller *et al.*, 1987).

Surface contamination

When material containing microorganisms is spilled or splashed and when droplets fall from pipettes during transfer of cultures the events may pass unnoticed. Specimen containers are often contaminated externally (Allen and Darrell, 1983).

Very small amounts of blood have been detected on laboratory surfaces (Beaumont, 1987; Evans *et al.*, 1990; Kennedy, 1997).

It was shown by Bond *et al.* (1981) that hepatitis B virus can survive for as long as 7 days in dried blood plasma.

Even if such contamination is noted and action taken disinfection may not be entirely effective.

TABLE 2.1 Sources of laboratory accidents

Source or contact	Number	%
Accident[a]	703	17.9
Animal or ectoparasite	659	17.8
Clinical specimen	287	7.3
Discarded glassware	46	1.2
Human autopsy	75	1.9
Intentional infection	19	0.5
Aerosol (known)	522	13.3
Work with agent	827	21.1
Others, unknown	783	20.0
Total	3921	

[a]See Table 2.2.

TABLE 2.2 Types of accidents preceding infections

Accident	Number	%
Spillage and splashes	188	26.7
Needle and syringe	177	25.2
Sharp objects, broken glass	112	15.9
Bite or scratch, animal or ectoparasite	95	13.5
Aspiration through pipette	92	13.1
Others or not known	39	5.5
Total	703	

Adapted from Pike (1976).

TABLE 2.3 Agent exposure/infection experience at the US National Animal Disease Center

Exposure	No. of exposures	No. of infections resulting
Syringe accidents		
Autoinoculation	38	3
Spray	8	—
Animal autopsy		
Laceration with instruments	12	2
Splash/spray	6	—
Conjunctival exposure	4	2
Mouth pipetting	6	—
Animal contact	11	2
Glassware accidents		
Lacerations	2	—
Dropped culture	6	—
Equipment failure	2	—
Other	8	—
Unknown (?aerosol)	25	25
Total	128	34

From Miller *et al.* (1987).
Reproduced by permission of the American Industrial Hygiene Association.

Routes of infection

Biological agents, in particular microorganisms, may enter the human body in several ways:

- through the lungs—inhalation;
- through the mouth—ingestion;
- by contact with the apparently unbroken skin and with mucous membranes;
- by injection, with hollow-bore needles and other sharps;
- through the conjunctivae;
- through the genitourinary tract;
- from animals (including arthropod) bites and scratches.

These routes are shown diagrammatically in Figure 2.1.

In laboratory-acquired infections the route may not be the same as when the disease is acquired naturally.

Through the lungs

In Pike's (1976) assessment of the sources of laboratory-acquired infections the 703 known accidents accounted for only 18% of 3921 infections. The mode of transmission in the other 82% was, as Pike remarked, a subject for speculation. In a growing number of reports the connections between the infected individuals and the causative organisms were, at the most, tenuous and often apparently non-existent. In some cases there was a history of harvesting viruses from eggs; in others certain pieces of equipment such as shaking machines, centrifuges and homogenizers were thought to have been involved in some way. Some of those infected were known to have worked with the organisms or with animals experimentally infected with them. Others had had no contact except that they worked in the same building or had visited it. Since about 1947, however, an

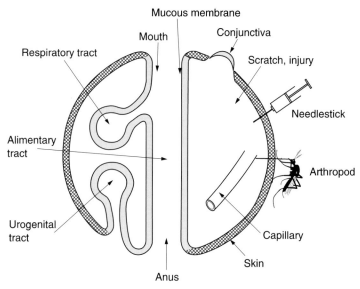

Figure 2.1 Routes of infection: the body's portals of entry of microbes. (From Mims, 1982, by permission of Academic Press)

increasing amount of evidence, deductive and experimental, indicated that many of these infections had been acquired by the inhalation of microorganisms released into the air during many of the technical procedures used to study them.

Aerosols, droplets and infected airborne particles

It has long been known that when a bubble bursts or a thin film of liquid is broken large numbers of small droplets are released. Similarly. if a liquid is squirted under pressure through a small hole, or a fine jet of liquid is allowed to impinge upon a solid surface, it becomes 'atomized' and a cloud of very small droplets collectively known as an aerosol is formed. As early as 1919 Fricke pointed out the hazards of 'small droplets' released during certain bacteriological activities. In 1934 Wells showed that if the liquid contained bacteria these would be distributed in the droplets and would remain viable for some time. Droplets produced in this way vary in size. The larger droplets, more than 0.1 mm in diameter, settle quickly and contaminate the surfaces on which they come to rest. The smaller droplets do not settle but evaporate very rapidly; Wells found that those with a diameter of 0.1 mm evaporated in 1.7 s and those with a diameter of 0.05 mm in 0.4 s. In addition, droplets may attract and absorb other, smaller particle in their vicinity The bacteria, and any other material in them, remain in a dried state as 'droplet nuclei', now usually referred to as infected airborne particles. Figure 2.2 shows, diagrammatically, the sequence of events (ISSA, 1998).

Table 2.4 shows the evaporation times and falling distances of droplets of different sizes (Wells, 1955; see also Gilchrist, 1995).

In addition, The smaller the droplet nuclei and size of dried particles the longer they will remain airborne (Green and Lane, 1964). They will be moved

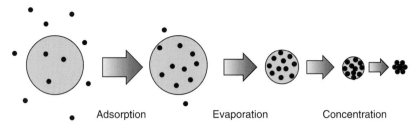

Adsorption   Evaporation   Concentration

Figure 2.2 Sequence of events in the formation of droplet nuclei. (ISSA, 1998, courtesy of the International Social Security Association)

TABLE 2.4 Evaporation time and falling distance of droplets based on time

Diameter of droplet (μm)	Evaporation time (s)	Distance fallen before evaporation (ft)
200	5.2	21.7
100	1.3	1.4
50	0.31	0.085
25	0.08	0.0053

Kennedy (1988), adapted from Wells (1934) and Gilchrist (1995).

around rooms and buildings by air currents generated by ventilation and the movements of people. Also, the smaller they are the greater their potential for travelling long distances. If the organisms are contained not in aqueous but in proteinaceous fluids, e.g. in sputum, mucus, serum, evaporation will be much slower as these materials tend to retain water. Such droplets will settle more rapidly; fewer will remain suspended in air and fewer infected airborne particles, available for wider dispersion, will be produced.

The term aerosol, long associated with liquids, was extended by Lacey and Dutkiewicz (1994) to include suspensions in air of any particles of biological origin such as organic dusts, which they termed 'bioaerosols'. In the context of this book these include lyophilized cultures, dried bacterial colonies, dried material on stoppers and caps of culture tubes and bottles, dried exudates, fungal and actinomycete spores released when cultures are opened, and also dusts from animal cages. All are sources of light particles which may contain viable organisms (Darlow, 1972).

It is now accepted that some of these droplets and infected airborne particles can initiate infection, although doubts persisted for many years (Andrewes, 1940). In a review of the epidemiology of airborne infection Langmuir (1961) mentioned several diseases that are known to be spread in the community by the inhalation of organisms dispersed in this way and it is of interest that some of them have also been responsible for those laboratory-associated infection where no accident or other cause could be demonstrated. These include tuberculosis, psittacosis, Q fever, pulmonary mycoses and, in special circumstances, brucellosis.

The size of the particles was found, experimentally, to influence infection. Lurie (1930) and Wells *et al.* (1948) showed that the smaller ones were capable of infecting experimental animals, but that the larger ones were not. To initiate infection it was necessary for the organisms to be able to reach the alveoli.

Larger particles are trapped in the mucus secreted by the upper respiratory tract and moved upwards by mucociliary escalation to the throat where they are swallowed (Mims, 1982). Hatch (1961) considered that the maximum size for this was 5 µm, but much depended on the density, shape and degree of aggregation of particles. Larger particles would be swallowed or trapped in the nose, although Lidwell (1970) found that larger particles, up to 10 µm, would penetrate as far as the bronchi if air was breathed in through the mouth instead of the nose. Lacey *et al.* (1972), who worked with the spores of actinomycetes and fungi, found that the optimal size for alveolar penetration was 0.2–0.4 µm. There is no ciliary escalation in the alveolar regions, but the alveoli are lined with macrophages which engulf particles that settle on their walls. (If tubercle bacilli reach the alveoli they can survive in these macrophages.) Most of the particles that are less than 1 µm in diameter, however, are not retained and are expelled on exhalation. The mechanism of retention—'deposition'—is described in detail by Parkes (1994).

It is now evident, however, that deposition, and hence infection, does not depend on size alone. Some microorganisms have a disposition to attach themselves to particular tissues. This is illustrated in Figure 2.3.

Aerosol production and dispersal in laboratories

It has been shown by a number of workers that many of the laboratory techniques, which use both simple and mechanical equipment, as well as common laboratory accidents, produce aerosols consisting of various sizes of particles. Most of these are considered later, in Chapter 4 which deals with the minimizing of aerosol production and of other hazards. They are therefore listed here without references to avoid repetition. They include use of bacteriologists'

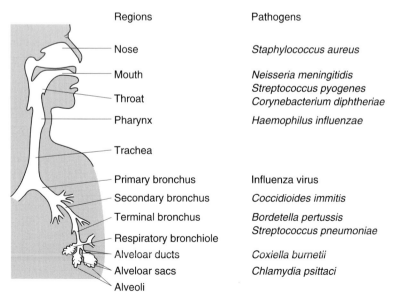

Figure 2.3 Sites of preferential attachment of some agents in the respiratory tract. (ISSA, 1998, courtesy of the International Social Security Association)

loops, pipettes, syringes and needles, opening tubes and bottles, use of centrifuges and blenders, harvesting of eggs and other virological procedures,
lyophilization and breakage of cultures. The techniques used to demonstrate
aerosols used bacteria, bacteriophages and radioactive materials and the particles released were counted with slit and cascade samplers, impingers and filters.
It was shown that some of the laboratory techniques produced particles that were
smaller than 5 μm and others produced larger ones. While it is not possible to be
precise about which activities produce which size particles, Tables 2.5 and 2.6
give a general picture.

It is clear, then, that ideal conditions exist in laboratories for the spread of
infection by airborne particles. Many microorganisms are maintained in aqueous
solutions and are frequently diluted for testing and counting. Paradoxically it is
the dilute suspensions that yield the most hazardous aerosol; droplets from these
contain very few organisms and when they dry the nuclei they leave are very
small and light. As pointed out above the sizes and weights of particles influence
the distance they travel on air currents. In laboratories more of these currents are
produced than in ordinary rooms. Bunsen burners, for example, produce considerable updrafts and any particles released at bench level are rapidly dispersed
around the laboratory. The operator himself may be protected by the updraft, but
other occupants of the room will not. Various other pieces of laboratory
equipment generate rapidly moving or convection currents. The current vogue in
laboratory design which insists on recycling air through various rooms may well
contribute to the dispersion of microorganisms, as it has in the conditions known
as humidifier fever and sick building syndrome (Collins *et al.*, 1997a). The
persistence of aerosols depends on local air currents. They are rapidly cleared
from rooms with good natural ventilation.

There are thus excellent conditions in laboratories for the dispersal and
inhalation of airborne particles, and even for their retention. Even the larger
particles and droplets, which do not evaporate, contribute to the hazards of
infection by contaminating surfaces; as indicated below, fingers may be contaminated in this way and microorganisms thus transferred to mouth and eyes.

Various factors can affect the character of an aerosol. A low energy input
yields large droplets (> 50 μl) but a high energy input yields small droplets
(< 10 μl). Temperature, humidity, the pH of the suspending medium and its
nutrient content are also important as is the porosity of any surface on which the
droplets settle. Drag, gravity, electrostatic and thermal conditions also have an

TABLE 2.5 Activities which may lead to
surface contamination by particles larger
than 5 μm

Opening containers
Pipettes—no visible spill
Test tube mixers
Opening lyophilized cultures
Centrifugation[a]

[a] Except tube breakage or wet screw cap.
Adapted from Kenny and Sable (1968) and Stern *et al.*
(1974).

TABLE 2.6 Activities which may lead to airborne contamination by releasing particles
smaller than 5 μm

Careful pouring
Fixed-volume automatic pipettors
Pipette mixing of liquid culture
Harvesting/dropping infected eggs
High speed blenders
Shaking machines
Dropping tubes or flasks of cultures
Pipette spills

Adapted from Kenny and Sable (1968) and Stern *et al.*
(1974).

effect on airborne particles. All of these, acting together, determine the trajectory of a particle. The distance travelled horizontally, from rest, is known as the stopping distance and the final vertical movement as the terminal velocity. Particles of about 50 μm or larger will not remain suspended very long in air, even when projected initially with a horizontal velocity of 1 m/s (Licht, 1972) as shown in Table 2.7.

Presumptive airborne infections: common-source outbreaks

Infections presumed to arise from the inhalation of infective airborne particles seem to be caused by a small number of agents and associated with a few laboratory activities. The numbers of individuals who contracted disease is, however, quite large.

A major incident involving brucella occurred at Michigan State University in 1938 and was reported by Newitt et al. (1939) and Huddleson and Munger (1940). There was a brucella research laboratory in the basement of the teaching laboratory building, but it was out of bounds to students. Nevertheless many students became infected. There were 45 clinical cases and 49 subclinical infections. One victim was a commercial traveller who visited the building twice. The organisms were probably dispersed by a centrifuge placed at the bottom of a stairwell and used to concentrate brucella suspensions. This could have produced a massive aerosol so that infective airborne particles were dispersed around the building.

Four other brucella infections probably arose from the inhalation of aerosols released during pipetting live cultures. In Cowan's (1951) case the worker was filling tubes for lyophilization. Spink (1956) reported the other three: two followed careless and one followed careful pipetting. A total of 60 cases were reported by Howe et al. (1947) and Trever et al. (1959) at one laboratory (Fort Detrick). Most of these were apparently airborne infections.

Q fever has a bad reputation for infecting people by the airborne route, even at considerable distance. This may be associated with the very low dose required to initiate infection (Tigertt et al., 1961). In 1940, in a period of less than 2 months, 15 of 153 people who worked in one building became infected (Hornibrook and Nelson, 1940). The laboratory where Q fever was being investigated was on the second floor; four of the people concerned worked on that floor, four worked in the basement and seven on the third floor. There were no cases on the

TABLE 2.7 Stopping distances, terminal velocities and downwards vertical distances travelled by particles of density 1 g/cm³ at different initial velocities

Particle size (μm)	Stopping distances (m)		Terminal velocity	Vertical downward distance travelled after 1 s (m)
	initial velocity = 0.1 m/s	initial velocity = 1.9 m/s		
1	3.54×10^{-7}	3.54×10^{-6}	3.47×10^{-6}	3.37×10^{-6}
10	3.08×10^{-5}	3.08×10^{-4}	3.02×10^{-3}	3.02×10^{-3}
50	7.70×10^{-4}	7.70×10^{-3}	7.55×10^{-2}	7.55×10^{-2}
100	3.08×10^{-3}	3.08×10^{-2}	3.00×10^{-1}	2.91×10^{-1}

After Licht (1972) and Kennedy (1988).

first (ground) floor. Another outbreak occurred in a US Army laboratory (Robbins and Rustigian, 1946). There were 20 cases in 3 months among staff and visitors. Another report (Commission on Acute Respiratory Diseases, 1946) tells of 16 cases spread through several rooms in different parts of another building. A much larger outbreak occurred in a single building in 1946 (Huebner, 1947). Altogether 47 people were affected, including some visitors. None of the staff who worked with the agent were infected: they were probably immune as a result of previous infections. The majority of victims worked on the same floor, but cases occurred on all five floors and among staff whose activities involved visiting all of them. Even some guinea pigs, previously serologically negative, became positive. All of these infections were associated with the harvesting, homogenizing and centrifuging of yolk sac material and all the evidence points to dispersal of infected airborne particles around the buildings by air currents.

An interesting outbreak ('Q fever down the drain') was reported by Stoker (1957). Five people were involved: one of them harvested yolk sacs; another was a histologist who entered the Q fever unit once; the third examined infected tissues in another laboratory; the other two worked in a room which was flooded when a drain was blocked with effluent from the Q fever unit. Blenders used for homogenizing yolk sac material had been filled with disinfectant and emptied down the sink. Coxiellas were recovered from the sink waste sludge.

Several infections with the agents of typhus of one kind or another have clearly been associated with aerosols or infected airborne particles. Gold and Fitzpatrick (1942) reported a case which followed an accident with a blender and in the same year Loffler and Mooser (1942) noted 11 that occurred after intranasal inoculation of mice (also associated with bubbling at the nares). In 1945 Silva and Kopciowska noted that two vaccinated workers escaped infection but six passers-by did not. Intranasal inoculation of animals was probably responsible for four cases reported by Van den Ende *et al.* (1943), but after the introduction of safety cabinets there were no more apparently airborne cases of that kind. Tullis *et al.* (1947) reported a case involving harvesting yolk sacs and Wright *et al.* (1968) noted one associated with the use of a blender and two who worked with the agents but had not had any accidents.

Eight cases of Venezuelan equine encephalitis reported by Lennette and Koprowski (1943) were probably caused by the inhalation of dust from mouse cages containing infected suckling mice. The mothers ate the young mice, and so contaminated the litter. The staff had to sort through the litter to recover uneaten mice. Four other infections, associated with blending egg cultures, were described by Koprowski and Cox (1947); two of the people affected worked elsewhere in the building. An airborne outbreak was reported by Slepushkin (1959). Some ampoules containing dried virus were dropped and broken in a hallway. No action was taken and 24 people who worked on the same floor, the one above and the one below were infected. Dispersal of particles was probably assisted by the opening and closing of many doors by people who wanted to know what had happened.

A number of other infections are worth mentioning in this context. McCoy (1930, 1934) reported 11 cases of psittacosis. Only two of those infected worked with the birds; the other nine worked in the same building. Three cases of louping ill among workers who had performed intranasal inoculations were recorded by Rivers and Schwenker (1934). A centrifuge accident led to four cases of glanders, with one death (Hunter, 1936). Airborne fungal spores have been responsible for some fungal infections according to Bush (1943). Infected dust from animal cages was probably responsible for the case of St Louis encephalitis (von Magnus, 1950). The three cases of Rocky Mountain spotted fever reported by Johnson and Kadull (1967) and the nine reported by Oster *et al.* (1977) were not associated with accidents or tick bites and were reasonably assumed to have been airborne infections. Cases of rabies, associated with the homogenization of infected brain material, were reported by Winkler *et al.* (1973) and Conomy *et al.* (1977). And finally, there is the anthrax incident in the former USSR, referred to on p. 10.

Other routes

Through the mouth

Microorganisms may be ingested as a result of eating, drinking and smoking in the laboratory, mouth pipetting and transfer to the mouth by the fingers or articles.

EATING, DRINKING AND SMOKING

These practices are quite properly prohibited in well-managed laboratories and it is difficult to find recent reports of infections that have been contracted in this way. Infections may arise from the consumption of contaminated food sent in for laboratory examination and the consumption of food brought into the laboratory and contaminated while it is there.

An example of the first was given by Pike (1979): a laboratory worker developed a streptococcal disease after tasting milk samples. An unpublished incident from our experience concerned a number of meat pies submitted for examination. Because of a numbering error they were all thought to be wholesome and some were eaten by members of the staff, who all developed salmonellosis.

The most likely, but unreported, event would be the contamination of food from laboratory benches, or while it is stored, pending the lunch break, in the laboratory refrigerator along with cultures and pathological material. To add to this hazard, the food may be eaten with contaminated fingers.

Only one incident involving smoking has been found: Lubarsch (1931) wrote of a man who smoked while working with anthrax and who became infected.

MOUTH PIPETTING

As long ago as 1915 both Paneth and Kisskalt warned of the hazards of pipetting by mouth. Paneth (1915) investigated 67 laboratory accidents, involving 45 infections and found that 40% of them resulted from mouth pipetting. He considered that there was one infection for every three known pipetting accidents. In Kisskalt's (1915) paper there is a reference to a physician who infected himself with typhoid fever in 1893 as a result of a mouth pipetting accident, and Schaefer (1950) considered that mouth pipetting was the chief source of laboratory infections with *Salmonella typhi*. Sulkin and Pike (1951) found that 34 of 1342 laboratory infections investigated between 1930 and 1950 were caused by mouth pipetting. In the report of Pike (1976) 92 (13%) of 703 known accidents that resulted in infection were associated with aspiration of infected material through pipettes. Later Pike (1978) identified 28 infections with *S. typhi*, six with other salmonellas and eight with shigellas, all as a result of mouth pipetting accidents. Other infections that have been reported include six cases of glanders in one year (Stewart, 1904); scarlet fever (Friedman, 1928); hepatitis (Sawyer *et al.*, 1944); brucellosis (Meyer, 1943); Coxsackie virus (Shaw *et al.*, 1950) and influenza (Cook, 1961). (Other hazards of mouth pipetting are discussed on p. 70.)

In 1977 Harrington and Shannon reported that 65% of 352 laboratories in England and Wales and 35% of 133 in Scotland still permitted mouth pipetting. The practice continues and we have even seen pasteur pipettes used for mouth pipetting of blood samples.

CONTAMINATED FINGERS OR ARTICLES

Fingers are frequently contaminated during laboratory manipulations, even by the most careful workers. Benches and equipment may be contaminated as a result of unrecognized spillage of cultures or blood, or by the deposition of airborne organisms (see p. 42). The organisms are picked up on the fingers or articles such as pens, pencils and labels and transferred, directly or indirectly, to the mouth.

There are several accounts of such 'direct contact' infections: Kisskalt (1929) wrote of a laboratory assistant who contaminated her fingers with a culture of cholera. She and a friend, who washed her linen, both died of the disease. Dried cultures on the outside of a flask were responsible for seven infections with one death according to Smith and Harrell (1948). A glassware cleaner contracted a streptococcal disease from unsterilized tubes (Sulkin and Pike, 1951). Newsom (1976a) mentions an infection with tubercle bacilli contracted from a culture that had merely been placed in disinfectant instead of being properly decontaminated. The case of typhoid (*Times*, 1977) mentioned on p. 18 was probably contracted in this way.

Through the skin and mucous membranes

The dry, horny outer layer of the skin offers considerable protection against the invasion of microorganisms, but is, in fact, rarely intact. Apart from obvious lesions, very small cuts and abrasions, not visible to the naked eye, offer portals of entry to the superficial blood vessels.

The term 'mucocutaneous' is used to describe exposures of the broken or apparently unbroken skin, and through the mucous membranes of the eyes. 'Percutaneous' exposure indicates penetration of the skin, e.g. by sharps objects such as hypodermic needles (see below).

CUTS, SCRATCHES AND OTHER LESIONS

Microorganisms may be picked up on the fingers and hands from contaminated benches and equipment and may enter the body through quite small, often inapparent lesions.

Hardy *et al.* (1929) referred to the skin as a portal of entry of *Brucella melitensis* and Meyer and Eddy (1941) reported a case of brucellosis in which the organisms entered through eczema lesions on the hands.

THROUGH THE CONJUNCTIVAE

Papp (1957) was able to transmit measles, mumps and rubella by swabbing human eyes with diluted saliva containing the viruses. Hogan and Zimmerman (1962) stated that the conjunctivae may be the site of primary lesions in tuberculosis and syphilis and that in tularaemia it may be the initial site of infection. Bond *et al.* (1982) described how hepatitis B infection occurred when the corneal surfaces of a chimpanzee were inoculated with 50 µl of HBsAg-positive plasma.

In laboratories the eyes seem to be particularly vulnerable to splashes (Baker *et al.* (1989). Infections reported include the agents of sporotrichosis (Fava, 1909; Wilder and McCullough, 1914); relapsing fever (Iwanowa, 1928), meningitis (*JAMA*, 1936), leptospira (Welcker, 1938), typhus (Gold and Fitzpatrick, 1942), Newcastle disease (Burnet, 1943; Yatom, 1946; Shimkin, 1946; Freyman and Bang, 1948; Gustafson and Moses, 1951; McCarthy, 1978; Mustaffa-Babjee *et al.*, 1976), trachoma (Smith, 1958), toxoplasmosis (Rawal *et al.* 1959; Field *et al.*, 1972), gonococcal conjunctivitis (Bruins and Tight, 1979; dengue (Melnick *et al.*, 1948), typhus, Wright *et al.*, 1968; Norazah *et al.*, 1995), Coxsackie B (Dietzman *et al.*, 1973); hepatitis B (Kew, 1973), acute haemorrhagic conjunctivitis (AHC) (Sasagawa *et al.*, 1976). The circumstances surrounding some of these are shown in Table 2.8 (Kennedy, 1988a).

The hand-to-eye route is less clearly documented as far as laboratory-acquired infections are concerned, but the potential is there. People touch their faces much more often than they realize. Flewett (1980) told the story of an ophthalmic unit where one member of the staff surreptitiously counted the number of times two others touched their faces (and presumably their eyes) in the course of half an hour. One did it 27 times and another rubbed his eyes 15 times. Hand-to-eye transmission could account for at least some of the 188 (27%) infections resulting from spills, sprays, etc. among Pike's (1976) total of 703 accidents.

Microscopes are potential source of eye infections in medical laboratories.

TABLE 2.8 Some laboratory-acquired infection where the conjunctiva appeared to be the portal of entry

Reference	Infection	Circumstances
McCarthy (1978)	Gonococcal eye infection	Spray in face while inoculating tube with syringe
Mustaffa-Babjee *et al.* (1976)	Newcastle virus conjunctivitis	Droplets in eye while grinding chicken tissue
Sasagawa *et al.* (1976)	AHC virus conjunctivitis	Needle came of syringe—droplets into eye
Smith (1958)	Trachoma virus	Needle came of syringe—spurt hit face
Kew (1973)	Hepatitis B virus (seroconversion)	Squirted HBsAg-positive blood into eye and rubbed it with hand

From Kennedy (1988).

There are three reports (Olcerst, 1987: Doyle *et al.*, 1989: and Paul *et al.*, 1989), all from industry, where such infections resulted from communal use.

Accidental inoculation

Infection may arise as the result of pricking, jabbing or cutting the skin with infected instruments or objects such as hypodermic needles, scalpels, and broken, contaminated glassware. Phillips (1969) ascertained that 148 (4%) of 3700 laboratory-acquired infections had resulted from accidental inoculations with hypodermic needles. Pike (1976) reported that of 703 infections resulting from known accidents 177 (25%) were associated with needle and syringe accidents but he did not say how many of these involved puncture with the needle. He also records that 112 (16%) followed injuries received from broken glass and sharp objects other than hypodermic needles.

Infections arising from needle-sticks and injuries from contaminated sharp instruments were discussed by Collins and Kennedy (1987) and include the following incidents (mentioned also in Chapter 1), all associated with laboratory, animal house or autopsy room activities: diphtheria (Mallory, 1913; Baldwin *et al.*, 1923; Hammerschmidt, 1924); gonococcal lymphangitis (Sears 1947); hae-molytic streptococci (Hawkey *et al.*, 1980); leptospirosis (Blumenberg, 1937; Welcker, 1938; Bertok *et al.*, 1960; Sarasin *et al.*, 1963); *Mycobacterium marinum* (Chappler *et al.*, 1977); mycoplasma (Hill, 1971); *Treponema pallidum* (Buschke, 1913; Graetz and Delbanco, 1914; Levaditi and Marie, 1919; Gahylle, 1924; Wakerlin, 1932); tuberculosis (Alderson, 1931; Borgen, 1953; Webber, 1956; Minkowitz, 1969; Sahn and Pierson, 1974); blastomycosis (Schwarz and Baum, 1951; Wilson *et al.*, 1955; Harrel and Curtis, 1959; Landay and Schwarz, 1971; Larsh and Schwarz, 1977); cryptococcosis (Glaser and Gordon, 1985); sporotrichosis (Thompson and Kaplan, 1977; Ishizaki *et al.*, 1979); Ebola fever (Emond *et al.*, 1977); hepatitis B (Callender *et al.*, 1982; Gerberding *et al.*, 1985; Grist and Emslie, 1987); Rocky Mountain spotted fever (Johnson and Kadull, 1967); HIV (CDC, 1988b) scrub typhus (Buckland *et al.*, 1945); malaria (Burne, 1970; Cannon *et al.*, 1972; Bouree and Fouquet, 1978; Bending and Maurice, 1980); toxoplasmosis (Strom, 1950–1951; Beverley *et al.*, 1955; van Soestbergen, 1957; Rawal, 1959), leishmaniasis (Knobloch and Demar, 1997). (Other hazards with syringes and needles are discussed on pp. 80–88.)

INJURIES ASSOCIATED WITH LABORATORY ANIMALS

Infection may follow when laboratory workers are bitten or scratched by experimental animals, including arthropods. Pike and Sulkin (1952) reported that 32 (15%) of 213 known accidents preceding infection were caused by the bites and scratches of laboratory animals. Later, Pike (1976) gave a figure of 95 (14%) injuries by animals and ectoparasites out of a total of 703 accidents. (See also p. 261 and Table 2.3.)

The increasing use of primates in laboratories has been a cause for concern, especially as simian B virus occurs in 1–3% of newly imported animals (Hartley, 1974). The virus is passed to humans by bites and scratches and has been responsible for a number of fatal infections. There were only three survivors of 24 cases reported (Bryan *et al.*, 1975). (See also Chapter 17.)

Material from foreign sources

Specimens and cultures from other countries, especially those in the tropics, may contain unexpected pathogens, even Hazard Group 4 agents, and should be regarded with suspicion (Chapter 11).

It is wise to open all such packages in a safety cabinet and treat the material under Level 3 containment conditions until the microbial content is identifed.

Reference, proficiency testing and external quality assurance materials

Specimens which bring into reference laboratories pathogens that may not normally be handled could be sources of infection through almost all of the above routes.

The classic example is typhoid fever acquired from such material in the USA (Blaser *et al.*, 1980; Holmes *et al.*, 1980; Blaser and Lofgren, 1981). Indeed, Blaser *et al.* (1980) have pointed to the laboratory as a reservoir of infection by *Salmonella typhi*. Jacobson *et al.* (1985) reported a case of Flexner dysentery acquired from a quality control specimen. Grist and Emslie (1985, 1991) reported three. Grist (personal communication) considers that most such infections are caused by shigellas. In the UK materials containing typhoid bacilli are not distributed as quality control specimens.

The (UK) Communicable Disease Surveillance Centre (CDSC, 1991) reported a *Brucella melitensis* infection acquired from a misidentified culture sent to a reference laboratory. Chin (1988) reported a case of laboratory-acquired diphtheria arising from an EQAS specimen.

External quality control materials are not above suspicion. All of five batches of immunoassay control sera of human origin tested gave positive results for anti-hepatitis C virus (Simmons *et al.*, 1990). An incident was reported (Anon., 1989) in which a pregnant laboratory worker developed hepatitis B after suffering a cut while handling quality control material which later gave a positive test result for hepatitis B virus. Jones *et al.* (1985) obtained positive results for HTLV III antibody when they tested some samples of Factor VIII-deficient plasma, and the Department of Health (DH 1985) warned of possible infection risk from human blood-based coagulation-factor deficient plasmas.

Stock cultures

Many laboratories maintain their own stock cultures, which are periodically subcultured. Infections arising from this procedure seem to be confined to salmonellas, especially *S. typhi*. Olson *et al.* (1961) found that a strain isolated 41 years earlier was still able to infect a worker. The CDC (1979a) reported 11 cases arising from stock cultures. Blaser and Lofgren (1981) told of a laboratory worker who handled a stock strain and transmitted it to two members of his family without becoming infected himself. Baumberg and Freeman (1971) reported a laboratory infection with an old strain of *S. typhimurium* long thought to be avirulent.

Vaccine production units

Workers in vaccine production laboratories may become infected with the agents used. Buckland *et al.* (1945) reported infections arising in a scrub typhus vaccine unit; Olle-Goig and Canela-Soler (1987) and Martin-Mazuelos *et al.* (1994) among staff in laboratories producing *Brucella melitensis* vaccines. A man who worked in a BCG production laboratory developed tuberculosis caused by that agent (Engbaek *et al.*, 1977).

Modern pharmaceutical and biotechnological operations are designed to protect workers against infection with vaccine strains (Beale, 1992; Collins and Beale, 1992; WHO, 1995).

Infectious dose

The dose or number of organisms required to initiate infection is obviously difficult to ascertain and it clearly depends on the route. Some information, accumulated by the National Institutes of Health, is shown in Table 2.9 (CDC, 1974b).

TABLE 2.9 Infectious doses for some diseases (25–50% volunteers)

Disease or agent	Route	Dose[a]
Scrub typhus	intradermal	3
Q fever	inhalation	10
Tularaemia	inhalation	10
Malaria	intravenous	10
Syphilis	intradermal	57
Shigella flexneri	ingestion	180
Anthrax	inhalation	$\geqslant 1300$
Typhoid	ingestion	10^5
Cholera	ingestion	10^8
Escherichia coli	ingestion	10^9
Shigellosis	ingestion	10^9
Measles	intranasal spray	0.2
Rhinovirus	nasal drops	$\geqslant 1$
Venezuelan equine encephalitis	subcutaneous	1
West Nile fever	intramuscular	1
Parainfluenza 1	nasal drops	$\geqslant 1.5$
Poliovirus 1	ingestion	2
Rubella	pharyngeal spray	> 10
Coxsackie A21	inhalation	> 18
Rubella	subcutaneous	30
Adenovirus 24	conjunctival swab	> 32
Rubella	nasal drops	60
Adenovirus 7	nasal drops	> 150
Respiratory syncytial virus	intranasal spray	$> 160–640$
Influenza A2	nasopharyngeal	> 790
SV-40 virus	nasopharyngeal	10 000

[a]Number of organisms or appropriate viral units. Adapted from CDC (1974).

Personnel

The laboratory worker and his clothing may spread infection unwittingly. There are the cholera cases mentioned above (p. 48) and the technician who acquired a brucella infection in the laboratory passed it on to his wife (Reuben *et al.*, 1991).

Contaminated laboratory clothing may also be a reservoir. There is some evidence (Wong and Nye, 1991) that laboratory overalls, especially their cuffs, are readily contaminated. Birnbaum and Grosche (1982) considered the transmission of infection by laboratory clothing and McKenzie (1992) drew attention to the potential dispersal of genetically-modified *Escherichia coli* by laboratory overalls, with the possibility of undesirable genetic recombination in the environment

Apart from their personal affairs, a heavy work load imposes stress on staff and may lead to short cuts, carelessness and poor technique and then to infection.

'Protocol drift' is not uncommon in laboratories where supervision is poor and standard operation procedures (SOPs) are not under continuous review. Evans *et al.* (1990) identified inappropriate behaviour, flawed techniques, mouth pipetting and failure to wear gloves as contributors to accidents and infections.

Deliberate infections

Apart from experiments on humans, e.g. self-inoculation in the 'interests of science', there have been attempts at suicide and at harming other people. Self-infection with tubercle bacilli has already been mentioned (p. 16), and there is a report (*Science Journal*, 1966) of a microbiologist who planted typhoid bacilli in food and infected 44 people.

Chapter 3
Hazard groups and containment levels

The information collected and published by many workers, and summarized in Chapters 1 and 2 indicates that some microorganisms are more hazardous than others. It became clear in the 1960s and early 1970s that some kind of hierarchical classification could separate those that could be regarded as harmless from those that needed much more care if they were to be handled safely. This classification has led to the recognition of what are now known as hazard (or risk) groups (or classes).

Such a classification lends itself to sets of safety measures of increasing complexity. As it is a waste of time and resources to take elaborate precautions when the risks are negligible but foolish to take none if they are considerable these precautions should be appropriate to the hazard group into which the organism being investigated is placed, and the techniques used. These sets of safety measures are given the same numbers as the hazard groups and are known as containment or biosafety levels.

Classification of microorganisms on the basis of hazard

The first classification on the basis of hazard was developed by US workers and passed through several steps of evolution from 1969 and was finally revised in 1976 and again in 1981 (CDC, 1976, 1981c) and was widely circulated within and outside the USA. It classified known microorganisms—the expression 'etiologic agent' is used throughout—into four classes (1–4) of increasing hazard.

In the United Kingdom a classification of pathogens into three categories was proposed by the Godber Working Party (DH, 1975). An alphabetical system was used to avoid confusion with the US system and because only pathogenic organisms were under consideration. One category—the most hazardous—was refined by the Dangerous Pathogens Advisory Group (DH, 1976) and the other two by the Howie Working Party (DH, 1978). The final classification, into three categories A, B and C, with the B category subdivided into B1 and B2 to accommodate hepatitis B material was incorporated in the *Code of Practice for the Prevention of Infection in Clinical Laboratories*—the Howie Code (DH, 1978).

In 1979 the participants in the World Health Organization's Special Programme on Safety Measures in Microbiology agreed a classification of agents

54

into risk groups that followed the US system, with additional criteria (WHO, 1979). This is followed in later WHO publications (WHO, 1993).

The UK system, which was never very satisfactory, was superseded by a numerical classification formulated by the Advisory Committee on Dangerous Pathogens (ACDP, 1984), which paralleled those of the USA and WHO.

In 1990 The European Community (EC) issued a directive on the protection of workers from the risks of exposure to biological agents at work (EC, 1990). The term 'biological agents' used includes microorganisms, both naturally occurring and those that are genetically modified, cell cultures, and human endoparasites, which are able to provoke infection, allergy or toxicity. The directive applied to all people who handled these agents, whether they worked in laboratories, in commercial production of materials from such agents, or otherwise came into contact with the agents in the course of their work. The requirements of this directive were incorporated into the (UK) *Control of Substances Hazardous to Health Regulations 1994* (COSHH) and to its Approved Code of Practice (HSE, (1995) and also to a new edition of the ACDP document (ACDP, 1995a).

The US, WHO and EC systems differ slightly in their wording but agree in principles; that of the US uses 'Classes' while the others use 'Groups'. They show an evolution: the later systems are more comprehensive, but that is of little account as the US has subsumed its classes into biosafety levels, as described below.

Group 1
USA   Agents that offer no or minimal hazard under ordinary conditions of handling.
WHO   An organism which is most unlikely to cause human disease.
EC   One that is unlikely to cause human disease.

Group 2
USA   Agents of ordinary potential hazard, including those that may produce disease of varying degrees of severity as a result of accidental laboratory infections.
WHO   Moderate individual risk, low community risk: a pathogen that can cause human or animal disease but is unlikely to be a serious hazard to laboratory workers, the community, livestock or the environment. Laboratory exposures may cause serious infection, but effective treatment and preventive measures are available and the risk of spread of infection is limited.
EC   One that can cause human disease and might be a hazard to workers; it is unlikely to spread in the community; effective prophylaxis or treatment usually available.

Group 3
USA   Agents that offer special hazards to laboratory workers.
WHO   High individual risk, low community risk; a pathogen that usually causes serious human or animal disease but does not ordinarily spread from one

infected individual to another. Effective treatment and preventive measures are available.

EC   One that can cause severe human disease and presents a serious hazard to workers; it may present a risk of spreading to the community but effective prophylaxis or treatment is usually available.

Group 4

USA   Agents that are extremely hazardous to laboratory workers or cause more serious epidemic disease.

WHO   High individual and community risk; a pathogen that usually causes serious human or animal disease and which may be readily transmitted from one individual to another, directly or indirectly. Effective treatment and preventive measures are not usually available.

EC   One that causes severe human disease and is a serious hazard to workers; it may present a high risk of spreading to the community; no effective prophylaxis or treatment is usually available.

Other countries introduced similar systems. That of Australia (first published in 1991) is now in the Australia/New Zealand Standard (AS/NZ, 1995) and that of Canada is in the laboratory safety guidelines first published in 1990 which has recently been revised (Health Canada, 1996).

It must be mentioned here that the groups and classes are variously labelled 'Hazard ...' or 'Risk ...'. Strictly speaking, a *hazard* is a potential to cause harm, while a *risk* is the probability that harm will be caused. In practice either term will suffice see Chapter 11.

Compilation of lists of microorganisms in the various groups

The compilation of these lists has been difficult and has generated much discussion and not a few disagreements. A comparison of eight lists (five European, before agreements made by the European Community – and those of Australia, Canada and the US) showed disagreements in the placing of 42 agents (Frommer *et al.*, 1989).

Committees convened to produce the lists have not always included, or consulted, microbiologists who are experienced in handling particular organisms and this has has been a cause of some concern. Infectious diseases are emotive subjects and public and political concerns may be overriding. The positions of the anthrax bacillus and rabies street virus are examples. Neither is particularly hazardous but both are placed in Group 3 in the EC list.

For details reference should be made to the published lists. Those of the EC (1990) and the ACDP (1995a) have recently been updated (HSE, 1998). For the USA see CDC/NIH (1993). Table 3.1 indicates the hazard groups (and containment levels—see below) into which the agents known to have caused laboratory-acquired infections and mentioned in this book have now been placed by the HSE (1998a).

Again, it seems natural to place 'new' pathogens and some that have enjoyed notoriety or publicity in higher categories than they deserve. Fortunately, common sense has prevailed and in the European Union (EC, 1990, 1993; see

TABLE 3.1 Hazard groups and containment levels of agents known to have caused laboratory-acquired infections

Agents	Hazard group/containment level
BACTERIA AND RICKETTSIAS	
Bacillus anthracis	3
Bordetella pertussis	2
Borrelia recurrentis	2
B. duttoni	2
Brucella abortus	3
B. melitensis	3
B. suis	3
Burkholderia mallei	3
B. pseudomallei	3
Campylobacter jejuni	2
C. pylori	2
Chlamydia psittaci	3
C. trachomatis	2
Clostridium botulinum	3
C. tetani	2
Corynebacterium diphtheriae	2
Coxiella burnetii	3
Erysipelothrix rhusiopathiae	2
Escherichia coli	2
E. coli O157 and other verotoxigenic strains	3
Francisella tularensis	3
Haemophilus ducreyi	2
H. influenzae	2
Helicobacter pylori	2
Leptospira spp.	2
Listeria monocytogenes	2
Mycobacterium tuberculosis	3
M. bovis	3
BCG	2
M. leprae	3
Neisseria gonorrhoeae	2
N. meningitidis	2
Pasteurella spp.	2
Rickettsia mooseri (*typhi*)	3
R. orientalis (*tsutsugamushi*)	3
R. prowazeki	3
R. rickettsii	3
Salmonella typhi	4
other serotypes	2
Serratia marcescens	2
Shigella dysenteriae	3
other spp.	2
Streptobacillus moniliformis	2
Treponema pallidum	2
Vibrio cholerae	2
V. parahaemolyticus	2
VIRUSES	
Adeno	2
Apeu	2*
Bebaru	2
Bhanja	3
Bluetongue	2*
Bunyanwera	2
Caraparu	2*

TABLE 3.1 (*Cont.*)

Agents	Hazard group/containment level
VIRUSES (*continued*)	
Catu	2*
Chikungunya	3
Colorado tick	2*
Coxsackie	2
Congo-Crimea	4
Dengue	3
Dugbe	3*
Eastern equine encephalitis	3
Ebola	4
Ganjam	
Germiston	3
Hanta	3
Hepatitis B	3
Herpes simiae B	3
Human immune deficiency	3
Hypr	3
Influenza	2
Issy-kul	3*
Japanese B encephalitis	3
Junin	4
Keystone	2*
Koutango	3*
Kunjin	2*
Kyasanur Forest	4
Lassa	4
Louping ill	3
Lymphocytic choriomeningitis	3
Machupo	4
Marburg	4
Marituba	2*
Mayoro	3
Modoc	2*
Mucambo	3
Muructucu	2*
Newcastle	2
Omsk	4
O'nyong-nyong	3
Oriboca	2*
Oropouche	3
Orungo	3*
Ossa	2*
Parvo B19	2
Piry	3
Pichende	2
Poliomyelitis	2
Powassan	3
Rabies	3
Rift Valley	3
Russian spring-summer	4
Sabia	4
St Louis encephalitis	3
Semliki Forest	3
Spondweni	3
Tacaribe	2*
Vaccinia	2
Variola	4

Venezuelan equine encephalitis	3
Vesicular stomatitis	2
Wesselbron	3
Western equine encephalitis	3
West Nile	3
Yaba	2
Yellow fever	3
Zika	2*

UNCLASSIFIED

Transmissible spongiform encephalopathy agents	3
New variant Creutzfeldt-Jakob agent	3

FUNGI

Blastomyces dermatitidis	3
Coccidioides immitis	3
Cryptococcus neoformans	2
Histoplasma capsulatum	3
Sporothrix schenckii	2
Trichophyton spp.	2

PARASITES

Cryptosporidium spp.	2
Leishmania braziliensis	3 M
L donovani	3 M
Naegleria fowleri	3
Plasmodium falciparum	3 M
other spp.	2
Schistosoma spp.	2
Trypanosma brucei rhodesiense	3 M
T. cruzi	3

Sources: COSHH Approved List ACOP (1994); ACDP (1994, 1995): *CDC/NIH (1993).
M = Microbiological safety cabinets not needed.

also ACDP, 1995) it is possible to obtain a certificate of exemption from some of the provisions of the *Control of Substances Hazardous to Health Regulations 1994* for work with certain agents in Group 3, where, e.g., the risk of airborne transmission is low. By the same token some agents, and under certain circumstances, the risk of infection is high, e.g. from heavy suspensions and through the apparently unbroken skin or mucosae. Under certain other circumstances, where the risk of airborne infection may be enhanced, they are placed in a 'mezzanine group', 2+. Both exemption candidates and 2+ agents are listed in Table 3.2.

In assigning biological agents to hazard groups care must also be taken not to concentrate on the obvious hazards and to overlook new developments which may not be widely reported. Although some organisms seem to infect almost everyone who handles them, others, once cheerfully regarded as harmless, have surprised a number of unfortunate victims. The hazards associated with *Francisella tularensis* are well known, but only about 10 years ago laboratory workers learned of those arising from certain manipulations with *Serratia marcescens*.

One obvious problem in assigning microorganisms to hazard groups according to risks to laboratory workers arises from their geographical and climatic distribution. An organism which offers no particular hazard to the community in one district may pose serious problems and require more precautions in another,

TABLE 3.2 Group 3 agents unlikely to present an airborne risk and Group 2+ agents, i.e., those that may offer an enhanced risk

Group 3 Exemption candidates	Group 2+ agents, supplementary measures
Escherichia coli (verotoxigenic strains)	*Borrelia bugdorferi*
Mycobacterium ulcerans	*B. duttoni,*
M. microti	*B. recurrentis*
Salmonella typhi	*Chlamydia trachomatis*
S. paratytyphi	*Clostridium botulinum*
Shigella dysenteriae	*Corynebacterium diphtheriae*
	Legionella pneumophila
Hepatitis B, C, D, E and G viruses	*Leptospira interrogans* (*canis,*
Human immunodeficiency virus	*icterohaemorrhagia, hebdomadis*)
Human T cell lymphotropic virus	*Treponema pallidum*
Simian immunodeficiency virus	*Vibrio cholerae,*
Agents of BSE, CJD, GSS and kuru including new variants	*V. el Tor*
	Neisseria meningitidis
Leishmania braziliensis	
L. donovani	*Cryptococcus neoformans*
Plasmodium falciparum	*Sporothrix schenkii*
Taenia solium	
Echinococcus granulosus	
E. vogelli	
E. multilocularis	

Adapted from ACDP (1995) and HSE (1998).

because of the presence of potential vectors and reservoirs of infection. The WHO recognized this, which is why it left the health authorities of member states to make their own lists. The incidence of infections with each microorganism in the community must also be considered. There is little point in placing an organism in a high risk category, requiring special precautions in the laboratory, if the workers are extensively exposed to during the 16 or so hours that they are outside it. The volume and concentration of the agent used are also relevant, as are the techniques used. Minimal precautions may be adequate for handling small volumes and low concentrations, but as the risks of working with large volumes and high concentrations are much greater, a higher level of precautions may be desirable.

Large scale culture of pathogens can be accomplished safely, as has been demonstrated in industry, but 'bucket bacteriology', practised in some educational and other establishments by scientists who have had no microbiological training could place many people at risk. There is nothing to prevent what the US system calls 'competent scientists' (not, note, 'competent microbiologists') from working with large volumes of some pathogens. Similarly, work with microorganisms maintained securely in culture vessels is much safer than work which involves aerosolization and some experiments involving the inoculation of animals. Other very important considerations are the availability of effective pre- and post-exposure vaccines and of antibiotics and chemotherapeutic agents.

It should not be assumed that an organism not listed in Groups 2, 3 or 4 is necessarily in Group 1. Taxonomic research often results in changes in specific and even generic names. Synonyms abound in microbiology. Another problem is 'guilt by association'—naming a genus followed by 'spp.' which infers that all members of that genus are in the same hazard group. This can be very misleading as it might imply that all the species in that genus are pathogenic.

Some of the organisms placed in Class or Group 1 are indeed hazardous as they or their spores may be allergenic.

Summary of criteria for assigning biological agents to hazard groups

(1) The past history of laboratory-acquired infections.
(2) The incidence of infection in the community.
(3) The dose required to initiate infection (if known).
(4) The route by which infection is acquired in the laboratory; this may not be the same as the 'natural' route.
(5) The presence of reservoirs and vectors in the district.
(6) The amounts and concentration of the agent used.
(7) The techniques employed, especially in respect of aerosol production and the likelihood of accidental release.
(8) The availability and effectiveness of prophylactics and treatment.

The hazard group notation is no longer used in the USA as the numbers equate with those of the US Biosafety Level. Duplication is therefore avoided. This has much to commend it.

Laboratory containment and biosafety levels

The safety measures that are essential for the protection of laboratory staff from infection increase in detail and complexity in parallel with the hazard groups. In the US and WHO systems that are termed 'Biosafety Levels' and in the EU 'Containment Levels'. Hazard Group 1 agents will require the minimum of safety measures, i.e. Level 1; Group 2 agents will require higher standards, and so on.

The word 'Containment' implies the sum total of measures to keep the agents in their containers, thus preventing them from escaping and infecting workers. Originally the US Public Health Service used the term 'Physical Containment', and thus the containment levels were abbreviated to P1, P2, etc. but since about 1993 this was dropped in favour of 'Biosafety Level. There is much to be said in favour of the term 'Biosafety Level.

The biosafety or containment levels specify the kind of 'containment', i.e. architectural, engineering, operational, equipment and technical requirements for work with microorganisms in each of the hazard groups. These have been published by various states and organizations and although there are differences in the wording (as with that of the hazard groups), there is general agreement in principle. We have attempted to collate published requirements or recommendations (EC, 1993; CDC/NIH, 1993; WHO, 1993; ACDP, 1995; AS/NZ, 1995; and Health Canada, 1996) and these are summarized in Table 3.3, which are, however, not all-inclusive. Local regulations should, of course, be observed and states that have not formulated their own would be advised to follow those of the WHO (1993).

TABLE 3.3 Summary of safety measures for work at Containment Levels 2, 3 and 4

	Level 2	*Level 3*	*Level 4*
Sites, buildings, engineering and facilities			
Laboratories separated from other activities in same building	If justified by risk assessment	Yes	Yes, preferably separate building
External windows	Closed during work	Lockable	Sealed, watertight and unbreakable
Internal windows so that occupants may be observed	Not necessary	Recommended	Yes
Handbasins	Yes	In each room	In each room
Showers	Not necessary	Recommended	Yes
Surfaces impermeable to water and cleaning agents	All work surfaces	All work surfaces and floors	All exposed surfaces
Surfaces impermeable to acids, bases, solvents and disinfectants	Recommended	Yes	Yes
Laboratories maintained at negative pressure relative to atmosphere	Not necessary	Yes	With gradient
HEPA filtration of intake and extract air	Not necessary	Extract air	Intake and extract air
Airlock access to laboratories	Not necessary	Recommended	Yes
Room sealable for decontamination	Not necessary	Yes	Yes
Separate effluent treatment	Not necessary	If indicated by risk assessment	Yes
Two-way intercom system	Not necessary	Yes	Yes
Equipment			
Laboratories to have own (dedicated) equipment	Not necessary	Yes	Yes
Microbiological safety cabinets	If indicated by risk assessment	Classes I and/or II	Class III
Autoclaves	In building	In room	Pass-through, double-ended
Centrifuges	Available	In room	In room
Operational measures			
Initial and annual tests for containment capability	Not necessary	Yes	Yes
Biohazard sign displayed	On all doors	On all doors	On all doors
Authorized access	Yes	Limited	Strictly limited
Validated disinfection and disposal methods	Yes	Yes	Yes
Emergency plans for spillages of infectious material	Yes	Yes	Yes
Safe storage of biological agents	Yes	In Level 3 room only	In Level 4 room only
Effective rodent and other vector control	Yes	Yes	Yes
Protective clothing to be worn	Standard overalls	Standard overalls	Full protection

Gloves to be worn	If indicated by risk assessment	Yes	Yes
Medical supervision	By occupational health service	By unit physician	By unit physician
Immunization	As for general public	As for general public and for agents used	As for general public and for agents used
Baseline sera	Not necessary	Recommended	Yes
Accident reporting	Yes	Yes	Yes
Two-person rule	Not necessary	Recommended	Yes
Supervision of maintenance and service personnel	Yes	Accompanied by staff member	Accompanied by staff member, after decontamination of room
Technical procedures			
Work with infectious materials	On open bench except if aerosol release is possible	In Class I or II microbiological safety cabinet	In Class III microbiological safety cabinet
Centrifugation	In closed containers	In sealable safety buckets	In sealable safety buckets
Use of 'sharps'	As authorized	Avoid	Banned except when especially authorized

Sources: Frommer *et al*. (1989), CDC/NIH (1993), ACDP (1995); Health Canada (1996).

The International Biohazard symbol

Large research institutions, where highly infectious material is handled, have had warning notices of various kinds for many years. In the 1970s the International Biohazard sign (Figure 3.1) was introduced. This is now used in most countries to identify materials, equipment and rooms which contain or are contaminated with hazardous microorganisms. The symbol is red, or black on a yellow background and usually includes the word 'Biohazard'. The notices may be purchased from laboratory suppliers in various sizes, suitable for screwing to doors, sticking to equipment and as adhesive tape.

Unfortunately, many people who do not work in microbiological laboratories do not understand either the symbol itself or the word 'biohazard'. It is

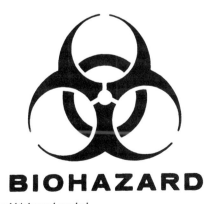

Figure 3.1 The international biohazard symbol

advisable, therefore, to supplement notices with additional information, e.g. 'Infectious hazard' or 'Danger of infection'.

These notices should be used sparingly and only to denote hazards from Hazard Groups 3 and 4 agents. If they are used too freely they lose their impact and become merely part of the laboratory scenery.

A problem which should be mentioned here is that although these classifications, both of organisms and laboratories, may be reasonable for clinical, pharmaceutical and biomedical research laboratories they are hardly applicable to many industrial, food science and agricultural laboratories. Some of the organisms in Hazard Group 2, requiring Level 2 containment (e.g. certain streptococci, enterobacters, proteus and pseudomonads) occur naturally in foods, and generally in the environment. To insist on Level 2 containment, for example to homogenize a sample in a laboratory but not in the adjacent kitchen or works canteen, is nonsensical.

It may well become necessary for different systems of classification to be applied: on the one hand to work with undoubted pathogens isolated in clinical laboratories; and on the other to opportunist or 'guilt by association' microorganisms normally present in foods and on plants.

Complications are likely to arise in industry as a result of a classification agreed by the Organization for Economic Cooperation and Development (OECD, 1992). In this there are still four levels but the first does not require containment as understood by most microbiologists. The others are containment levels CL1, CL2 and CL3. As these four levels equate fairly with Hazard Groups 1–4 respectively, it follows that the numbering systems for groups of organisms will be out of step with containment levels, e.g. organisms in Hazard Group 3 will require OECD Containment Level 2, which is absurd. While this system is unlikely to affect clinical laboratories it could pose problems in commerce during the transitional stages of a microbial product from laboratory to pilot plant and thence to large scale production, all of which are likely to take place on the same premises.

Chapter 4

Equipment- and technique-related hazards

It is now quite clear that many laboratory-acquired infections are related to the use of particular items of equipment or particular techniques or both. Some of these have already been mentioned in Chapter 2. Since the 1950s a considerable amount of work has been done by a number of people, aimed at assessing the hazards presented to microbiologists and others who handle infectious material by the tools and practices of their trade. This has led to a better understanding of the principles of the spread of laboratory-acquired infections and has pointed to ways of minimizing these hazards, in some cases eliminating some of them altogether, and to the furtherance of 'good laboratory practice'. Some of this work and the lessons that may be learned from it are discussed in this chapter.

The inoculating loop

For many years wire loops, initially made of platinum, and recently of nicrome, have been used to transfer cultures and make microscopical preparations. There were early reports, e.g. by Fricke (1919), that these procedures dispersed micro-organisms into the air or on working surfaces, but it was not until the 1950s that scientific investigations were made into the possibility that laboratory infections might be caused by improper use of these simple instruments.

Various investigations were carried out by Anderson *et al.* (1952), Wedum (1953), Reitman and Wedum (1956) and Phillips and Reitman (1956). The results of these investigations suggested that certain precautions should be taken and these have been reviewed and improved by a number of other workers (Morris, 1960; Chatigny, 1961; Darlow, 1969, 1972; Collins, 1972, 1974, 1976; Collins *et al.*, 1995).

Loops of various sizes, some completely closed, some unclosed, and on shanks of varying length are found in laboratories. These factors, and the ways in which loops are used, contribute to the formation of aerosols by spontaneous discharge, flaming and inexpert use.

Spontaneous discharge; good and bad loops

Large and badly-made loops readily shed their loads, either spontaneously or as a result of vibration during transfer. The surface tension of most liquids used in microbiology does not allow films (loopsful) of a large area or volume to be retained. Similarly, loops which are incompletely closed impose strains

65

on the films of liquid which they hold and the films break readily. An aerosol is produced when a loopful discharges spontaneously. In the experiments of Anderson *et al.* (1952) suspensions containing about 10^9 *Serratia indica* per ml were used and films in inoculating loops were burst by touching them. An average of 0.2 colonies of the organisms was recovered per operation. One colony would represent about 10 organisms. There was considerable variation, however, and allowing for this and the small volume of air that could be sampled the results demonstrated a serious contamination and infection hazard from large or poorly-made loops.

The optimal size of a loop appears to be about 2–3 mm internal diameter and it must be completely closed. Welded loops are available commercially, and so are loops made by forming the centre of a length of wire around a rod of suitable diameter and twisting the remainder into a spiral.

A loop on the end of a long wire tends to vibrate and will readily discharge its contents. Platinum wire does not vibrate as much as nicrome wire but is expensive. In their experiments Anderson *et al.* recovered an average of 0.6 colonies per operation from charged loops that were made to vibrate. If a loop contains a drop, rather than a film, much greater contamination of surfaces, as well as aerosols, would result.

Loops with shanks not longer than 5–6 cm are recommended (Collins, 1974, 1993; HSE, 1991a) as vibration is minimized. It is not true that long shanks are necessary to make subcultures from tubes or bottles to avoid contaminating the loop holder. Good technicians learnt long ago that inclining the tube not only brings the fluid nearer to the open end, but also minimizes 'fall in' by airborne contaminants.

Loops should be expected to have a short life. When they become bent, or encrusted with carbonized material they should be replaced.

Loop holders

It is surprising that loops sealed into the ends of glass rods still persist in some places. They are a hazard to the worker as the glass frequently shatters when held in the flame, so there is a temptation not to flame the glass, although it may well be contaminated. Aluminium alloy and steel holders are much safer and more satisfactory and are not expensive.

Plastic loops

Pre-sterilized plastic loops in packets of 50 are available in several sizes, holding between 1 and 10 µl. They are completely closed, and do not vibrate. They are more rigid than wire loops and are therefore most convenient for handling viscous material such as sputum. As they do not need flaming another risk is obviated (see below) and they are very useful for work in safety cabinets, where, as indicated in Chapter 5, bunsen burners should not be used. After use, the plastic loops are discarded into disinfectant.

Alternatives to loops

For some procedures there are alternatives to loops. Wooden sticks (swab sticks) and throat swabs are convenient for handling faeces and sputum, e.g. for microscopical preparations and primary inoculation of liquid media, or of solid media before looping out (Collins, 1972).

Flaming loops

The spattering which is visible and audible when a loop charged with wet or proteinaceous material is held in a bunsen flame has long been of concern to bacteriologists and was noted by Fricke (1919). Small droplets can be seen, carried clear of the flame. These may be carried upwards by the hot air stream rising around the bunsen (Morris, 1960). It was thought that larger particles might contaminate the bench, but later work, by Harvey *et al.* (1976), suggests that this may not be so. They collected and cultured 500 samples of inspissated salmonella culture material and 571 of inspissated shigella culture material that had been ejected from loops during flaming and failed to recover either organism.

There is little evidence that large amounts of aerosols are generated in this way. In the experiments of Wedum (1953) and of Phillips and Reitman (1956), in which loops charged with broth cultures were held in various parts of a bunsen flame, the numbers of colonies grown from air samples around the bunsen varied from none to 0.3 per operation.

However minimal these hazards may be it seems wise to take some precautions when organisms in the higher risk groups are cultured. Several methods and pieces of equipment have been devised. The alcohol-sand flask is an American innovation. A conical flask is three-quarters filled with sand and 70% alcohol added to give a 2–3 cm layer above the sand. The contaminated loops are cleaned by pushing them into the sand and rotating them, before they are flamed. The alcohol-sand flask is autoclaved and replaced regularly. An alternative (Collins, 1974, 1976) is a bolt-head flask of water gently boiling on a Thermomantle or Simmerstat. Before they are flamed contaminated loops are held in the boiling water for a few seconds to kill vegetative organisms and remove inoculum.

Various kinds of 'hooded bunsens' have been developed and two are particularly suitable for bacteriological work. That of Darlow (1959) can be made in the laboratory workshop to fit any size bunsen burner. Two 'micro-incinerators' (such as those of Kampff (unpublished) and Allen (1977)) are available commercially (Figure 4.1). Material ejected in the flame is contained and incinerated on the wall of the metal or glass tube.

Electrically operated 'microincinerators' ('electric bunsens') are also on the market. Impatient workers find that these, and the microincinerators take longer than ordinary bunsens to make loops red hot. This is usually as a result of lack of experience on the part of the workers. It is important to flame not only the loop but the rest of the wire and that part of the holder that has been inside the specimen or culture tube. Some of these devices have yet to be evaluated.

Microscopic preparations and slide agglutinations

When a loopful of a liquid culture is spread on a slide or a suspension is made on a slide from a solid culture small droplets may be broadcast, particularly if the loop is wielded energetically. When the loop is withdrawn from the drop more small droplets may be scattered, and aerosols may be formed. This was

(a)

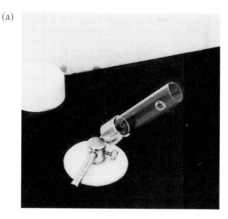

(b)

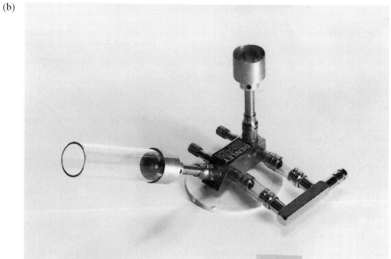

Figure 4.1 Microincinerators (a) gas, Kampff (Horwell); (b) gas, Allen (Denly)

demonstrated by Hirschbruck and Forthman (cited by Fricke, 1919) who made smears on cover glasses placed on the surface of culture media which they afterwards incubated. Price (1976) sampled the bench on which slide agglutinations with salmonellas and shigellas were performed. He used swabs and contact plates and sampled the bench after each session during which 18–200 slide agglutinations were done. Salmonellas were recovered from as many as 28 of 30 samplings and shigellas from 15 of 22. Aerosol formation during slide agglutination tests was also studied by Reitman and Wedum (1956) who recovered an average of 0.3 colonies per operation from the air during 60 slide agglutinations.

Gentle movements, particularly when the loop is raised from the slide, will reduce the numbers of droplets splashed and aerosols formed. Collins and Lyne (1976) suggested using a drop of a saturated solution of mercuric chloride instead of saline for making preparations of mycobacteria. The organisms are killed rapidly. Price (1976) tried this for slide agglutinations but found that suspensions autoagglutinated. He then experimented with 10% formalin in saline and found a marked reduction in the recovery of salmonellas and shigellas from the bench.

Work of this nature with particularly hazardous organisms should be done in a safety cabinet, but once microscopical preparations have been made the slides may be brought out of the cabinet to dry, fix and stain. The hazard from droplets and aerosols is then past (but is replaced by that of contamination of the fingers).

The hot versus cold loop

It is common practice to sterilize a loop in a bunsen flame and then plunge it into a culture. Even with a short pause between the two operations a sizzling noise is heard. Anderson *et al.* (1952) showed that aerosols could be created in this way, although the amount generated depended on the volume of air above the culture in the container. The greater this volume the more aerosol was produced. With 100 ml of culture in a 250 ml flask and a hot loop an average of 8.7 colonies per operation were grown, but with a cold loop the average number was only 0.8. They also found that when a hot loop was agitated in the culture, more aerosol was formed. The neck of the container and the plug or cap were likely to be contaminated.

We were trained to employ two loops. One is in use while the other, after flaming, cools on a rack next to the bunsen (later, on the bunsen pilot switch). This practice is still observed in some laboratories and has much to commend it.

Plating cultures

Sweeping a charged loop across the surface of a petri dish of solid medium may generate aerosols unless the surface of the medium is smooth. If the medium contains the remains of air bubbles or other irregularities the loop will vibrate as it catches on them. This was demonstrated by Wedum (1953) and Reitman and Wedum (1956). When a loopful of broth culture was streaked on smooth agar the air sampler yielded from 0.06 to 4.6 colonies per operation depending on the skill of the technician. With rough agar, the average number of colonies was 25.

An alternative to a loop—the glass spreader—reduced the number of particles released from smooth agar to the level of that of the best technician (0.06 colonies) and on rough agar to 8.7 colonies per operation.

The catalase test

The traditional catalase test in which a loopful of organisms is added to a drop of peroxide on a slide results in much bubbling and dispersal of aerosols (Lennox and Ackerman, 1986). The tube method (Collins, 1974) is safer. A mixture of peroxide and Tween 80 is added to the culture in a tube or bottle and the cap replaced. Another safe method uses capillary tubing containing peroxide. The tip of this is touched on the colony and if catalase is present small bubbles rise in the tube and remain there. Another method employs a cover glass. A drop of peroxide is placed on a cover glass which is inverted over the colonies on a petri dish culture.

Summary of precautions

Short, fully-closed loops in proper loopholders, or plastic loops should be used and glass spreaders should be considered. Gentle movements are necessary to avoid broadcasting droplets and aerosols. A suitable bactericidal liquid should be used for microscopical preparations and slide agglutinations. Work with organisms that are known to cause infection by the airborne route should be done in a safety cabinet.

Using pipettes

Infectious hazards associated with pipettes fall into five groups:

(1) aspiration into the mouth, i.e. mouth pipetting;
(2) inhalation of aerosols through the lumen of the pipette;
(3) transfer to the mouth by fingers contaminated by the proximal end of the pipette;
(4) contamination of the environment, e.g. the air, the bench and equipment;
(5) injuries sustained from sharp or broken contaminated pipettes.

Mouth pipetting

Pipettes have been used since the beginning of the nineteenth century but no-one knows who 'invented' the practice of transferring fluids by sucking them up in tubes held in the mouth. Generations of students and scientists have used them in this way and it is not surprising that accidents have occurred in which toxic or corrosive fluids have been aspirated into the mouth. It was quite natural, however, for the early bacteriologists to use mouth pipetting to transfer cultures of microorganisms from one vessel to another.

The custom of plugging the mouth ends of pipettes with cotton wool was introduced in the late nineteenth century to avoid contamination of cultures from the mouth, not to protect the mouth from the culture. It would be unrealistic to assume that all, or even the majority, of pipette-associated infections were caused by unplugged pipettes, so one must conclude that the plug is no barrier to aspiration. Even well-made plugs are not effective against violent sucking. Very tight plugs, which encourage strong suction, may suddenly come out into the operator's mouth, followed by the contents of the pipette.

Paneth (1915) suggested that instead of pipetting by mouth, rubber 'balloons' (teats) could be used. These teats, of various sizes, and also lengths of rubber tubing connecting the pipette to a mouth piece were used by some workers for many years, but it was not until the middle of this century that pipetting devices began to appear on the market (Wedum, 1950) although Fricke (1919) lists 23 references to such devices. Even after 1950, and in spite of reports of pipette associated infections these 'pipettors' did not meet with much favour among many laboratory workers. In 1961 Phillips reported that 63 (62%) of the 102 laboratories he visited permitted mouth pipetting. Some 15 years later Harrington and Shannon (1977) surveyed safety in British medical laboratories and reported that mouth pipetting was practised in 229 (65%) of 352 laboratories in England and Wales and in 47 (35%) of 133 in Scotland.

Even in the 1980s mouth pipetting was observed in some US laboratories (Evans *et al.*, 1990).

Aspiration of a culture into the mouth is an accident to be remembered and should always be reported. There are other hazards of mouth pipetting, however, that may pass unnoticed, and never recorded as they do not constitute accidents.

BANNING MOUTH PIPETTING, AND OBJECTIONS TO BANS

A great deal of work has been done and much has been written on the hazards of mouth pipetting. Paneth (1915) calculated that 22 of the cases of laboratory-acquired typhoid fever reported by Kisskalt (1915) were the result of mouth pipetting. Since then, Reitman and Wedum (1956), Morris (1960), Phillips (1961), Darlow (1969, 1972), Phillips and Bailey (1966), Moore (1971) and Collins (1980a) have all stressed the risks associated with this practice. But although it has been expressly banned by various organizations (e.g. DH, 1972, 1978; NIH, 1978; WHO, 1993; ACDP, 1990, 1995), it is unfortunate that little is being done, in many places, to enforce the ban. There was not much difference between the numbers of laboratories where mouth pipetting was condoned in the 1950s (Phillips, 1961) and in the late 1970s (Harrington and Shannon, 1977). Our experiences in visiting laboratories bears this out. In 1980 and in 1986 one of us (CHC) saw laboratory workers mouth pipetting blood with pasteur pipettes! One hears complaints that the laboratory is 'too busy', that pipetting devices 'waste time' and are 'expensive' and 'difficult to work with'. All those objections seem to fall apart when someone in such a laboratory becomes infected. In the UK, where there are still strong feelings about the risks of hepatitis B and HIV, it is interesting that there is so little concern about mouth pipetting, particularly of blood, serum and dilutions of both. What is equally disturbing is when pronouncements are made that mouth pipetting is acceptable 'in certain circumstances' such as the collection of capillary blood from infants. One such counsel (DH, 1980), later withdrawn, invoked an assessment of the hazards of mouth pipetting (Collins, 1980a) and of the dangers of 'special circumstances' becoming 'general circumstances'. Both in turn, generated strong feelings (Correspondence, *IMLS Gazette,* 1980).

MODERN ALTERNATIVES TO MOUTH PIPETTING

As indicated above, the rubber teat has been available and has been used by many bacteriologists for over half a century. The official instructions for testing milk in the 1930s included using teats on 1 ml pipettes for making dilution of that harmless fluid.

A great many of the objections to rubber teats, at least since the Second World War, have stemmed from the lack of instruction in their use. Few teachers, and until 1964 no standard textbooks, gave directions. The following is cited from Collins (1964) and repeated in subsequent editions of Collins *et al.* (1995).

'Choose teats with a capacity greater than that of the pipettes for which they are intended, i.e. a 1 ml teat for Pasteur pipettes, a 2 ml teat for 1 ml pipette, otherwise the teat must be used fully compressed, which is tiring. Most beginners compress the teat completely, then suck up the liquid and try to hold it at the mark while transferring it. This is unsatisfactory and leads to spilling and inaccuracy. Compress the teat just enough to suck the liquid a little way past the mark on the pipette. Withdraw the pipette from the liquid, press the teat slightly to bring the fluid to the mark and then release it. The correct volume is now held in the pipette without tiring the thumb and without risking loss. To discharge the pipette, press the teat slowly and gently and then release it in the same way. Violent operation usually fails to eject all the liquid; bubbles are sucked back and aerosols are formed.'

A large number of devices that are more sophisticated than simple rubber teats are now available. Broadly speaking there are four kinds of these:

(1) rubber bulbs with valves that control suction and dispensing;
(2) syringe-like machines that hold pipettes more rigidly than rubber bulbs and have a plunger operated by a rack and pinion or a lever;
(3) electrically operated pumps fitted with flexible tubes in which pipettes can be inserted;
(4) mechanical plunger devices which take small plastic pipette tips and are capable of repeatedly delivering very small volumes with great accuracy.

Some of these are shown in Figure 4.2.

It is not easy to give advice on the relative merits of the various devices. That which suits one operator, or is best for one purpose may not be suitable for others. Choice should therefore be made by the operators, not by managers or administrators who will not use them. None of those in categories 1, 2 and 4

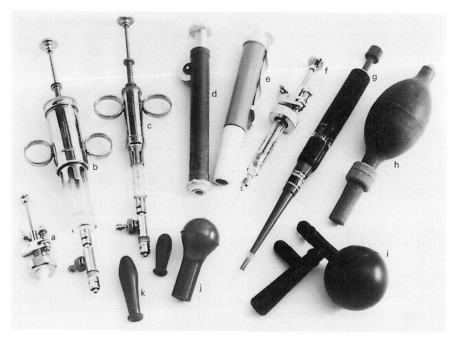

Figure 4.2 Pipetting devices in use in a UK laboratory (a) MicroRepette (Jencons). (b) (c) Acurette (Jencons). (d) Pipump (Payne). (e) Sarpette (Sarsted). (f) Repette (Jencons). (g) Finn-pipette (Jencons). (h) Aspirette (Jencons). (i) Saffron (Payne). (j) Tapered bulb for disposable pipettes (Sterilin). (k) Rubber teats. (Other companies supply these or similar articles). (Photo: ada-p)

above is expensive, and it should be possible for several different models to be available. What is necessary is some system of instruction in their use and in their maintenance.

A few years ago there were complaints that some of those in (2) above actually contributed to hazards in the laboratory. It was alleged that they allowed pipettes to leak and that the force necessary to insert the pipette sometimes caused it to break and to cut the hand of the operator. As this was not our experience, some of the offending devices were examined. In two that undoubtedly permitted leakage the insides of the rubber cones that hold the pipettes were found to be rough, with cuts in the surfaces. It was then noted that several of the pipettes in use in that laboratory had broken and chipped ends. These had damaged the cones when the pipettes were pushed into them. In another model the plastic barrel surrounding the pipette holder was cracked, expanded when a pipette was pushed in, and did not hold it tightly enough to prevent leakage. Another leakage was traced to an ill-fitting piston. It had hardened and had shrunk away from the barrel. Hardening and deterioration of the rubber cones, with consequent loss of elasticity, was observed in two pipettors which had been associated with broken pipettes.

It was obvious in all these cases that it was not the devices themselves that were responsible for the hazards, but poor laboratory management. All of those seen had been in use for some time and had not been inspected. These pipettors should not be expected to last for ever, but maintenance, including the application of silicone grease and rubber preservative, will prolong their lives and ensure that they work properly. Chipped and broken pipettes should be discarded. They can cause cut fingers anyway. It helps to wet the ends of pipettes with water or disinfectant before pushing them into these pipettors.

INHALATION OF AEROSOLS

This is a hazard that is not fully appreciated, although the risks were pointed out over 30 years ago.

When a column of liquid is sucked up in a pipette the surface of the liquid is under reduced pressure and is agitated. Aerosols are formed and these could be aspirated into the mouth. Bloom (1960) experimented with unplugged pipettes and aspirated tritium oxide, using a modified syringe to apply suction. Measurements of tritium oxide in the air in the syringe showed that after each aspiration 5–70 μl of the solution was present.

Similar investigations were made by Phillips and Bailey (1966) who used *Serratia marcescens* and *Bacillus subtilis*. They used a 10 ml syringe to take 10 ml amounts of culture into pipettes. Rinses of the syringe after 10 such aspirations, which were plated on agar, revealed the presence of organisms that had passed into it from the fluid in the pipette in the absence of any overt aspiration of fluid. The experiments were repeated 120 times for each of the two organisms. In 41 of the experiments with *S. marcescens* and 69 with *B. subtilis*, 1–300 organisms were recovered from the pipette.

The experiments of Bloom and of Phillips and Bailey were conducted with unplugged pipettes and were used as a strong argument for the cotton wool plug. Current knowledge of air filtration suggests, however, that these plugs are not an effective barrier against infected airborne particles except perhaps at atmospheric pressure. Such particles might be aspirated through the average cotton wool plug by the suction necessary to fill the pipette. This hazard is also present when lengths of rubber tubing are used between pipette and mouth.

It may also be argued that these aerosols would enter teats and pipetting aids. This is undoubtedly true, but they would not thereby gain access to the mouth. The question of contamination of these devices is raised below.

ORAL CONTAMINATION

This is another hazard that is neglected, although attention has been drawn to it frequently. During ordinary mouth pipetting operations the finger is placed over the proximal end of the pipette to contain the contents and to ensure controlled release. The finger may be contaminated from the bench or equipment, as described elsewhere in this book, and this action may result in oral contamination. Mouthpieces on the end of lengths of rubber tubing attached to pipettes are also likely to become contaminated. Although the finger is not placed over the end of the mouthpiece, the latter has many opportunities of becoming contaminated when it is placed on the bench or in the pocket of the worker's laboratory overall.

Contamination of the laboratory environment

The air, the benches, equipment, the hands and arms of the laboratory worker may become contaminated during pipetting operations. These hazards have been investigated, or have been discussed by a number of workers (Anderson *et al.*, 1952; Wedum, 1953; Reitman and Phillips, 1955; Reitman and Wedum, 1956; Morris, 1960; Phillips, 1961; Darlow, 1969, 1972).

THE FALLING DROP

There must be very few laboratory workers who have not observed, with varying degrees of alarm, a drop of culture fluid gather on the end of a pipette and then fall on to the bench. Many workers would suppose that the drop, having reached the bench, contaminates only that small area with which it is in contact and that mopping up with a suitable disinfectant is all that is required. This, unfortunately, is not always the case. Much depends on the height from which the drop falls and the nature of the surface it strikes.

Anderson *et al.* (1952) demonstrated this in a series of experiments in which drops were allowed to fall from heights of 3 inches and 12 inches on stainless steel, painted wood, a commercial bench-top material, a dry hand towel, a hand towel wet with phenol, a paper towel, wrapping paper and a pan of 5% phenol. Air around the experimental area was sampled at the time the drops were falling and for a few seconds afterwards. Aerosols, detected by the sampling apparatus, were greatest when drops fell 12 inches on to stainless steel, painted wood, and the commercial bench-top, all very hard materials; but as many colonies developed from the dry hand towel experiment as from the bench-top material. There were markedly fewer colonies in the experiments using the absorbent materials, the phenol-soaked towel and the pan of phenol. The difference between the dry towel and the disinfectant-soaked towel were surprising as many workers used the former, expecting the drops to be absorbed, instead of splattering. Anderson and his colleagues observed what happens to the towel material under a low power microscope. When the drop fell on the dry towel there was a considerable and rapid movement of the fibres which persisted for some time; on the wet towel the movement was much less. It is presumed that it is this movement that disperses the aerosols. Similar results were obtained in a series of experiments by Reitman and Wedum (1956).

According to Darlow (1972) when a drop falls on to a shallow liquid film, such as that occurring on moist agar in a petri dish there is a 'coronet-shaped upsurge of droplets' (Figure 4.3). Some of the droplets are small enough to constitute aerosols; some may be large enough to fall and repeat the process.

Although the results of Anderson *et al.* indicate that fewer aerosols are formed when a drop falls on a paper towel than on one soaked in phenol many American workers still use, and recommend working over, a disinfectant-soaked cloth. Darlow suggested that the towel should be moistened, not soaked, and this seems to be more in keeping with experimental findings. In the UK, working on wet surfaces is unpopular, and dry absorbent paper or filter paper, and especially the very absorbent proprietary bench covering are used.

Apart from this precaution, overcoming the hazard of the falling drop is a matter of training and experience. It is never preventable.

THE LAST DROP IN THE PIPETTE

Pipettes used by chemists are calibrated 'to deliver' and the last drop remains in the tip of the instrument. Pipettes used by bacteriologists are usually calibrated 'to contain' and the last drop is blown out. It is this last drop that may disperse an abundance of aerosols.

This has been demonstrated by high-speed photography (Figure 4.4). When the last drop was blown out bubbles were formed and burst and a spray of about 15 000 droplets was formed. Many of these were under 10 μm in diameter—the

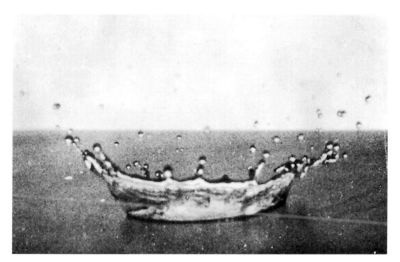

Figure 4.3 The falling drop. Formation of a 'coronet' produced by the impact of a drop falling from a pipette on to a thin film of liquid on a small surface. The release of tiny droplets can be seen. (Reprinted from Darlow, 1972, with permission of the publisher, Academic Press Ltd)

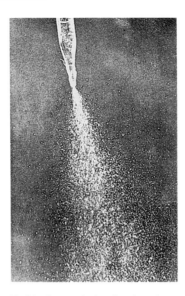

Figure 4.4 Aerosol produced by blowing out the last drop in a pipette

size at which they are likely to dry and leave behind very light infectious droplet nuclei. It was also shown that when 1 ml of a culture was blown out into a petri dish, not only was an aerosol formed but droplets bounced out of the dish on to the bench. Anderson *et al.* (1952) observed bubbles bursting at the tips of pipettes. Reitman and Phillips (1955) compared the effect of blowing out the last drop gently, when bubbles formed at the end of the pipette, with leaving the last drop so that no bubbles formed; there was a 66% reduction in the numbers of colony forming units.

The operator has a choice, then, of a slight inaccuracy and greater safety, or greater accuracy and more personal risk. Fortunately, 1 ml and 10 ml 'delivery' pipettes are now readily available commercially, so this particular hazard may be avoided by allowing the contents of the pipette to drain down the side of the tube or flask.

MIXING AND TRANSFER OF FLUID CULTURES WITH PIPETTES

When liquid cultures are transferred from one container to another, and dilutions are made, it is customary to mix the contents of each tube by sucking and blowing with the pipette. Unless this is done gently there is considerable bubbling and frothing, resulting in the formation of aerosols. Anderson *et al.* (1952) compared the recovery of airborne organisms when mixing was done with and without bubbling. Mixing without bubbling achieved a 75% reduction in colony forming units. When the cultures were mixed by sucking up the fluid and then allowing it to run back by gravity the reduction was 100%.

Reitman and Phillips (1955) also showed that aerosols are produced when cultures are transferred by pipetting and that the amount of aerosol increases with the size of the inoculum and container. When 2 ml of culture was pipetted into 100 ml of broth in a 500 ml flask twice as many colony forming units were recovered as when two drops of culture were added to 10 ml of broth in a 50 ml tube. Adding 2 ml of the culture diluted 1/10 to 100 ml of broth in a 500 ml flask, however, yielded no colonies on the sampling plates.

It is apparent that safe transfer and mixing are possible if some care and patience are used and a little more time is taken over the operation. Kenny and Sable (1968) showed that a 100% reduction in aerosol formation could be achieved by using a tube (Vortex) mixer instead of a pipette (p. 93).

CONTAMINATION FROM THE OUTSIDES OF PIPETTES

When a pipette is dipped into a culture the outside of the distal end becomes contaminated. If that end of the pipette is then touched against the rim of another vessel, including the rim of a discard jar, then the part touched becomes contaminated. This is a not very obvious hazard but could be the cause of unexplained infections if the rims and tops of the flasks, tubes, or jars are handled by an unsuspecting person.

CONTAMINATION OF TEATS AND PIPETTING DEVICES

Infected fluids and aerosols may be aspirated into rubber teats, bulbs and pipetting devices in the same way as the mouth. Most of these aids can be rinsed out with an appropriate disinfectant (one which will not combine with or be retained by the rubber or plastic). Even if aspiration of infected material is not evident it is good practice to disinfect teats, bulbs and pipettors in this way.

Discarding infected pipettes

Contaminated pipettes should always be discarded into disinfectant solution which is prepared daily. It is folly to discard them into dry jars or pans in the expectation that someone will eventually collect and autoclave them. Jars or pans may be used. Jars, preferably of rubber or polypropylene, as these can be autoclaved, should be tall enough to contain enough disinfectant to ensure that the pipettes are completely submerged. Tall jars offer problems to short people who are unable to reach them and who may have to slide the pipette over the rim of the jar, which will contaminate it, as described above. Long pipettes should not be discarded into short jars (Figure 4.5). The upper parts of the lumen will not be disinfected and the jar will be easily knocked over, as it will if jars are placed on the floor besides the worker

A solution was offered by Darlow (personal communication). Rubber jars with square ends are supported at an angle (Figure 4.6). Pipettes can be placed gently into the disinfectant, which is safer than dropping them in and possibly ejecting aerosols through the top end. Ideally, of course, bubbles should be avoided, but this is usually impossible. These jars are convenient for use in safety cabinets, where tall jars cannot be used.

Pasteur pipettes allow short jars to be used, but these must still be tall enough to allow the pipettes to be completely submerged. The jars should be made of autoclavable material.

If pans, e.g. catheter trays, are preferred they should be deep, so that the contents do not spill when they are moved. They should be made of enamel,

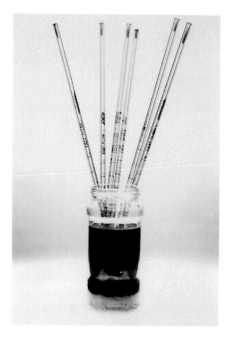

Figure 4.5 Long pipettes in a short disposal jar. Much of the pipettes are not in contact with the disinfectant. (Photo ada-p)

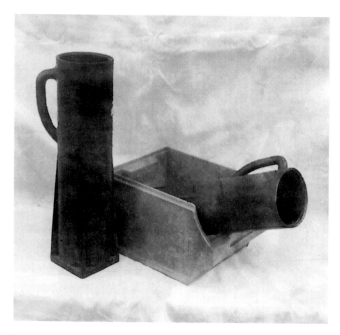

Figure 4.6 Pipette jars. Rubber and polypropylene are safer than glass. Sloping jars are safer and more convenient than those that are used upright

stainless steel or polypropylene so that they can be autoclaved. There may be problems in filling discarded pipettes with disinfectant.

Whichever containers are chosen there remains the need for discipline in their use. They must not be overfilled. One often sees 'art forms' where serried ranks of pipettes, especially pasteur pipettes, appear to grow out of discard jars. Most of the pipettes discarded in this way have no contact with the disinfectant (Figure 4.7). Pasteur pipettes may be safely discarded into the containers used for syringes and needles (see p. 84).

Final treatment and disposal of contaminated pipettes are considered in Chapter 7.

Injuries from pipettes

Injuries to fingers from the broken and chipped ends of graduated pipettes are mentioned above and may be prevented by discarding such articles. A greater

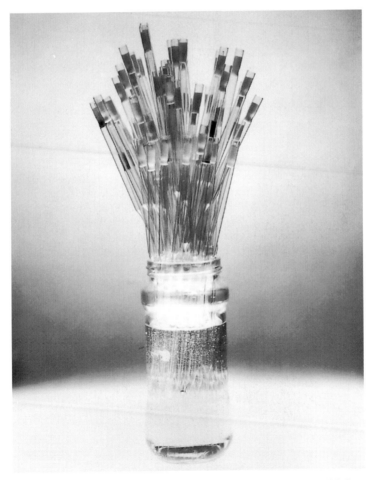

Figure 4.7 Misuse of a pipette disposal jar. Many of these pipettes never reach the disinfectant. (Photo ada-p)

hazard is the glass pasteur pipette, with its fragile, sharp, capillary end. Regrettably, stabbing of the hands and fingers with these pipettes, which may contain microorganisms at the time, is all too common an accident. Soft plastic pasteur pipettes of various sizes, some with integral teats are now on the market. They are supplied in small packs and may be obtained already sterilized. They are much safer than glass pasteur pipettes for work with hazardous microorganisms and for separating serum.

Summary of precautions

The ban on mouth pipetting, and of rubber tubes with mouthpieces, should be enforced with vigour. Laboratory workers should receive training in the use of teats, and pipetting devices should be standard laboratory equipment. Care should be taken to avoid accidental loss of drops from the end of the pipette. The last drop should not be blown out, and when the pipette is used for mixing fluids bubbling should be avoided. Pipettes should be discarded into disinfectant in such a way that the rim of the discard jar is not contaminated and the pipettes are completely submerged. Pipetting devices should be inspected regularly and properly maintained. Chipped and broken pipettes should be thrown away and plastic instead of glass pasteur pipettes used for hazardous materials.

Hypodermic needles and syringes

The hypodermic syringe and its hollow-bore needle seem to be the most hazardous pieces of equipment in common use. At least three surveys of equipment-related infection have shown that about one-quarter of overt accidents which resulted in infection were caused by these instruments. Sulkin and Pike (1951) incriminated them in 26.5% of 215 such accidents; Pike et al. (1965) in 24.5% of 371; and Pike (1976) in 25.2% of 703.

There are at least three ways in which infections can arise; from injection of the operator or colleague, from contamination of fingers and the environment, and from the inhalation of aerosols. Phillips (1969) who investigated reports of 3700 infections (not just accidents) noted that 1.2% of them were caused by injection and 4% by the other methods.

Accidental inoculation: 'needle-stick'

Collins and Kennedy (1987) reviewed 'needle-stick' accidents among health-care workers and identified about 20 infections arising from them (Table 4.1).

At present the main fears seem to be about HIV and hepatitis B.

Many needle-stick accidents occur when the needle is being disconnected from the syringe so that blood may be discharged into its specimen container gently to avoid haemolysis. It is now general policy in the UK (British Medical Association; BMA, 1990) not to disconnect needles from syringes, but to dispose of the whole unit into appropriate containers (see below and p. 84). A popular alternative to the needle and syringe is the vacuum collection outfit.

Most early reports are of inoculations that occurred during experiments with animals. A difficult animal or an inexperienced handler or inoculator can result in any one of them receiving an injection.

TABLE 4.1 Agents known to have caused infections as a result of needlestick and sharps injuries in health-care workers[*]

Brucella spp.	Ebola virus
Cryptococcus neoformans	Hepatitis B virus
Corynebacterium diphtheriae (cutaneous)	Herpes viruses
Leptospira spp.	Human immunodeficiency virus
Mycobacterium marinum	Lassa virus
Mycobacterium tuberculosis	
Mycoplasma spp.	*Blastomyces dermatitidis*
Neisseria gonorrhoeae (cutaneous)	*Cryptococcus neoformans*
Staphylococcus aureus	*Sporotrichum schenckii*
Streptococcus pyogenes	
Treponema pallidum	*Leishmania* spp.
	Plasmodium spp.
Rickettsia rickettsii	*Trypanosoma* spp.
Rickettsia tsutugamushi	

[*] Including laboratory staff.
From Collins and Kennedy (1987) and incidents reported since then.

The increasing use of rubber gloves outside or inside Class III biological safety cabinets has resulted in several cases of operators inoculating themselves when they were using syringes to transfer infected material. Even the most experienced workers may suffer in this way. Emond *et al.* (1977) reported a near-fatal case of Ebola fever contracted from a minute finger prick. There is little doubt that the thick gloves, necessarily worn for such work do lessen tactile sensitivity, and hamper movements.

Syringe and needle assemblies are often used instead of pipettes. As the former offer the greatest hazard they should not be used unless the needle is replaced by a cannula or piece of plastic tubing. There are cheap and effective gadgets for the removal of septum caps so that conventional pipettes may be used to sample contents.

Contamination from leaking syringes

Some syringe plungers do not fit the barrels very well and infected material may leak along the barrel and contaminate the hands of the user. Even with well-fitting plungers there may be some capillary action, especially if the same syringe is used several times.

Disposable plastic syringes are widely used at present and as they come already sterilized it may not be reasonable to test them before use. If it is, filling them with sterile water, blocking the ends and applying pressure to the plungers may demonstrate leakage or capillary action.

Adjusting the volume in a syringe

When a syringe has been filled it is usual to adjust the volume and remove air bubbles by holding the syringe vertically and squirting fluid and bubbles into a wad of cotton wool. Unless this wad is soaked in disinfectant (e.g. 70% alcohol) the fingers may be contaminated. Fluids spread rapidly through dry cotton wool. Phillips (1961) described a much better method which he observed in Australia. A 25 ml screw-capped bottle was filled with cotton wool which was soaked with

70% alcohol. The needle was inserted into the bottle to adjust the volume in the syringe. This method also minimized the risk of self inoculation. If this excellent precaution is not taken the operator should wear gloves.

Animal inoculation

Contamination of animal handlers, bedding and cages may occur unless certain precautions are taken before and after inoculation, particularly by the intra-dermal route. This was shown by Wedum (1953) and Hanel and Alg (1955). All injection sites were shown to be contaminated, due to leakage, but a 30% reduction in organisms resulted from swabbing the site of inoculation with disinfectant before and after injection. (See also Production of aerosols and Virology procedures, below.)

Production of aerosols

Aerosols are produced during several manipulations with syringes and needles. These include withdrawing the needle from a vaccine bottle with a septum cap, or through a rubber stopper, accidental discharge of contents and certain procedures peculiar to virology. They were investigated by Anderson *et al.* (1952), Wedum (1953) and Hanel and Alg (1955) using sieve samplers and bench swabs, with *Serratia indica* and coliphage T-3.

WITHDRAWING THE NEEDLE FROM A VACCINE BOTTLE

Two events occur: high speed photography shows that the needle vibrates, throwing off liquid from its surface in the form of aerosols: the fine thread of liquid drawn out through the stopper by the tip of the needle breaks up into a 'string of beads' (Darlow, 1972) as shown in Figure 4.8. The smaller of the beads became aerosols. The larger ones fall and contaminate the bench. Anderson *et al.* (1952), Wedum (1953) and Hanel and Alg (1955) showed that

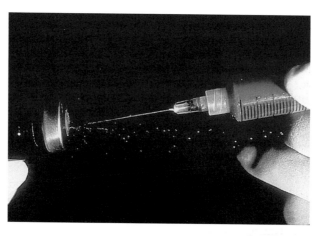

Figure 4.8 Withdrawing a hypodermic needle through a septum cap gives a fine thread of fluid which breaks up into an aerosol

there was a substantial reduction (95%) in organisms recovered when the needle and bottle cap were wrapped in cotton wool soaked in disinfectant, while the needle was withdrawn. A further reduction (99%) was obtained if no air was pushed into the bottle before fluid was withdrawn, i.e. when the contents of the bottle were at atmospheric pressure. Reitman et al. (1954) used a syringe and needle and vaccine bottles to make 10-fold dilutions. They recovered 2.3 coliphage particles per operation without the disinfectant soaked wad but none at all when they used it.

It is wise to wear gloves to hold the wool swab.

ACCIDENTAL DISCHARGE

This usually occurs when the needle does not fit tightly on the butt of the syringe. The needle flies off, or if it is in an animal or a stopper, separates violently from the syringe. In simulated accidents of this kind in a room of volume 500 m^3 in which 0.5 ml of culture was released Hanel and Alg (1955) recovered an average of 235 colonies per plate during a 10-min sieve sampling with the room ventilation off. When the room was ventilated at 11 changes of air per hour an average of 124 colonies per plate were recovered. There was, however, wider dispersion of aerosol in the room when it was being ventilated.

This hazard may be avoided entirely if Luer-Lok syringes are used. In these the needle locks on to the butt and cannot be pulled or pushed off. They are more expensive than disposable or ordinary glass syringes but are so much safer. They are more popular in the USA than in Europe.

VIROLOGY PROCEDURES

Hypodermic needles and syringes are used in virology for a number of procedures. Reitman et al. (1954) investigated the release of aerosols in several of these using coliphage T-3.

The intranasal inoculation of mice yielded few particles recovered per operation with dilution of the inoculum. For example, 27 phage particles were recovered when 1.5 ml containing 1.5×10^8 were inoculated into each of 10 mice, but 0.1 particles per operation when the same experiments were done with a 10^3 dose. Intracerebral inoculation yielded fewer aerosols; only 1.1 particles were recovered per operation when 10 mice were injected with 3.3×10^7 phage particles. Swabbing with 70% alcohol before and after, and surrounding the needle with an alcohol-soaked swab reduced this to 0.2 particles per operation.

When a needle and syringe were used to harvest allantoic fluids from batches of five eggs containing an average of 11.1×10^7 phage particles per ml the recovery was 5.6 particles per operation. In a similar experiment, harvesting amniotic fluid from eggs containing an average of 23.3×10^7 particles the recovery was only 1.0 particle per operation.

Capillary blood sampling

Various kinds of lancing devices are used for this operation, and the instruments are usually disposable. Apart from the hazard to patients when, usually for economic reasons, these lancets are re-used, the operator is also at risk from needle-stick injury. The Medical Devices Agency (MDA, 1997, 1998) has evaluated a number of these devices. The reports include safety considerations.

(It is worth noting here that an alternative to the syringe and needle technique for drawing capillary blood has been examined by Fonseca *et al.* (1997). This uses an erbium YAG laser.)

Discarding contaminated needles and syringes

DISPOSABLES

Disposable syringes and needles are easiest to discard. The needle should never be recapped—a hazardous procedure (Collins and Kennedy, 1987; BMA, 1990) as shown in Figure 4.9.

The best way is to place them in one of the commercially available receptacles that satisfy national standards, e.g. in the UK BS 7320 (BS, 1990b). These containers (Figure 4.10) hold both articles so there is no need to disconnect

(a)

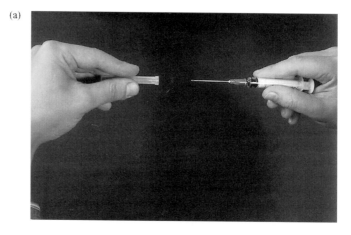

(b)

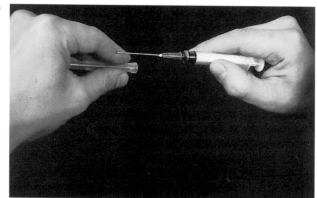

Figure 4.9 The hazard of resheathing a hypodermic needle. (a) The operator aims the needle towards the sheath and (b) misses, jabbing the hand that holds the cap. (Courtesy of the British Medical Association)

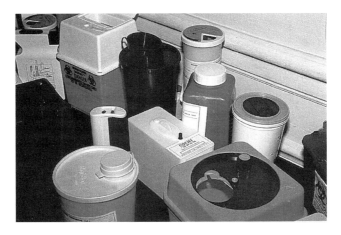

Figure 4.10 Used needle ('sharps') and syringe containers. (Courtesy of M. V. Couson, Institut de Recherche et Sécurité, Paris, France).

them. Needles cannot penetrate the heavy-duty plastic of which they are made. Containers for needles only are sometimes made of thin card and it is not uncommon to see hypodermic needles sticking out through their sides. Anglim *et al.* (1995) reported an outbreak of needle-stick injuries in hospitals that used fibreboard containers.

An inexpensive alternative is to drop needles, or needles and syringes, into half-gallon sized plastic bottles such as those used for retailing orange juice or domestic detergents. Used syringe and needle containers should be autoclaved and/or incinerated (Chapter 7).

RE-USABLES

If needles are removed from re-usable syringes in air, and/or the plunger is withdrawn from the barrel aerosols may be formed. It is best to fill the syringe slowly with disinfectant by withdrawing the plunger with the needle fully immersed in the fluid. The needle should then be disconnected under the surface of the disinfectant with forceps, and the plunger withdrawn so that all three parts are covered with disinfectant and there are no air bubbles.

The final disposal of hypodermic needles and syringes is described in Chapter 7.

Summary of precautions

Care is needed in the choice of syringes. They should not leak past the barrel. Luer-Lok syringes are safest to use. Training and practice are essential to avoid accidental inoculation. Adjustment of volumes should be done with the needle in a swab soaked in disinfectant. A disinfectant-soaked swab should enclose the needle shaft and cap of any bottle from which fluid is to be extracted. Used needles should not be recapped. Disposable needles and syringes should not be disconnected but discarded into special containers. Reusables may be dismantled while totally submerged in disinfectant.

Centrifugation

Reitman and Wedum (1956) and Reitman and Phillips (1956) showed that most operations used at that time in centrifugation released varying amounts of aerosols.

The number of centrifuge accidents known to have caused infection, however, is small. Of a total of 595 accidents of all kinds only 11 were attributable to centrifuges (Sulkin and Pike, 1951, 1965; Phillips, 1961; Pike et al., 1965). A single accident, however, can involve a large number of people. One was known to have led to the infection of 94 individuals with *Brucella melitensis* (Huddleson and Munger, 1940) and another to 122 infections with *Coxiella burnetii* (Huebner, 1947). Not all of these illnesses were associated with traditional centrifuges. Some of the machines were continuous-flow devices.

The nature of these accidents, all of which preceded infections by the airborne route, suggests strongly that inapparent or unrecognized events involving centrifugation might be responsible for some of the 80% of infections which could not be attributed to any personal accident.

Dispersal of material from centrifuges

When a centrifuge rotor revolves at speed a stream of air at high velocity may issue from between the bowl and lid and from the ventilation ports. In unpublished observations made on older and traditional types of centrifuge made in the 1970s we recorded air speeds of up to 8 m/s within a few centimetres of the lid and ports. Smoke test showed considerable turbulence in the air round the machine. Later experiments, with more modern machines by Collins and Gunthorpe (1981) showed air speeds of 0.2–0.4 m/s around the machine, with 3.0 m/s at the lid fastener and 5.0 m/s at the vent (see p. 89).

If droplets of infected materal are released within the bowl they will be comminuted by impact with the moving parts and the wall and will issue on the air stream. This may happen if tubes break in the centrifuge—an obvious accident—or if fluid escapes in some other way from centrifuge tubes. Inspection of the bowl of a centrifuge, or of the wall behind it will reveal, in some laboratories, evidence of this kind of contamination.

BROKEN TUBES IN THE CENTRIFUGE

In their experiments on aerosol dispersal Reitman and Phillips (1956) recovered 118 viable particles of *Serratia indica* per ft^3 of room air sampled over 10 min when a tube containing 500 ml of broth culture was broken at normal centrifugation speed. This kind of centrifuge accident is not uncommon and is often attributable to poor laboratory management and staff training. A tube may break because it is cracked or flawed, or because there are fragments of glass in the bucket from a previous accident which etch the bottom of the tube when it is under centrifugal stress. Buckets may not be placed correctly in their trunnions, and 'spin off' when the machine is started suddenly, or in some cases when at high speeds. This has happened when centrifuges have been placed on high benches, where short people cannot see into them to fit buckets and trunnions properly in the rotor. Another relatively common event is bucket failure when buckets have become corroded as a result of poor maintenance. When this happens it is salutory to examine the surviving buckets. In all of these accidents the centrifuge tube will be shattered and its contents dispersed. Massive aerosol formation is the result.

DISPERSION NOT RESULTING FROM ACCIDENTS

It was the dirty streaks on the wall behind their centrifuge that prompted the investigations of Whitwell *et al.* (1957). They used several bacteriological and chemical indicators and found that a fine spray of liquid was broadcast when the centrifuge operated, even though they used screw-capped tubes. They found that the rims of the tubes became contaminated during uncapping and recapping and shaking (see also pp. 96). Some of the contaminating fluid found its way between the threads of the tubes and caps. During centrifugation this fluid was thrown outside the tube and escaped from the angle head of the machine through the lid and the bearings.

Wedum (1964a) and Darlow (1969) have pointed out that angle head centrifuges are more prone to disperse aerosols than are the swing-out variety. When the angle head rotates the fluid level swings through more than 90° and if the tube is too full it will overflow.

Even if the tube is capped, the fluid may leak under the centrifugal force imposed on it. When Burmeister *et al.* (1962) were investigating laboratory infections with plague they found that fluid containing the organisms remained on the lip of the centrifuge tube after decanting before recentrifugation. This hazard was also noted by Hellman (1969). That centrifugation does not deposit all organisms is pointed out by Morris (1960) who cited the personal observations of W. R. Bale: the supernatant fluid of a culture of *Escherichia coli* which had been centrifuged at 3500 rev/min for 30 min still contained enough organisms to produce an infectious aerosol when decanted. Improper use of the centrifuge, such as abrupt starting and stopping, and failure to balance the tubes may also displace liquid out of the tube. This will then rapidly become aerosolized by the rotor and air movements and will emerge with air stream. Kenny and Sable (1968) found that when a culture is spilt onto a spinning centrifuge rotor large numbers of aerosol particles are generated, many in the 3–5 µm range. They considered that the numbers and sizes of particles containing brucella, tularaemia, Q fever and Venezuelan equine encephalitis agents broadcast in this way could cause infections.

Prevention of dispersal

Aside from the obvious precautions of following manufacturers' instructions, care, good maintenance and avoiding the hazardous practices described above, two courses of action may be taken to prevent the accidental dispersal of material from centrifuges. These are containment of the centrifuge tube in sealed buckets or rotors and containment and filtration of air emitted from the machines by placing them in specially constructed cabinets or enclosures.

SEALED BUCKETS (SAFETY CUPS) AND ROTORS

The sealed centrifuge bucket, known in the USA as a safety cup, is designed to retain the contents of the centrifuge tube if it breaks or its contents leak or otherwise escape. Such buckets have been on the market since the 1950s (Reitman and Wedum, 1956; Chatigny, 1961). Phillips (1961) found various types in use in the USA, Australia and Sweden, although not many of the laboratories he visited (12 of 111) used them.

These buckets are made of heavy gauge aluminium alloy or steel and some have polycarbonate caps so the contents may be seen. It is important that they are not just 'screw-capped tubes' otherwise they may leak, as described by Whitwell *et al.* (1957) and above. In most models there is an O-ring seal. The cap fits into, not onto, the body so the screw thread is inside and any fluid which gets into the thread will be centrifuged back inside the bucket (Figure 4.11).

If a centrifuge tube leaks or breaks inside a sealed bucket a large amount of aerosol will be formed, and as it is contained it will be under pressure. Sealed buckets used for centrifuging tubercle bacilli and similar material should be opened inside a safety cabinet.

Sealed rotors are sometimes offered instead of sealed buckets for traditional centrifuges. They have the disadvantage that if one centrifuge tube breaks all the others are contaminated. With sealed buckets this does not happen. In addition, the seals are more difficult to maintain and the rotor caps, being large, are more likely to be distorted and therefore to leak. It is worth noting here that one of

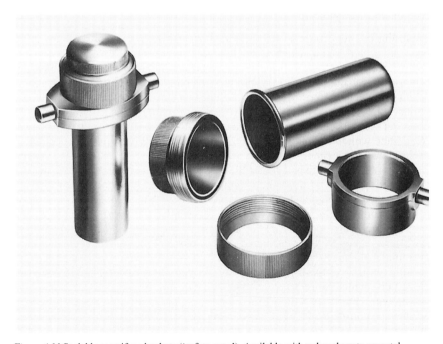

Figure 4.11 Sealable centrifuge buckets ('safety cups'). Available with polycarbonate or metal screw-in caps (MSE)

cases of laboratory-acquired tuberculosis reported by Grist (1983) was associated with a leaking rotor seal.

TESTING SEALED BUCKETS

The British Standard (BS 4402, 1982b) specifies filling sealable buckets with sodium fluorescein and inverting them on filter paper in a container under a negative pressure of 30 mmHg for 3 min. Sealable rotors may be tested by placing filter paper around the inside of the centrifuge bowl, filling the rotors with the fluorescein and centrifuging at a high speed. The paper is then examined by ultraviolet light.

Although this is a rapid and convenient method, Harper (1984) found that it is not as sensitive as a biological test. It does not tell us what happens outside the centrifuge when a tube breaks and a sealed bucket or rotor fails to contain its contents. Harper used deliberately cracked bottles containing *Bacillus globigii* and stood them in the buckets on ball bearings. A cyclone air sampler was placed near the centrifuge and after the tubes had broken the inside of the bowl was swabbed. Seven (27%) of 26 models failed this test and generated aerosols when the bottles broke. More sealed rotors than sealed buckets failed. There were problems with the seals and Harper recommended that buckets should have an O-ring, be of stainless steel rather than aluminium, and that the caps should screw in, not screw on. Plastic caps may not tell the truth—it may be difficult to see through them. If buckets are dislodged while rotating their plastic caps may be fractured. Some plastic caps cannot be autoclaved.

CONTAINING THE CENTRIFUGE

Enclosing the centrifuge so that aerosols emitted are not widely dispersed has been advocated and questioned for about 25 years. Gibson (1955) placed a centrifuge in a cupboard fitted with ultraviolet lights. Reitman and Wedum (1956) illustrated a centrifuge whose top was covered by what is now known as a Class III safety cabinet. Lind (1959) placed a centrifuge in an enclosure with a window. During his worldwide survey of safety precautions Phillips (1961) observed several centrifuges in closed (Class III) safety cabinets, some of which were fitted with ultraviolet light and time switches to prevent premature opening of the centrifuge cabinet.

Darlow (1972) and Evans *et al.* (1972) built a safety cabinet (Class III) around a standard trolley-type centrifuge. Morris and Everall (1972) tried ducting the air from the centrifuge ventilation ports to a safety cabinet, but found that if the velocity and volume of the ducted air exceeded the exhaust capacity of the cabinet much of the ducted air escaped from the cabinet. Gervin and Willis (1973) and Hencke (1973) described various closed and open cabinet assemblies over ultracentrifuges and also a large (28 × 4 × 7 ft high) ventilated cabinet constructed of an aluminium frame and acrylic sheeting fitted with a row of glove ports which housed a centrifuge and preparation assembly. A traditional trolley-type centrifuge was adapted by Hall (1975) by ducting air from the exhaust port through a HEPA filter with the aid of a 'blower' (exhaust fan), both of which could be built onto the machine.

It is noteworthy that in many of these observations and recommendations the centrifuges, whether they were of the traditional or high-speed types, were enclosed in or covered by specially adapted Class III safety cabinets (glove boxes). That this is a safe and satisfactory procedure was demonstrated by Chatigny *et al.* (1979). The rotor of a high-speed centrifuge was weakened and loaded with a bacterial culture. It was then run to destruction. Test bacteria leaked from the vacuum chamber as a result of damage, but were not found outside the cabinet.

Centrifuges in Class I (open-fronted) safety cabinets

It is unfortunate that the concept of enclosing a centrifuge in a safety cabinet was misinterpreted because in clinical laboratories the latter term usually means a Class I, open-fronted cabinet. The experiments reported by Morris and Everall (1972) stimulated one of us (CHC) to test the velocity of air emitted from several centrifuges. Collins (1974) concluded that the pull of the cabinet exhaust may not overcome the discharge velocity of the air from the centrifuge and that the turbulence of air within the cabinet would allow air—and aerosols—to escape into the room.

In spite of the obvious hazards the doctrine of centrifuges in (Class I) safety cabinets continued to be propagated—at least in the UK, even some at courses of instruction for safety officers. This prompted Collins and Gunthorpe (1981) to test the effect of placing a modern bench centrifuge in a modern microbiological safety cabinet that satisfied the requirements of the (then) British Standard (BS 5726, 1979). Air flow from the loaded centrifuge, operated at 3000 rev/min, and before it was placed in the cabinet, varied from 0.2–3.0 m/s around the lid, and was 5.0 m/s from the ventilation port. Air flow into the empty cabinet was 0.85 m/s at all points on the working face. When the centrifuge was placed in the cabinet, but was not working the air flow into the cabinet was disturbed and varied between 0.7 and 1.0 m/s at different parts of the face. Smoke tests showed turbulence around the machine. The centrifuge was then run at 3000 rev/min. Air flow into the cabinet then varied between 0.1 m/s at some parts of the face and 1.0 m/s at others. Smoke tests showed gross air turbulence within the cabinet and some escape of smoke at one part of the working face.

It was concluded that running centrifuges in Class I safety cabinets is a hazardous practice. Similar experiments (unpublished) with Class II cabinets have given comparable results.

There is, of course, no need to place traditional centrifuges in Class I cabinets. As indicated above, sealed centrifuge buckets provide a safe alternative.

Centrifuges for special purposes

Centrifuges have been designed for washing blood cells for serological investigations, concentrating and preparing films of fluids for cytological examination and making blood films for microscopy. It became apparent that some of these machines were capable of dispersing aerosols and droplets which contaminated the bench and surrounding areas. Rutter and Evans (1972) detected blood and bacterial aerosols ejected from a microhaematcrit centrifuge when the tubes leaked.

The problem was investigated in detail by Harper (1981, 1984) who tested several machines with suspensions of *Bacillus globigii*. He operated them in a

Class III safety cabinet under controlled conditions, using settle plates and air sampling equipment. All the machines originally tested produced aerosols. When sealed containers were supplied by the manufacturers, or HEPA filters were fitted, the hazards were considerably reduced. It is encouraging to learn that manufacturers are incorporating safety features into the design of some new equipment.

Summary of precautions

Care should be taken that centrifuge tubes are not cracked or flawed, or they may break under the stress of centrifugation. Tubes should not be more than three-quarters full, especially if angle centrifuges are used. Tubes should preferably be capped and they and the buckets should be balanced carefully to avoid vibration which might lead to breakage. Material containing agents that are particularly likely to cause laboratory infections should be centrifuged, capped, in sealed centrifuge buckets which are subsequently opened in a safety cabinet.

Guidelines for mechanical safety are given by the International Federation of Clinical Chemistry (IFCC, 1990).

Blending, homogenizing and shaking

Many microbiological investigations require material to be blended or homo-genized to obtain smooth suspensions. Microbial suspensions and cultures frequently need to be shaken to obtain an even distribution of microorganisms. It became apparent during the late 1940s and early 1950s that some of these operations dispersed aerosols and droplets and could therefore be sources of laboratory-acquired infections.

High speed blenders and homogenizers

These words refer to the same machines on opposite sides of the Atlantic. The most commonly used model consists of a metal bowl or cylinder through the base of which there is a spindle fitted with cutting blades on the inside and a connection on the underside for an electric motor. The propeller-like blades rotate at a high speed. The top of the bowl or cylinder usually has a tightly fitting cap. The best known is the Waring blender.

Smadel (1951) drew attention to the hazards arising from the use and misuse of the Waring blender and described the precautions taken when using it in his laboratory. These included a method of removing fluid from the bowl without liberating aerosols; operating the blender in a 'sterile' room, which could be decontaminated; a plastic cover over the machine during operation; pre-use servicing; inspection and a trial run with saline; and prompt autoclaving after use. The Waring blender was also investigated by Anderson *et al.* (1952), who homogenized 100 ml amounts of a culture of *Serratia indica*. When the cap was removed immediately after a 2-min run a sieve sampler nearby collected more than 2100 organisms (viable units) per operation. When the cap was removed 5 min after running the yield was between 306 and 629 depending on the type of cap (plastic or screw). Removing the cap 30 min after running gave counts of between 40 and 50 organisms. Sampling during use yielded, for each operation, an average of 521 organisms with a plastic cap and 18 with a screw cap. Anderson and his colleagues decided that with the design of the blender (at that time) it was not possible to prevent leakage. They recommended operation in a ventilated bacteriological cabinet.

Further work with the blender by Reitman *et al.* (1953) established that aerosols were also released if the gaskets were missing or faulty and if the bearings were worn or the drive shaft was loose. A few years later Reitman and Wedum (1956) found that removing a tight-fitting cover immediately after mixing a *S. indica* culture gave too many colonies to count on the plates in a sieve sampler. Removing the cover after 1 hour gave between five and 33 colonies (15 operations). Sampling during use, with a screw cap but no gasket gave between 0 and 31 colonies (10 operations), with a rubber gasket but worn bearings between 12 and 126 (10 operations); and with a loose plastic cover between 77 and 1246 (15 operations).

The large amount of energy used in these blenders and the heat generated results in an increased pressure in the bowl. When the cap is removed any aerosols and particles suspended in the air above the homogenate are dispersed violently. Andersen (1958) and Hilleman and Taylor (1958) proposed safer high speed blender designs and an outcome is a container (Waring AS-1; Figure 4.12) which allows the safe removal of contents and also has other safety features.

The precautions described by Smadel in 1951 (see above) are still sound. The plastic cover he recommends might be replaced by a towel soaked in disinfectant, and the blender should certainly be opened in a safety cabinet after standing for as long as practicable once blending has ceased. Some

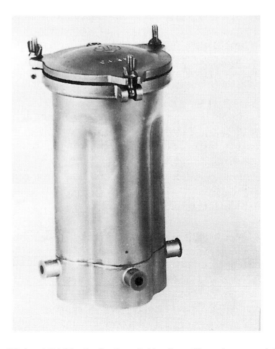

Figure 4.12 The Waring AS-1 blender for the safe blending of hazardous materials (Christison)

workers have suggested that blenders should be operated in safety cabinets. But as with centrifuges, the velocity of particles issuing from a defective blender may exceed that of the inflowing air in an open-fronted cabinet. Extremely hazardous material should be blended in a totally enclosed (Class III) safety cabinet.

The Colworth Stomacher

An entirely new approach to the problems of homogenizing food for microbiological examination was made by Sharpe (1976). This is the Colworth Stomacher. Material to be homogenized is placed in a stout plastic bag and positioned in the open end. When the door is closed rubber pads compress the mouth of the bag and prevent leakage during homogenizing. When the machine is switched on two paddles, mounted side by side and operated through rubber connecting rods, alternately pound the contents of the bag against the door. The action is thorough but gentle. No reports of tests or evaluations have been found, but in the UK the machine has largely replaced blenders in food science laboratories and is increasingly used in pathology and biomedical research establishments. Various safety devices are built in and burst bags seem to be rare. Nevertheless, it seems advisable to use two bags, the inner one being self-sealing or heat sealed, when infectious materials, e.g. egg embryos, tissues and faeces, are homogenized. The bags should be opened in a microbiological safety cabinet.

Other devices

Some blenders and 'macerators' have blades on the ends of spindles that are permanently attached to electric motors. A glass container is clamped underneath the machine, with the blades immersed in the contents. A screw cap may or may not be provided. Apart from the risk of dispersing aerosols and splashes, breakage of the glass container offers a considerable hazard. If these machines are used then large, tough plastic boxes should be inverted over them.

Hand blenders known as Griffiths tubes or tissue grinders are used for small pieces of tissue or fungal growths (Figure 4.13). A heavy duty glass tube is constricted near its closed end and a pestle, which may be of stainless steel or PTFE-covered glass is ground into the constriction. Some liquid and the tissue are placed in the tube and the pestle rotated by hand to macerate the material. These tubes sometimes break. The contents may be dispersed, and the hand holding them cut by the glass. The operator should wear stout gloves, hold the tube in a wad of cotton soaked in disinfectant, and work in a microbiological safety cabinet.

Magnetic stirrers act gently but their action may result in wet caps or plugs. After stirring, the bottles or flasks should be opened in a biological safety cabinet. Vortex stirrers also mix without violent agitation and bubbling, and Stern et al. (1974) found that no aerosols were produced during their operation. The cap, however, may be contaminated. Sonicators can generate the same hazards as blenders. Aerosols may escape through loosely fitting covers. Reitman and Wedum (1956) suggested fitting larger O-rings and a rubber diaphragm through which material could be extracted with a needle and syringe (an additional hazard).

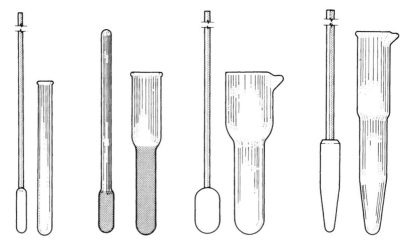

Figure 4.13 Glass/PTFE tissue homogenizers (Camlab)

Sonicators should be used in enclosed (Class III) microbiological safety cabinets.

Reciprocating shakers

These vary from small tube shakers to large flask or bottle culture shakers. Unless the caps or other closures are secure the contents may splash out, or the bottles leak so that the outside becomes contaminated. Chatigny (1961) recommended placing shakers in microbiological safety cabinets to avoid dispersal of aerosols into the room. As an alternative Wedum (1964) suggested placing them in leak-proof boxes fitted with a window and fibreglass filters. Stern *et al.* (1974) studied the custom of shaking stool suspensions in these machines and noted that large amounts of aerosols were produced inside the containers. These persisted for some time. A very large number of organisms were recovered from the air around the shaker when the container was opened an hour after shaking had ceased. Collins (1974) advised placing bottles containing material to be shaken in self-sealing plastic bags. Earlier, Collins (1959) found no advantage in shaking sputum homogenates, either in obtaining more positive cultures or reducing contamination of media.

Summary of precautions

Careful choice of equipment and a high level of maintenance are essential. Blenders should be inspected before use, especially O-rings, gaskets and spindle seals. High speed blenders and shakers should be covered with a plastic box or a disinfectant-soaked towel during use and opened in a Class I safety cabinet. The longer the delay between operating and opening the safer is the process. Very hazardous material should be blended or shaken in a Class III safety cabinet. Glass bowls, and domestic equipment should be discouraged. Small glass devices should be held in a disinfectant-soaked cloth in gloved hands.

Opening cultures and ampoules

If there is a film of liquid between two surfaces and those surfaces are pulled apart the film will be violently ruptured and aerosols will be formed. Dried material, e.g. fungal spores and dried bacteria on the rims of containers, may disperse into the atmosphere if they are disturbed.

Cotton wool plugged tubes

One would expect that removing dry cotton wool plugs from test tube cultures would release no organisms and this was demonstrated by Anderson *et al.* (1952). When the plug was wetted, however, as might happen when a culture tube falls over or is carelessly handled, organisms are released into the air. When wet plugs were removed from test tubes containing 5 ml amounts of cultures of *Serratia indica* a sieve sampler picked up between seven and 10 organisms per operation. The length of the tube seemed to influence dispersal, however, because an average of 2.5 organisms per operation were collected when dry plugs were removed from 15 ml centrifuge tubes containing 10 ml of culture. Centrifuging generated aerosols within these tubes, as 6.4 organisms per operation were collected when the dry plugs were removed after centrifugation.

The release of organisms from centrifuge tubes after centrifuging was also investigated by Reitman and Phillips (1956). Removing cotton wool plugs from 100 tubes containing a culture of *S. indica*, yielded, in 10 separate tests, an average of 2.3 viable units per operation. The same experiment, using rubber caps, yielded none. In another experiment 80 rubber caps were removed in 10 tests and an average of 0.2 units per operation were recovered.

It is unlikely that substituting plugs of foam or expanded plastic material for cotton wool would reduce these hazards. The only obvious precaution against dispersal of aerosols is careful handling to avoid wetting the plugs. Hazardous materials should be handled in a safety cabinet.

Push-in and screw-in closures

Corks and rubber bungs are now rarely used for culture tubes (although the latter persist in some virology tissue culture laboratories). Plastic plugs which push or screw into specimen collection tubes are common. A large film of liquid is likely to be trapped between the tube and any rubber or plastic closure which fits inside its rim, especially if the container is shaken or falls over. It is very difficult to open these containers gently. Abrupt movement releases aerosols and visible sprays (Collins, 1974) and the fingers are likely to be contaminated. These closures should be avoided, not only in culture work but also for the collection of blood which may well contain hepatitis virus (see Chapter 12). One way of dealing with the problem is to wear disposable gloves and to open the container by gripping the closures through a strip of paper which is wrapped round both the closure and the top of the container. Paper and cap may then be discarded into disinfectant, and if necessary, a fresh cap used.

Screw-capped bottles

Although these have replaced cotton wool plugged test tubes and flasks in many laboratories, they are not without risk.

A film of liquid may be present between the rim and the cap liner. Sometimes the film may extend across the whole orifice. When such films are broken (see above) aerosols are generated (Figure 4.14).

Anderson *et al.* (1952) investigated the release of organisms from screw-capped bottles containing 100 ml amounts of culture. The caps were removed immediately after shaking the contents and an average of eight particles were recovered per operation. Waiting 30 s after shaking yielded an average of 11 particles per operation.

In 1957 Tomlinson reported a series of experiments in which he opened screw-capped 20 ml bottles containing cultures of '*Chromobacterium prodigiosum*' (*Serratia marcescens*). He ensured that the rims of the bottles were wet, i.e. there was a film of culture between the rims and the rubber liners of the cap. A slit sampler was sited 6 ft away and collected 9–11 colonies in 2 min, 14–20 colonies in 5–7 min and 7–10 colonies in 72–92 min after opening the bottles.

A reasonable precaution is to unscrew the cap slightly and then wait a second or two before removing it. Bottles containing hazardous material should be opened in a safety cabinet.

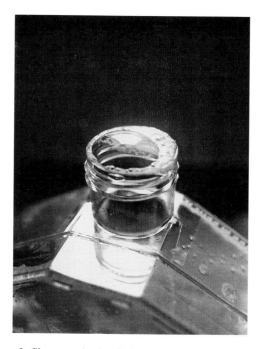

Figure 4.14 Rupture of a film across the rim of a bottle releases aerosols. (ISSA (1998), courtesy of the International Social Security Association

Petri dishes

There are two hazards associated with opening petri dishes. Water of syneresis often collects in the lid and it may contain many microorganisms. This was noticed by Fricke in 1919. Harvey *et al.* (1976) found salmonellas in 29/136 (20%) of samples from dishes used to culture those organisms. The numbers of salmonellas present in the fluid varied between 16 and 136 per ml. The liquid may form a film between the lid and the rim of the inverted dish. When the lid is opened and the film is broken aerosols are dispersed. Vented petri dishes, which have nibs so that the lid touches the rim at only three places, reduce this hazard (Collins, 1974).

The other hazard is from fungal spores (Hanel and Kruse, 1967). Disturbing the growth by opening the dish may result in the dispersal of very large numbers of spores. The spores of even 'harmless' fungi, may be allergenic. The spores of mycelial bacteria released in this way may also offer a health risk. To prevent accidental dispersion of spores, e.g. if the dish is dropped, the two parts should be taped together. Opening and manipulating such cultures are best done in Class I or Class II safety cabinets.

Smelling ('sniffing') cultures

Cultures of some microorganisms are said to have distinctive odours and the practice of smelling them is not uncommon. As the act of opening a culture to smell it may generate aerosols this is a hazardous procedure. Grammon-Cupillard *et al.* (1996) reported three cases of brucellosis that resulted from sniffing cultures.

Dried materials

Darlow (1972) and Collins (1974) noted that dried deposits are sometimes seen on and just inside the rims of culture tubes, and on their caps and other closures. These may contain microorganisms and they are dispersed when the tubes are opened. This is a hazard with the trisodium phosphate method for culturing tubercle bacilli from sputum.

LYOPHILIZED CULTURES

Microorganisms and materials containing them are frequently freeze-dried for storage and transport. Opening ampoules of freeze-dried (lyophilized) material can be hazardous. Fine dry powders are easily dispersed into the atmosphere by the rush of air into the evacuated tube or ampoule when it is broken open to retrieve the contents. This hazard has been emphasized by (among others) Smadel (1951), Reitman *et al.* (1954), Reitman and Wedum (1956), Darlow (1972), Collins (1974), Collins *et al.* (1995). Several of these have recommended methods which minimize or prevent dispersal, including wrapping the ampoule in alcohol-soaked cotton wool before breaking it at a file scratch. Most culture collections isssue instructions for the safe opening of their ampoules with each consignment of cultures.

Summary of precautions

The release of aerosols and splashes containing microorganisms when cultures containing them are opened seems almost inevitable. The hazards may be minimized by careful choice of containers and closures, avoiding the wetting of plugs and caps by culture fluids, using vented petri dishes, and opening containers of especially hazardous materials in appropriate safety cabinets. Lyophilized cultures should be opened according to the directions issued by type culture collections.

Pouring infectious material

Pouring off the supernatant fluid after centrifuging cultures of bacteria, sputum homogenates and clinical specimens is common practice. These fluids, which may still contain microorganisms (see p. 87), are usually poured into disinfectant in the hope that any microorganisms they contain will be killed. Two hazards can arise: production of aerosols, and contamination of the outside of the tube from which the material is poured.

When one liquid is poured into another the impact may cause some of the poured liquid to bounce into the air. As the last of the poured liquid hits the surface of the other liquid a central fountain—the 'Rayleigh jet'—is produced and the breaking of its surface film releases particles into the air in much the same way as described above under the hazards of the falling drop. If liquids containing microorganisms are poured into disinfectants it is therefore possible for aerosols and droplets that have had no contact with the disinfectant to be released and to contaminate the air and local surfaces.

The rim of a tube or bottle from which liquids are poured will become contaminated. Sometimes a visible drop remains on the outside of the rim and this may run down and contaminate the outside of the tube and therefore the fingers of the worker.

Precautions

Both of these hazards can be minimized. Infected fluids should be poured into a funnel, the end of which is below the surface of disinfectant in a beaker. The top of the funnel should be only slightly larger than that of the beaker so it rests securely; both should be made of metal or polypropylene so that they can be handled and autoclaved safely (Figure 4.15). After use some more disinfectant should be poured through the funnel.

Small strips of blotting paper should be available to wipe the rims of tubes after pouring, e.g. after serum separation, and to remove external drops of liquid. The ends of the strips should be dipped into disinfectant before use.

Breakage and spillage

Breakage of culture tubes and glass petri dishes may result in contamination of local surfaces as well as release of aerosols. Aerosols are generated when petri dish cultures are dropped (Barbeito *et al.*, 1961) but fewer aerosols are released

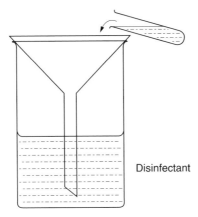

Figure 4.15 A safe way to pour infectious material into, e.g., disinfectant, avoiding splashing and aerosols

when cultures in plastic petri dishes are dropped than with similar accidents with glass dishes. Spillage of cultures causes local contamination but less aerosol. Methods for dealing with such accidents are given in Chapter 7.

Hazards from other equipment and materials

'Sharps'

Injuries from sharp instruments and materials (other than from hollow-bore needles) are not uncommon in laboratories, and may become infected. Kennedy (1988) made extracts from a hospital laboratory accident book covering a 10-year period. Sharp objects that caused skin injuries are listed in Table 4.2.

Accidental inoculation with hypodermic needles, other sharp instruments, pasteur pipettes and broken glass may be reduced, if not entirely avoided by replacing such hazardous equipment with inherently safer articles. Needles may be replaced by cannulas, glass pasteur pipettes by the soft plastic types with integral bulbs, and other glass equipment by that made with rigid plastics or break-resistant glass. All re-usable glassware, especially pipettes, should be examined critically before it leaves the preparation room for chips and rough adges. Used sharp objects and broken glass should be discarded into standard issue sharps containers (p. 84).

TABLE 4.2 Sharp objects that have caused skin injuries in clinical laboratories

Glass fragments	Metal tube rack
Broken glass slides	Edge of locker
Whole glass slides	Autoclaving containers
Glass pasteur pipettes	Stapling machine
Glass test tubes	Centrifuge component
Glass capillary tubes	Blood cell counter component
Scalpels	Edge of seat
Insides of metal sharps bins	
Metal sealing rings of vials	

After Kennedy (1988).

Ultrasonic devices

These are used in many laboratories for cleaning glassware. Turner *et al.* (1975) demonstrated aerosol production and table top contamination (from splashes and drips) by one device. This suggests that articles destined for ultrasonic cleaning should first be properly decontaminated.

ELISA equipment

Harper (1983) has shown that some enzyme-linked immunoassay (ELISA) equipment contaminates the environment.

Liquid nitrogen

Liquid nitrogen in Dewar vessels is known to have been contaminated—and the contaminants preserved in a viable state—when ampoules have broken in them. Ampoules and bottles should be stored over, i.e. in the gaseous phase, not submerged in liquid nitrogen. If the liquid finds its way into an imperfectly sealed ampoule it will expand rapidly to its gaseous phase when the ampoule is taken out of the freezer, causing it to explode and disperse its contents. Schafer *et al.* (1976) reported shattered ampoules in which vesicular stomatitis virus had been stored under nitrogen. The virus was recovered from the liquid nitrogen.

Water-baths

The common laboratory water-bath is not without fault. Harvey *et al.* (1976) recovered salmonellas from water-baths used for enrichment at 43°C. The heated block 'incubators' are safer.

Autoclaves and incinerators

Some autoclaves have released infected aerosols into laboratories and incinerators have released infected airborne particles into the atmosphere (Barbeito and Brookey, 1976). (See Chapter 7.)

Flow cytometer/cell sorter

These instruments produce a stream of droplets as part of their normal function. The jet orifice is 100 µm in diameter and the droplets are produced at a rate of 19 000/s. The stream pases through a 'steam catcher' and the sorted droplets are deflected into collection vessels on either side (Merrill, 1981). There is thus a potential for aerosol dispersion.

Cryostat microtomes

When tissues are subjected to a blast of fluorocarbon freezing spray an aerosol is generated (Vetter, 1977). The velocity of the spray varies with the distance from the actuator but at 2 cm it can be between 17 and 52 m/s depending on the internal pressure of the pack. The mass median diameter of particles is between 60 and 300 µm, and the impact can easily dislodge infectious particles from the tissues. Cases of Mantoux skin test conversion associated with tuberculous lung tissue that was precooled by a freezing spray have been reported (Anon., 1981; Duray et al., 1981).

Laboratory request forms

Fears have been expressed about contamination of laboratory request forms. In well-managed laboratories the forms are always separated from the specimens, e.g. in compartmentalized plastic bags, but in others senders are allowed to wrap the forms around the specimen containers—the outside of which may well be contaminated (Allen and Darrell, 1983). Chattopadhyay and Thomas (1978) recovered Staphylococcus aureus, S. albus and Escherichia coli from request forms. These organisms could, of course, have been derived from the hands, etc. of those who handled them rather than from specimens. Pattison et al. (1974) pointed to a possible association between endemic hepatitis in the laboratory and computer card handling.

Films and smears for microscopy

The infectious nature of blood and other material spread on slides for micro-scopical examination is often discussed in laboratories. Dankhert et al. (1976) thought that blood and marrow smears might be a reservoir of hepatitis B (see Chapter 12). Kohn (1976) drew attention to the inconsistencies between the precautions required for tubed blood and those (if any) for blood films. In fact, little information and even less guidance is available.

Buffered formalin may be useful for decontaminating blood films. This is made by dissolving 22.75 g of $NaH_2PO_4H_2O$ and 32.5 g of Na_2HPO_4 in 450 ml of distilled water and adding 500 ml of formalin (which is a 37–40% solution in water of formaldehyde gas). Malarial parasites may be recognized on blood films treated in this way (ACDP, 1990) and it should take care of HIV and HBV; but such films are not suitable for differential white cell counts. Although 70% ethanol or isopropanol will probably kill both viruses there seems to be no information about the action of methanol, used for fixing and staining blood films for haematological investigations. This is an area that requires scientific investigation rather than opinions.

Apart from the possibility that microorganisms may be liberated from thick, dried sputum smears if they are disturbed, well-made smears that are not touched or allowed to come into contact with other articles are quite safe to handle (e.g. with forceps), even if staining does not kill all organisms or viruses on them. Tubercle bacilli may even survive heat fixation but not after the smears have been stained with auramine phenol (Allen, 981). Possible contamination of oil-immersion lenses may be avoided by using cover glasses.

Cover glasses are always placed on 'wet films' of faeces, etc. examined for parasites and laboratory workers have learnt to handle them with care.

Automated equipment

Automated equipment used for infectious or potentially infectious material (e.g. blood) should be of the closed type to avoid dispersion of droplets and aerosols.

Effluents should be collected in closed bottles or discharged at least 25 cm into the waste plumbing system.

The sampling probes of some automated equipment are sharp because they are required to sample through septum caps. They offer a real hazard that is not often appreciated. Probes should be wiped with tissues held in gloved hands and the tissues discarded into colour-coded bags or other containers.

Testing for environmental contamination

It may be necessary or desirable to test surfaces and air for the presence of microorganisms released during microbiological activities.

Surfaces

Surfaces may be sampled using contact (RODAC) plates. These are small petri dishes, filled to the brim with selective or non-selective agar media so that there is a slight meniscus. Recently, flexible versions have been made available for sampling irregular surfaces. They are inverted over and gently pressed on the surface to be sampled. The cover is then replaced and they are incubated. Viable bacteria picked up on the culture media develop into countable colonies.

Irregular surfaces may also be sampled with cotton wool or alginate swabs which should first be wetted with quarter-strength Ringer solution. After brisk swabbing the cotton wool swabs are rubbed on agar media or squeezed into broth. Alginate swabs are dissolved in sodium hexametaphosphate solution which is then plated.

Both methods lend themselves to quantitative as well as qualitative assessment of contamination, and to search for specific organisms. Technical details are given by Collins et al. (1995).

Detection of blood

Major blood spillages and splashes are obvious, but surfaces may also be contaminated with very small amounts of blood, not visible to the naked eye. Even these may contain large numbers of virus particles (p. 153) or microorganisms; for example Bond et al. (1984) showed that hepatitis B virus can survive in dried blood plasma (under experimental conditions) for over a week.

Table 4.3 lists the surfaces in clinical laboratories found to be contaminated with blood (Kennedy, 1997).

Methods for the detection of inapparent blood contamination have been investigated and reviewed by Kennedy (1988, 1997) and Kennedy et al. (1988).

The Kastel–Meyer test for blood (Culliford, 1981; Gaensslen, 1983), used in forensic investigations, is not suitable for routine laboratory use but the various haemoglobin test strips and kits may be used to test for blood in surface swab rinses and will detect very small amounts of blood. Table 4.4 (Kennedy, 1997) indicates the sensitivity of some of these. False positive reactions may be caused by oxidising agents such as hydrogen peroxide and sodium hypochlorite (Beaumont, 1987).

Hepatitis B surface antigen (HBsAg) has been detected on contaminated surfaces by testing swab rinses by a radioimmunoassay technique (Seder et al.,

TABLE 4.3 Surface blood contamination in clinical laboratories

Lauer *et al.* (1979)
  Outer surface of sample container
  Gloves and bare hands
  Ballpoint pens and felt-tipped markers
  Reagent container
  Surface of cell counter
  Blood film spreader
Holton and Prince (1986)
  Outside of specimen tubes
  Gloves worn for venepuncture
  Needle holder used for venepuncture
  Working surfaces
Kennedy *et al.* (1988)
  Outside of specimen tubes
  Disposable gloves
  Bench surface
  Floor
  Analytical equipment
  Inside of discard bucket
  Computer keyboard

From Kennedy (1997).

TABLE 4.4 Sensitivities of reagents for testing for blood on surfaces

Test	Sensitivity	Reference
Kastel-Meyer	Blood diluted 1:10^6	Gaensslen (1983)
Hemastix[1]	Blood diluted 1:10^5	Beaumont (1987)
Chemstrip 9[2]	About red cells per high power field	Daum *et al.* (1988)
Multistix 10SG[3]		
Combur Test[4]	10 red cells/µl	Cole *et al.* (1992)
nephroPHAN[5]		
Combi screen[6]		

Suppliers: 1 and 3, Bayer Diagnostics; 2 and 4, Boehringer-Mannheim Diagnostics; 5, Chemopol UK; 6, Cambridge Selfcare Diagnostics.
From Kennedy (1997).

1975) and by Palmer *et al.* (1991) using commercial assay kits. HBsAG was detected at a concentration of 0.125 IU per ml.

Airborne contamination

SETTLE PLATES

For the assessment of aerial contamination settle plates are the simplest method. A number of petri dishes, containing appropriate selective or non-selective media, are exposed, media side up for specified periods as close as possible to the equipment or procedure. They are then incubated, the colonies counted and organisms identified.

IMPINGERS

For sampling large volumes of air impingers may be used. Air, at a measured rate, is pulled through the jet it impinges upon a known volume of a liquid when microorganisms are captured. Viable counts are then made on the liquid.

The all-glass Porton impingers (Figure 4.16) sample particles between 0.5 and 18 µm and less than 50% of particles will enter the liquid (May and Harper, 1957). Thus it is reasonable to assume that the majority of particles collected are capable of entering the human alveolar system.

IMPACTORS

In impactors, e.g. slit and cascade samplers, an air stream through a slit is directed on solid culture contained in a petri dish or held on a plastic strip. These are then incubated and the colonies are counted. In the slit sampler (e.g. Casella (Figure 4.17) and Reynier, USA) the plates of culture media revolve beneath a slit half their diameter in length in a chamber through which air is drawn at a predetermined volume per minute. The prototype of this instrument (Bourdillon *et al.*, 1941) was shown to be about 96% efficient in collecting aerosols consisting of single *Staphylococcus albus* cells but only 1/200 times as efficient as a settle plate in collecting larger particles. Again the particles collected are of a size capable of entering the human alveolar regions.

In the cascade sampler (Andersen, 1958) the air passes through a series of graded sized holes in metal plates sited over and covering the same area as the media plates. This instrument allows the relative sizes as well as the numbers of viable particles to be determined. Figure 4.18 illustrates a modern version of this device.

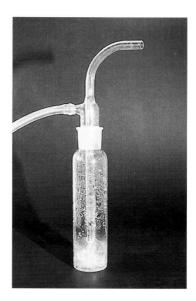

Figure 4.16 The all-glass Porton impingers. (CAMR. Courtesy of the Director, Centre for Applied Microbiology and Research, Porton)

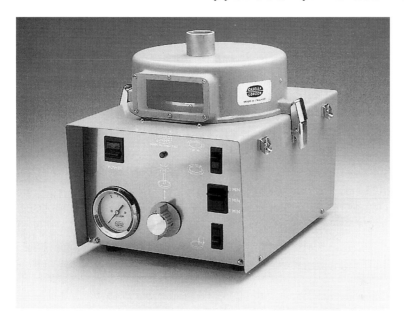

Figure 4.17 Slit-air sampler (Casella)

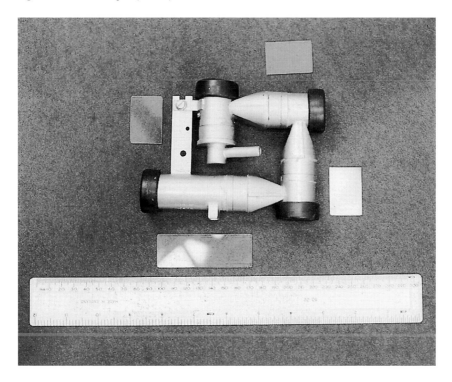

Figure 4.18 Cascade impactor. (CAMR. Courtesy of the Director, Centre for Applied Microbiology and Research, Porton)

Hand-held, battery-operated impactor samplers are now available. The Surface Air System (SAS) uses contact plates and the Biotest Centrifugal Air Sampler (RCS) impacts air on plastic strips (Figure 4.19). In general these devices give results comparable with those of slit samplers but there have been problems of correlation. The papers of Nakhla and Cummings (1981), Clark *et al.* (1981), Casewell *et al.* (1984, 1986) and Lach (1985) should be consulted.

FILTRATION METHODS

There are several samplers that depend on the filtration of measured volumes of air through cellulose ester filters of known pore size (Figure 4.20). The

(a)

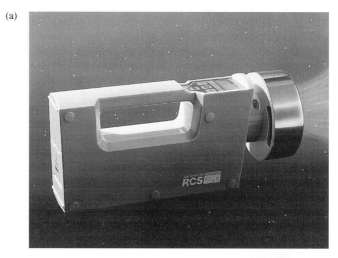

(b)

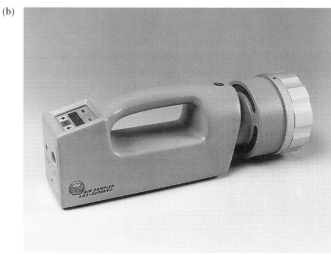

Figure 4.19 Hand-held impactors (a) Surface air sampler (SAS), (b) Centrifugal air sampler (RCS, Biotest)

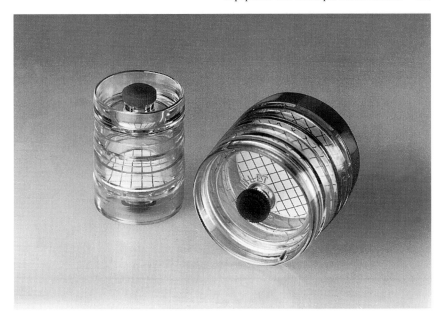

Figure 4.20 Membrane filter (Millipore)

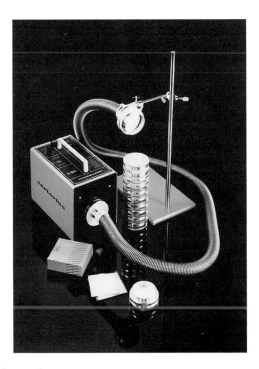

Figure 4.21 Sartorius sampler

membrane is then placed on the surface of culture media, incubated and the colonies counted. A disadvantage is that the air stream may dehydrate the organisms and render them non-viable. This is overcome in the Sartorius instrument (Figure 4.21) which uses moist gelatin filters.

The relative advantages of these various samplers have been assessed by Hambleton *et al*. (1992). Table 4.5 is reproduced from their paper. (See also Crook, 1995.)

Indicator systems

Shinton *et al*. (1982) agreed that biological tests are the most sensitive for the detection of aerosols or potentially infected airborne droplets, but suggested that a chemical marker could be used as test material and its presence determined by examining under ultraviolet light sheets of filter paper placed around the test area. Harper (1983) found that this method was not as sensitive as spore suspensions. It failed to detect the smaller particles that could be retained in the lungs and initiate infection (see also p. 41). Kennedy (1985) and Kennedy *et al*. (1988) studied the use of 'double', i.e. combined biological and chemical tracers.

TABLE 4.5 Characteristics of commonly used air sampling devices

Type	Flow rate (l/min)	Advantages	Disadvantages
Impactors		*No sample manipulation*	*Semiquantitative, not suitable for high concentrations (> 10 organisms/litre)*
Casella slit	30–700	Efficient, easy to use	Static, bulky
Andersen	27	Particle size information	Difficult to assemble
SAS Cherwell	180	Portable, easy to use, directional	Inefficient at small particle sizes (< 5 µm)
RCS Biotest	40	Portable, easy to use, directional	Inefficient at small particle sizes (< 5 µm)
Cascade	175	Portable, particle size information	Low volume sample; processing may be necessary
Impingers		*Suitable for high concentrations (> 10 organisms/l)*	*Sample processing necessary; not suitable for low concentrations (< 10 organisms/l)*
Porton	11	Easy to use, small	Fragile, sample evaporation, violent sampling
May 3-stage	55	Particle size information, gentle sampling	Fragile, standardized manufacture difficult
Others			
Cyclone (impinger)	750	Suitable for wide range of concentrations	No particle size information
Personal filter samplers	1–4	Suitable for high concentrations; estimates worker exposure	Low volume; sample recovery and processing difficulties
Settle plates (impactors)	NA	Easy to use	Inefficient, qualitative

Reproduced from *Trends in Biotechnology* **10**, pp. 192–9, Hambleton, P., Bennett, A.M. & Leaver, G. Biosafety monitoring devices for biotechnology processes. (1992) with permission of Elsevier Trends Journals.

Airborne blood

Very small droplets of blood, aerosolized blood and particles of dried blood may be detected by the sampling methods described above, using filter papers instead of culture media and testing these, or the fluid in impingers with a haemoglobin test kit or (for HBaAg) by a radioimmunoassay technique (see Bond *et al.*, 1977).

Good microbiological practice

The precautions described in this chapter can all be included in the term 'good microbiological practice' and will undoubtedly do much to minimize the dispersion of microorganisms and contact between them and the worker. It is obvious, however, that 100% containment cannot be achieved, even with the best possible technique and equipment. For the additional and necessary protection against aerosols and infected airborne particles further containment in microbiological safety cabinets is essential and is the subject of the next chapter.

Chapter 5

Microbiological safety cabinets

Microbiological safety cabinets 'are designed to capture and retain infected airborne particles released in the course of certain manipulations and to protect the laboratory worker from infection which may arise from inhaling them' (Collins, 1974). Some types of cabinet offer additional protection to workers by means of a physical barrier between them and the infected material. As well as offering protection to the workers, some types of cabinet also offer protection to the material being worked on against contaminating airborne particles. The limitations of the protection offered by microbiological safety cabinets to workers and the possible inherent hazards of these cabinets are considered later.

Although intrinsically effective microbiological safety cabinets have been available since about 1958 and in common use for only about half of that time, they have had, until recently in our experience, an unrivalled record of poor installation and general misuse. In addition, some poorly designed and even frankly unsafe cabinets have been manufactured and sold for laboratory use. Some problems arose because there was little agreement about the terms which were used to describe these devices. Names included inoculating hoods or boxes, glove boxes, safety hoods or benches, clean air cabinets, safety work stations, exhaust protective cabinets, laminar flow cabinets and biological safety cabinets. A few years ago a portmanteau phrase, 'protective air enclosures', which, like 'hood', is vague and capable of several interpretations, has been introduced by engineers. The phrases should be discarded in favour of the now generally accepted term. They were (and still are, especially by engineers and 'design teams') frequently confused with chemical fume cupboards and little or no distinction seems to have been made between cabinets designed to protect the worker from infection and those designed solely to protect the work from contamination.

It is hardly surprising that either the incorrect equipment or the incorrect facilities have sometimes been fitted where laboratory workers requested safety cabinets by that or any of the other names, or when one or other of these expressions appeared in design specifications.

The evolution of microbiological safety cabinets, and the lessons learnt by both engineers and microbiologists, have been described in some detail in earlier editions of this book and will not be repeated here. They led to a better understanding of the functions of the cabinets and of the behaviour of airflows in and around them, and then to the formulation and official adoption of national standards for construction, installation and performance. Those in the English

110

language include the US National Sanitation Foundation Standard 49 (NSF, 1983), British Standard 5726 (BS 5726 Parts 1–4: 1992), and Australian Standards AS 2252, Parts 1 and 2 (AS 2252.1: 1994; AS 2252.2: 1994) and AS 2647 (AS 2647: 1994). Recently, a draft European standard, on the performance criteria for microbiological safety cabinets, prEN 12469, has been published (CEN, 1998). BS 5726 and prEN 12469 will be revised later on.

Even though the situation has improved markedly, there is no cause for complacency. Ineffective cabinets are still available in some parts of the world (see below); good cabinets may be badly installed or poorly maintained, and there is frequently a lack of instruction in their use (see p. 205).

Types of microbiological safety cabinets

There are basically three types of microbiological safety cabinets, generally known as Classes I, II and III. Flexible film isolators are in essence a variety of the Class III cabinet.

Class I cabinets

A Class I cabinet is shown in cross-section in Figure 5.1. The operator sits at the cabinet, works with hands inside and looks at what is being done through the transparent screen. Any aerosols released from the material being handled are entrained in a current of air that passes in at the front of the cabinet. This sweeps the aerosols up through the filters which remove all or most of the organisms (see below). The filtered air then passes through the fan, which maintains the airflow, and is exhausted to atmosphere, where any particles or organisms that have not been retained on the filter are so diluted that they are no longer likely to cause infection if inhaled. In some installations, instead of

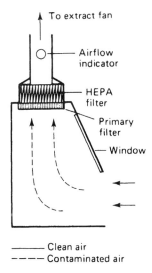

Figure 5.1 Class I microbiological safety cabinet

being exhausted to atmosphere, the effluent air passes through two HEPA filters before being returned to the laboratory. The advantages and disadvantages of disposal to atmosphere and recirculation of effluent air are discussed below. Whatever method is chosen, a minimum airflow of 0.7 m/s must be maintained through the front of the cabinet; modern cabinets have airflow indicators and warning devices. The filters must be changed when the airflow falls below this level.

Class II cabinets

The Class II cabinet (Figure 5.2) is a more complicated piece of air engineering and is unfortunately sometimes still called a laminar flow cabinet (e.g., see AS 2252.2: 1994) but as this term is also used for clean air cabinets which do not protect the worker (see p. 115) it should be avoided. In the Class II cabinet about 70% of the air is recirculated within the cabinet through HEPA filters so that the working area is bathed in clean (almost sterile) air. This down-flowing air entrains any aerosols produced in the course of the work and these are removed by the filters. Some of the air (about 30%) is exhausted to atmosphere and is replaced by a 'curtain' of room air which enters at the working face. This prevents the escape of any particles or aerosols released in the cabinet.

There are other types of Class II cabinets, with different airflows and exhaust systems including double filtration of effluent air and return to the laboratory (see below). Some types of Class II cabinets may also be used for work with cytotoxic drugs, but these are not considered here.

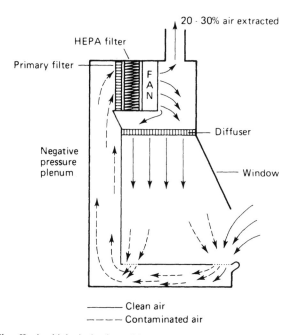

Figure 5.2 Class II microbiological safety cabinet

Class III cabinets

The Class III cabinet is totally enclosed and designed to be pressure-tight. The operator works with gloves which are sealed into the front of the cabinet by removable gaskets. Even if by accident one glove becomes totally detached from its mounting, the cabinet fails safe because aerosols are retained within the carcase by an air stream of at least 0.7 m/s that is drawn through the opening. Air enters through a HEPA filter at the rear or side of the cabinet (thus protecting the work from airborne microbial contamination) and is exhausted to atmosphere through one or (usually) two filters (Figure 5.3). Originally, material was placed in and removed from these cabinets by opening the front viewing panel or the glove panel. Both of these were fastened down by very effective clamps onto rubber gaskets. Dunk tanks containing disinfectant (Figure 5.4) were then fitted and goods passed in and out in sealed containers (Evans *et al.*, 1972). Air locks were also used for transfer of materials. These cabinets are assembled into 'production lines' in some laboratories. A series of sealable transfer ports between the cabinets enables them to be used individually or for sequential processing of materials. The last cabinet in the line communicates with an interlocking double-door autoclave, so that no material can leave without being sterilized.

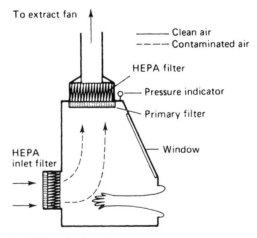

Figure 5.3 Class III microbiological safety cabinet

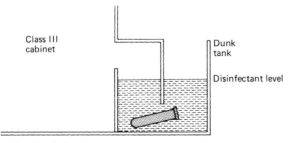

Figure 5.4 Principle of a 'dunk-tank' attached to a Class III safety cabinet to enable materials to be removed through a disinfectant bath

Flexible film isolators

Another method for placing effective barriers between the laboratory worker and dangerous pathogens with which he is working is the negative pressure flexible film isolator which can be considered, in some circumstances, as a reasonable alternative to a microbiological safety cabinet.

Flexible film isolators have been used for the management of gnotobiotic animals (Trexler and Reynold, 1957) and to protect patients with immunological deficiencies from microorganisms in the environment (Goldman *et al.*, 1976). Similar devices under negative pressure have been used to isolate, nurse and transport patients with highly infectious diseases (Trexler *et al.*, 1977; Isaacson *et al.*, 1978; Emond, 1978). They may also be used for performing potentially hazardous autopsies (Trexler and Gilmour, 1983). Plastic 'safety hoods' for work with bacteria were described by Phillips *et al.* as long ago as 1955 and the marriage of these two technologies (van der Groen *et al.*, 1980) has produced an isolator in which a variety of microbiological and clinical pathology tests can be performed

The isolator consists of a heavy duty plastic envelope, held in a metal frame on a metal trolley. The sides are sloping and may be fitted with semirigid plastic viewing panels. Flexible sleeves, with glove fittings, are welded into the envelope, allowing up to four operators to work. There is a large supply port at one end and a smaller one at the other. These allow apparatus to be placed into the isolator. Infectious material in sealed containers may be 'bagged' in and out so that it need not be opened on the open laboratory bench. The ports also allow several isolators to be connected together, one e.g. containing an incubator. A long plastic sleeve external to the isolator enables small objects to be placed in a refrigerator on the base of the trolley. A microscope can be placed inside the envelope with its eyepieces sealed into the plastic film. Sealable plastic cones allow electricity or other services to be led into the envelope. One electric motor drives both the supply and exhaust fans. Air enters through one HEPA filter and after circulating is exhausted through another one. The envelope is maintained at a constant negative pressure by dampers which respond to changes in pressure, e.g. by the operator's movements. They are under the control of the operators and there are manual controls as well. The manometer which indicates the negative pressure (20 Pa) is visible to the operator.

Exhaust air may be returned to the room or ducted out of a window through a flexible hose. In the laboratory of van der Groen and his colleagues (van der Groen *et al.*, 1980) it is ducted to a Class I safety cabinet. Collins and Yates (1982) ducted it into the exhaust system of a disconnected safety cabinet, giving a thimble system. If an isolator is mounted on a trolley, the castors must be capable of being locked securely to prevent movement when the isolator is in use (ACDP, 1985).

Van der Groen used one of these isolators in a maximum containment laboratory and they are obviously of great value in field work where it would not be possible to erect Class III cabinets. They could also save considerably on the costs of maintaining Containment Level 4 laboratories, as they could be used in almost any clinical laboratory for exclusion diagnosis, thus reducing the numbers of specimens that are sent to the specialist laboratories. Using an isolator for occasional work with Hazard Group 3 pathogens would give the staff sufficient experience to test specimens from patients who were suspected of having, for example, one of the viral haemorrhagic fevers. A flexible film isolator in a Level 3 Containment Laboratory for work with Hazard Group 3 pathogens and for less hazardous work has been found to be easy and practicable to use (Collins and Yates, 1982), but as a matter of convenience we would not wish to use the isolator for work with tuberculous material on a regular basis.

General maintenance and changing filters offer no problems to laboratory staff. Guidance on the use, testing and maintenance of these isolators is given by ACDP (1985).

Laminar flow (clean air) cabinets

Laminar flow, clean air cabinets or clean air work stations are mentioned here because, as has been said before, they are sometimes confused with microbiological safety cabinets. Air enters through HEPA filters (often of a lower standard than those used in safety cabinets) and passes horizontally across the working surface and into the room. These cabinets are widely used in pharmacies for preparing sterile solutions and in microbiological laboratories for pouring and tubing culture media. They do not protect the operator, however. Any aerosols released in a horizontal laminar flow cabinet will be blown into the operator's face.

Factors affecting the performance of safety cabinets

Air must enter a Class I safety cabinet at a velocity sufficient to retain within the working area any infectious particles that are released in the course of the work. This velocity must not be so great that turbulence is caused within the cabinet or some air may spill out around the edges of the open front.

The 1950s saw the beginning of a number of investigations into the rate of air flow into safety cabinets necessary to capture and retain airborne particles. Opinions and experience yielded figures that varied between 0.25 and 1.0 m/s (Wedum, 1953; Soltorovsky *et al.*, 1953; Williams and Lidwell, 1957; Chatigny, 1961; Newsom, 1979a). Other work showed that the airflow into any given cabinet varied considerably according to its place in a room in relation to fitments, furniture and other equipment, the normal ventilation and 'make-up' air movements (see p. 117), disturbances in air currents caused by apparatus that generated heat, and cross-draughts caused by the movement and activities of people in the room (Chatigny and Clinger, 1969; Rake, 1978; Clark and Mullen, 1978; Newsom, 1979a,b, and others, reviewed in previous editions of this book). Tests on many cabinets in different laboratories, both in the USA and the UK revealed unacceptably low airflows, some intrinsic to the cabinets, others related to room air movements mentioned above (Barkley, 1972; Newsom, 1979a,b; Collins, unpublished, 1972-1978).

As indicated above, the 1979 the British Standard (BS 5726, 1979) settled for an inflow of 0.7–1.0 m/s for Class I cabinets and 0.4 m/s for the down-flowing air stream of Class II cabinets. These figures were retained in the later standard (BS 5726: 1992) and there is general agreement with this among other standards.

Siting cabinets in rooms

The positions of cabinets in rooms is therefore important. The main problems are caused by draughts from doors and windows and the movement of people. It is difficult to prevent the occasional opening of a door; locking it may cause local problems (but see p. 220 on design of Containment Level 3 laboratories); and although windows are usually closed while work is done in safety cabinets they can cause convection draughts if there is a large temperature difference between room and the outside air. Possible sites for cabinets in a room are shown in Figure 5.5.

A is a poor site, as it is near to the door and airflow into the cabinet will be disturbed every time the door is opened and someone walks past the cabinet into the room. Site B is not much better, as it is almost in a direct line between door and window, although no-one is likely to walk past it. Its left side is also close to the wall and airflow into it on that side may be affected by the 'skin effect', i.e. the slowing down of air when it passes parallel and close to a surface. Air passing across the window may be cooled, and will meet warm air from the rest of the room at the cabinet face, when turbulence may result. Site C is better and Site D is best of all. If two cabinets are required in the same room, sites C and D would be satisfactory, but they should not be too close together, or one may disturb the airflow of the other. One of us (CHC) remembers a laboratory where a Class I cabinet was placed next to a Class II cabinet. When the former was in use it extracted air from the latter and rendered it quite ineffective. Recently, we

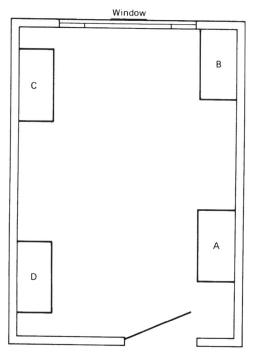

Figure 5.5 Possible sites for safety cabinets in relation to cross-draughts from door and window. A is bad; B is poor; C is better. D is best

had a similar experience with an unusually efficient fume cupboard that compromised the airflow in an adjacent Class I safety cabinet. The British Standard (BS, 5726:1992) now recommends distances between cabinets and side walls and between opposite cabinets. It also provides for other problems of siting, such as architectural features.

Care must also be taken in siting any other equipment that might generate air currents, e.g. fans and heaters. Mechanical room ventilation may be a problem if (rarely) it is efficient, but this can be overcome by linking it to the electric circuits of the cabinets so that either, but not both are extracting air from the room at any one time. Alternatively baffles may be fitted to air inlets and outlets to avoid conflicting air currents near to the cabinet. Tests with smoke generators (see below) will establish the directions of air currents in rooms.

The design of a mechanically-ventilated laboratory may produce excessive turbulence and draughts which can jeopardise the containment of Class I and II cabinets. Air supplied from ceiling-mounted diffusers may be especially troublesome. On-site commissioning tests (see p. 131) always need to be done, and it may be necessary to make adjustments to the air supply and exhaust systems in order to achieve, and to maintain, adequate operator protection (Clark *et al.*, 1990).

These considerations apply to open-fronted cabinets. The containment of Class III cabinets, which are in any case usually operated in more controlled environments, and flexible film isolators is not likely to be reduced by air movements within a room. Nevertheless, on-site commissioning tests (see p. 131) should be done before such cabinets are put into service.

The Advisory Committee on Dangerous Pathogens (ACDP, 1985) advises that adequate space should be provided for flexible film isolators and that this is particularly important when gloves are fitted to more than one side.

Make-up air

When a Class I cabinet is in use it moves about $80-90$ m^3 of air out of the room each minute. Replacement (technically 'make-up') air must be provided. If there is insufficient make-up air, the ability of a cabinet to entrain aerosols is compromised. Make-up air may come from the building ventilation system inlet if the outlet is blocked off. It should not be brought in directly from outside the building because of possible differences in temperature and the turbulence which might affect the airflow into the cabinet. Usually it finds its way in from the corridors or other rooms, through cracks and under doors. If it cannot do this the amount of air in the room may become insufficient for the cabinet to operate properly. It is therefore good practice to provide transfer grilles in the internal walls or in the doors. This problem of ventilating rooms containing safety cabinets is also considered in Chapter 10.

Testing airflows

The presence and direction of air currents and draughts are determined with 'smoke'. This may indeed be from burning material in a device like that used by bee keepers, but is usually a chemical which produces a dense, visible vapour. Titanium tetrachloride is commonly used. If a cotton wool-tipped stick, e.g. a throat swab, is dipped into this liquid and then waved in the air a white cloud is formed which responds to quite small air movements. Commercial airflow testers are more convenient. They are small glass tubes, sealed at each end. Both ends are broken off with the gadget provided and a rubber bulb fitted to one end. Pressing the bulb to pass air through the tube causes it to emit white smoke. These methods are suitable for ascertaining air movements indoors. A water fog airflow visualization method is described by Kennedy (1987).

To measure airflows an anemometer is required. Small vane anemometers, timed by a stopwatch, are useful for occasional work but for serious activities electronic models, with a direct reading scale are essential. Two are shown in Figure 5.6. The electronic vane type has a diameter of about 10 cm. It has a satisfactory time constant and responds rapidly enough to show the changes in velocity that are constantly occurring when air is passing into a Class I safety cabinet. Hot wire or thermistor anemometers may be used but they may show very rapid fluctuations and need damping (Newsom, 1976a). Both can be connected to chart recorders.

(a)

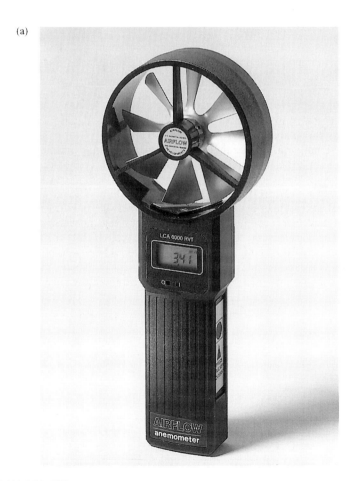

Figure 5.6 (a) LCA 6000 anemometer

(b)

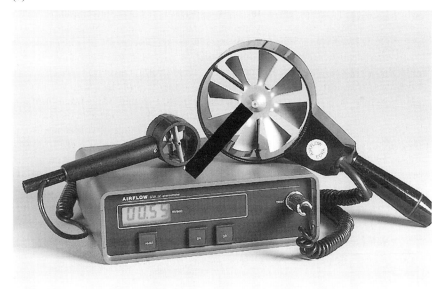

Figure 5.6 (b) EDRA5 anemometer (Air Flow Developments Ltd)

It is necessary to measure the airflow into a Class I cabinet at at least five places in the plane of the working face (Figure 5.7) An average is then calculated, but at no place should there be a reading that differs from the mean by more than 20%. If there is such a difference there will be turbulence within the cabinet. Usually some piece of equipment, inside or outside the cabinet, or the operator's body profile, is influencing the airflow. BS 5726: 1992 specifies an inward airflow between 0.7 and 1.0 m/s. Lower airflows cannot be relied on to retain aerosols produced by normal microbiological work; higher airflows create turbulence that may cause particles to be ejected from the open front.

Although airflows into Class I cabinets are usually much the same at all points on the working face this is not true for Class II cabinets, where the flow is greater at the bottom than at the top. In these cabinets, the average inward flow

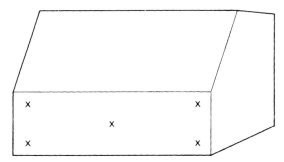

Figure 5.7 Testing airflow into a Class I safety cabinet. Anemometer readings should be taken at five places, marked with an X, in the plane of the working face with no-one working at the cabinet

can be calculated by measuring the velocity of air leaving the exhaust and the area of the exhaust vent. From this the volumetric rate of air discharge is found and this is also the amount entering the cabinet. Divided by the area of the working face it gives the average velocity. A rough and ready way, suitable for day-to-day use, requires a sheet of plywood or metal which can be fitted over the working face. In the centre of this an aperture is made which is 20 × 25 mm. The inward velocity of air through this is measured and the average velocity over the whole face calculated from this figure and the area of the working face. Whichever way is used a check should also be made with smoke to ensure that air is in fact entering the cabinet all the way round its perimeter and not just at the lower edge.

The downward velocity of air in a Class II cabinet should be measured with an anemometer at eight points in the horizontal plane 100 mm above the top edge of the working face (Figure 5.8). No reading should differ from the mean by more than 20%. BS 5726 (1992) specifies an inward airflow of 0.4 m/s and mean downward flow between 0.25 and 0.5 m/s. It is usual, when testing airflows with an anemometer, to observe or record the readings at each position for several minutes, because of possible fluctuations.

To measure the airflow through a Class III cabinet the gloves should be removed and readings taken at each glove port. Measurements should also be taken at the inlet filter face when the gloves are attached. BS 5726:1992 specifies an inward flow at each open glove of at least 0.7 m/s over a period of 5 min. At the inlet filter face it should be not less than 6 m³/min with the cabinet at a negative pressure of at least 200 Pa. Recommended airflows for each class of cabinet are shown in Table 5.1.

These tests should be done frequently even on cabinets fitted with airflow devices and airflow failure alarm systems.

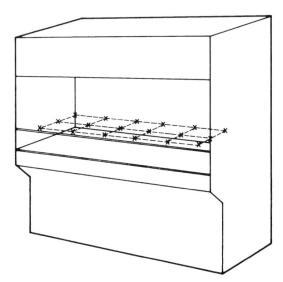

Figure 5.8 Testing the vertical airflow in a Class II safety cabinet. Anemometer readings should be taken at points marked X on an imaginary grid 6 inches within the cabinet walls and just above the level of the glass window

TABLE 5.1 Mean airflows (m/s) for microbiological safety cabinets according to British Standard 5726 (1992)

	Class I	Class II	Class III
Inflow at working face	$0.7–1.0^a$	0.4	—
Downflow	—	0.25–0.5	—
Inflow at glove ports	—	—	0.75
Inflow at filter	—	—	6 m^3/min

[a]With unused filters.
Data from BS 5726 with permission of the British Standards Institution.

Airflow indicators

Although anemometers are essential for the regular checking of cabinet airflows it would be tedious to use them every time a cabinet is operated. A built-in indicator is therefore useful so that the worker can see what is happening in the cabinet at all times. It is important that the operator can see the indicator from a normal sitting position, merely by raising the eyes. The operator can see easily if it is safe to start work, and can stop any time the indicator falls below the 'safe' level. Manometers, which indicate the pressure drop across the filters, are popular with engineers but are not a great deal of use to laboratory workers. If fitted, they are usually out of sight of the operator, and the fluid in them has been known to dry up. Alarm systems that give audible warning to the operator if the airflow falls below the recommended setting are now fitted to most safety cabinets.

Treatment and disposal of cabinet air

Air from safety cabinets must be treated to remove as many viable microorganisms as possible and then be discharged in such a way that if some organisms do escape there is little or no likelihood that they will initiate infections. These objectives are usually achieved by passing the air through high-efficiency particulate air (HEPA) filters that will remove 99.997% of particles and then ducting it to the outside of the building to ensure a high dilution with normal air.

Ultraviolet treatment has been considered, as has incineration. The former was shown by Newson and Walsingham (1974) to be ineffective. The latter was very expensive to operate and was uncertain (Barbeito and Gremillion, 1968; Chatigny et al., 1970).

AIR FILTRATION

Bacteriological tests on slagwool and glass fibre filters were described by Tejerson and Cherry (1947) who measured the penetration of Bacillus subtilis spores generated by a Collison nebulizer, thus initiating filter-testing procedures which follow much the same lines today. The modern HEPA filters were developed in the late 1940s and are made of glass fibre paper about 60 μm thick. The fibres vary from 0.4 to 1.4 μm in diameter. A sheet of this material about 18 m^2 in area is pleated around aluminium spacers into a cuboid pack with about 6.5 mm between pleats. The pack is then sealed into a metal box with a resilient synthetic rubber compound. This amount of glass fibre makes a filter

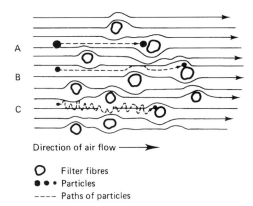

Direction of air flow ⟶

○   Filter fibres
● ● •   Particles
- - - -   Paths of particles

Figure 5.9 Capture of particles by filters. Very large particles cannot enter the filter web. Those that can may not follow the airflow because of their inertia (A). They continue in their original direction, hit a fibre and are trapped. Smaller particles (B) have less inertia, follow the flow lines until they pass near enough to a fibre to be trapped. Very small particles (C) assume Brownian motion and deviate from flow lines. Eventually they touch a fibre and are trapped. (Adapted from Newsom, 1976)

about 600 mm square by 300 mm deep, but HEPA filters are available in other sizes.

The fibres of the filter make up three-dimensional webs which remove particles from air flowing through them by inertia, interception and diffusion. Figure 5.9 (Newsom, 1976) shows this diagrammatically. Air changes direction as it meets a fibre, to flow around it. Large particles do not follow this change of direction because of their inertia. They continue in their original direction, hit the fibre and are trapped. Smaller particles have less inertia and follow the flow line. Sooner or later they will pass near to a fibre. If they approach one closer than half their diameter they will be intercepted and retained. Still smaller particles assume a Brownian movement which causes them to deviate from the flow lines and again, sooner or later they will touch a fibre and stick to it. Once a particle touches a fibre it is held to it by electrostatic (van der Waals) forces, and becomes very diffficult to dislodge.

The combination of these mechanisms retains even submicrometre particles (Harstad *et al.*, 1967) and explains the efficiency of HEPA filters. Viruses are usually attached to larger particles, anyway. Paradoxically the filters increase in efficiency as they become loaded. A new filter will pass about 1700 m³/h with a pressure drop of 25 mm WG. It will collect about 500 g of particulates before reaching 76 mm WG when it should be changed. This will be indicated by the drop in airflow (see airflow indicators, p. 118).

TESTING NEW FILTERS

HEPA filters are tested by challenging them with particulate matter at an airflow equal or greater than that expected in normal use. The apparatus, which is about 8 m long, is shown diagrammatically in Figure 5.10. It consists of a tunnel through which air is drawn by a fan. Test particles are released and dried in the chamber A, and air containing them passes through the first part of the tunnel where there is a sample port D into which a probe is inserted to count the

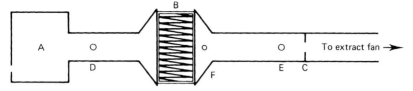

Figure 5.10 Principle of a filter test rig. (A) Nebulizing chamber. (B) Filter under test. (C) Adjustable diaphragm to control airflow. (D) Sample port to measure challenge dose. (E) Sample port to measure penetration. (F) Sample port to scan filter for locating position of leaks

number of particles per unit volume. The air then passes through the test filter B and the number of particles which are not removed are counted by a probe in sample port E. Another sample port F permits scanning of the filter to identify the positions of any leaks. The pressure drop across the test filter is measured by a manometer and air velocity in the tunnel is measured and controlled by an iris damper.

Challenge doses may consist of monodispersed spores of *Bacillus subtilis*, var. *globigii*, vaporized sodium chloride or dioctyl phthalate (DOP). The spores are released by a Collison nebulizer and counted by using a glass impinger upstream of the filter (D) and by a slit sampler downstream (E). Sodium chloride and DOP are generated by heat in special and rather expensive devices. Sodium chloride is estimated at each sampling port by a flame photometer and DOP by a particle counter. The challenge doses are predetermined and the three methods, variously used in different places and for different local standards give acceptably similar results. A filter suitable for microbiological safety cabinets should have a sodium chloride or DOP penetration not exceeding 0.003% when tested according to British Standard 3928 (BS, 1962). Testing the filters in cabinets in laboratories is described on p. 134.

ROUGHING OR PREFILTERS

In safety cabinets HEPA filters are usually protected by coarser filters, which remove dust and other particles down to about 5 μm. These are much cheaper than HEPA filters and prolong their lives.

There is a provisional European standard (CEN prEN 1822, 1995) for HEPA and other filters.

CARE OF FILTERS

A very high standard is maintained by filter manufacturers and is required by manufacturers of safety cabinets. Filters are very fragile, and although they satisfy the standards when they leave the manufacturer there is no guarantee that they will stand up to rough, or even 'normal', handling during transport. Changing filters in cabinets (see p. 143) is often left to unskilled individuals or people who equate this task with the less exacting technique of changing filters in air conditioning and industrial plants. One of us (CHC) has seen a number of filters that have being damaged before or during fitting. In addition, spontaneous leaks may arise in filters during use, either in the glass fibre or because of ageing and

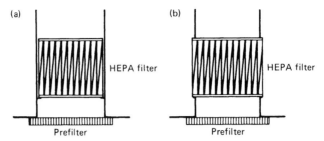

Figure 5.11 Position of HEPA filter in a Class I and Class III safety cabinet: (a) is wrong as the filter is inside the trunking and air may leak past it; (b) is right as the filter forms part of the trunking

cracking of the cement seal. These hazards indicate that great care is necessary in the use of filters, not only in maintenance but in the disposal of cabinet air.

Position of filters

In pre-BS 5726 Class I cabinets the prefilters were usually above the plenum and were removed by dismantling the assembly above the cabinet. Or they were inside the plenum and could be removed by opening a panel which was usually bolted down on a gasket. The HEPA filters were also inside the plenum or in a box above it (Figure 5.11a).

BS 5726 (1992), requires the prefilter to be accessible from the inside the cabinet (Figure 5.11a) and it is usually just pushed or clipped into place. The HEPA filter must be part of the external wall above the cabinet and not fitted within the plenum or ducting (Figure 5.11b). This is to prevent any contaminated air by-passing the filter as occasionally happened in earlier models when the seating or gaskets that held it deteriorated or the filter was badly fitted.

Ducting cabinet effluents to atmosphere

A 'good' HEPA filter, which retains 99.997% of particles, may therefore allow three of every 100 000 organisms in an aerosol burst in a cabinet. Exhaust air may then contain one organism in about 3 m³. Cabinet air is usually exhausted at about $8.5 \, \text{m}^3/\text{min}$ and during aerosol bursts, three organisms would be released into the atmosphere each minute, although, of course, aerosols are not being released all the time that a cabinet is in use. The dilution factor when these organisms leave the cabinet exhaust into the open air is enormous. Air outside a building is not still and movement contributes to dilution. It is extremely unlikely that any individual in the vicinity would breathe in enough organisms to initiate infection, even with Q fever, which is said to require as few as 10 (Wedum *et al.*, 1972). Even if some air containing effluent blew into an adjacent window it is most unlikely that it would contain an infective dose of microorganisms, as it would be diluted even further.

There is, nevertheless, a belief that air from safety cabinets should be ducted to a considerable height above the building. This height seems to be determined arbitrarily by national or local authorities and their inspectors. Various estimates, between 3 m and half the height of the building, have been cited to us but no

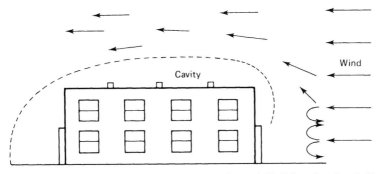

Figure 5.12 The 'cavity' of comparatively still air over a flat-roofed building when the wind is blowing. Particles (and vapours) released into the cavity may not be dispersed and may be drawn into the building by ventilation intakes

printed rules or regulations seem to be available. This principle arises from confusion between the nature of the effluent from fume cupboards and micro-biological safety cabinets. One contains very large numbers of molecules, the other very small numbers of comparatively much larger particles.

When wind blows against a building a 'cavity' of fairly still air is created on the leeward side. This 'cavity' may extend back over a flat roof, and its size and shape is influenced by the shape of the roof and the size and location of other buildings (Figure 5.12). Any fumes released into the 'cavity' are dispersed slowly and may be captured by an air intake on the roof. This happened, in the experience of one of us (CHC), when acetanilide, legitimately released in a fume cupboard, was brought back into another part of the building by the ventilation system. Ideally, toxic and smelly fumes should be ducted above the 'cavity'. This is not easy; the size and shape of the 'cavity' alter with changing wind direction and velocity, but it need not trouble those who install microbiological safety cabinets. Even if microorganisms are released into the 'cavity' the dilution will be so great that they will be in small numbers, and unlike molecules of chemicals, they are likely to be removed during the tempering (filtration, washing, etc.) of air that is taken into buildings to be circulated among its occupants.

Nevertheless, it is not prudent to discharge the effluents from microbiological safety cabinets near to open windows, especially of hospital wards, or near to ventilation system intakes. While the actual risk of infection may be negligible, nevertheless an infection risk may be perceived with great concern by some people and it is best to avoid such situations. It is advisable to see where the effluent is likely to go by doing smoke tests with the high volume generators used by engineers. The methods described on p. 117 are not suitable for use in the open air.

Disposal of cabinet air into the building ventilation system

Ducting air from a safety cabinet into a building ventilation system poses a number of problems. The building ventilation must be a 'total loss' system, i.e., there must be no possibility of recirculation into any other room. Non-return valves are necessary to prevent this if the main exhaust fans fail. The pull of the fans must be adequate to ensure the correct face velocity at the cabinet; or if the

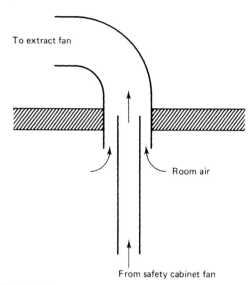

To extract fan

Room air

From safety cabinet fan

Figure 5.13 A 'thimble' unit. The extract system removes air from both the room and the cabinet

cabinet has its own fan (as, for example, a Class II cabinet) the cabinet air should enter the room exhaust duct by a thimble unit (Figure 5.13) and that should be the only exhaust duct from the room. The thimble ensures that air is exhausted continually from the room, whether the cabinet is in use or not. When the cabinet fan is switched on the building exhaust must be capable of accepting the cabinet exhaust and some room air, otherwise at least some cabinet air will be discharged back into the room.

An unbroken connection between the cabinet exhaust fan and the building exhaust fan is highly undesirable. The least efficient fan will merely act as a partial obstruction to the airflow. A warning device is needed to tell anyone who is working at the cabinet when the building exhaust fan fails or is switched off.

This method of disposing of cabinet air has little to commend it for Class I cabinets, but may be useful for Class II cabinets.

Recirculation of filtered cabinet air

The recirculation of air from Class I cabinets back into the room is the simplest and cheapest method of disposal and is therefore seized upon eagerly by designers and others who are not themselves at risk. Apart from cost, the reasons advanced for this measure arise from misunderstandings about the efficiency of filters, from bad laboratory design and, the most fatuous of all, from claims that ducting the effluent out of building would 'spoil the elevation'.

The reasons why filters cannot be relied upon entirely to protect laboratory workers are given above. Although good laboratory practices do not usually generate aerosols containing more than about 10^5 organisms, errors and accidents do occur and larger bursts may be expected from time to time. A faulty filter (see above) will increase the risk considerably. There is also the possibility that room air contaminated in this way can be uncontrollably transferred to other rooms and corridors.

Double filtration—passing cabinet air through two HEPA filters in series—has been advocated for laboratories that are so poorly designed that the air cannot be ducted to atmosphere (e.g. where a laboratory is buried deep inside a large building). The argument is based on theoretical grounds. If three in every 100 000 organisms get through the first filter in a series of two good HEPA filters, the likelihood of any of these escapees getting through the second filter is vanishingly small.

It is sometimes claimed that there are 'exceptional cirumstances' that which make it difficult to exhaust the air to atmosphere. It is difficult to understand the nature of these circumstances when all that is required is a reallocation of rooms, unless one accepts that there are two subspecies of *Homo sapiens*—one that must have windows and one that need not. Although the British Standard (BS 5726, 1992) offers the alternative of exhaust to atmosphere or to the room through two filters the ACDP (1995) prefers the first option, and we agree with them.

Engineers and administrators sometimes argue in favour of recirculation because of the cost of dumping expensively warmed air. It is something that they have to come to terms with. Except in large research institutions the amount of warm air lost from a microbiological safety cabinet is not very great compared with that lost through open doors and windows, and wasted by overheating some rooms.

There is another aspect of recirculation which its advocates (but not the ACDP!) have overlooked. It is necessary to fumigate cabinets with formaldehyde. As it is necessary to run the fan to get the formaldehyde into the filter, and to purge the cabinet after treatment, the gas will render the room uninhabitable and unless the room is sealed formaldehyde will escape and cause inconvenience and discomfort to people in the vicinity. Exposure to formaldehyde is known to be hazardous (HSE, 1981c, 1992). Anyone who has disinfected rooms with formaldehyde, which is very pervasive, knows the problems and risks involved, including the provision of appropriate respirators (ordinary gas masks will not do) and training in their use. Decontamination of such cabinets presents problems (see p. 140).

One of us (CHC) has met the 'elevation-spoiling' argument on several occasions. Two are worth reporting here. A laboratory wished to project two pieces of rectangular cabinet exhaust ducting, each 100 mm by 80 mm, about 300 mm from the top of the window of a room quite high up a building which had no openable windows. When objections were made the elevation was examined. It was noted that the ducts would be barely visible from the ground and that there was a large mushroom baffle of an axial ventilating fan in the middle of an office window on a lower floor. The point was well taken that ducts for the safety of one group of people 'spoiled the elevation' less than an extractor fan for the comfort of others, and the exhausts were installed. On the other occasion the designers claimed to have adequate and satisfying evidence that it was quite safe to recirculate to the laboratory the air from a safety cabinet to be installed for tuberculosis bacteriology. They were unwilling, however, to reveal the provenance of this evidence and the laboratory staff remained unconvinced. Fortunately the design of the building suggested a compromise. A short and unobtrusive length of trunking was proposed to take the cabinet air to the room of one member of the design team, who, until then had insisted that the air was safe to breathe. The elevation of the building was duly 'spoiled' by ducting the cabinet air through a wall!

The Howie Code (DH, 1978) stated categorically that safety cabinets 'must not circulate air into the same room, corridor or any other room'. This conclusion was reached by a group of people who used safety cabinets, had studied the problems involved and who had taken pains to obtain advice from other recognized experts. This code's successor (HSE, 1991) rather ducks the issue and BS 5726 (1992) specifically permits recirculation through two exhaust filters. On balance, we believe that when Hazard Group 3 organisms are being handled in a cabinet, the safety of the workers will be maximal if the effluent is ducted outside the building.

Exhaust fans (blowers) and outlets

It is most important that the exhaust fan should be at the distal end of the trunking to ensure negative pressure, so that any leaks will be into and not out of that trunking. Exceptions are allowed in BS 5726 (1992) for trunking less than 2 m in length, when the fan may be fitted in the cabinet. This is the thin end of a very long wedge. One of us (CHC) has encountered a newly installed cabinet with an integral fan designed for 2 m of trunking, which was expected to deal with over 20 m of trunking. Airflow at the working face of the cabinet was barely detectable.

Each Class I cabinet must have its own separate trunking and exhaust fan. Although it may be permissible, or desirable, to duct fume cupboards to a common extract system this is a bad principle for Class I safety cabinets. We have seen several installations in which the trunking for two or more cabinets has been combined into a single exhaust system. None has been satisfactory. It is not good practice, as it may be with fume cupboards, to have safety cabinets exhausting all the time, whether in use or not. Running a cabinet unnecessarily shortens the life of the expensive HEPA filters.

The size, or rating, of the extractor fan depends on the length of trunking. Theoretically, if the trunking is very long (and it should not be; see below) then a higher rated fan will give the necessary face velocity at the cabinet. Unfortunately, this is not always considered and it can, in any case, be very expensive. Cabinet manufacturers, who are now skilled at their trade, and who are in business to make money, provide the right fan for a short length of trunking (with few bends). This is usually a standard model. Unless the manufacturer knows that the trunking is to be very long, this is what he will supply. There is, then, a sound argument—supported by the philosophy of BS 5726 (1992)—in favour of purchasing a complete installation, rather than a cabinet and fan and relying on local labour to install them. Cabinet installations and maintenance require as much specialized knowledge as do sterilizers, centrifuges and refrigerators, but are frequently left to people who are meeting them for the first time or who confuse them with fume cupboards. We know of two places where the fans were ingeniously installed the wrong way round and blew air into the cabinets.

Class I cabinets require only one fan. In some installations, where a fan incorporated in the cabinet has failed to push enough air through the trunking to give a satisfactory face velocity another fan has been fitted at the distal end of the trunking, or even somewhere along its length. This is most unsatisfactory. The least efficient fan merely acts as an obstruction to the passage of air to the other one. If cabinets with integral fans are to be converted to work efficiently (e.g. with more than 2 m of trunking) then the integral fan should be removed.

Class II cabinets necessarily have integral fans, to recirculate up to 70% of the air inside them. These fans may be competent to push the 30% or so exhaust air through a short length of trunking to the outside of the building, but mostly they need assistance. The cabinet exhaust duct should then vent into a thimble unit (see p. 126) which is connected via ducting to an extract fan. The latter must be capable of removing more air than the cabinet exhaust delivers, i.e. take some room air as well, or cabinet air will remain in the room. On no account should the cabinet exhaust be connected directly to the ducting. Apart from the reasons given above, for Class I cabinets, this would upset the balance of recirculated and dumped air in a Class II cabinet and render it ineffective for either product or operator protection or both.

It may be necessary to protect the exhaust outlet from rain, and also from birds, which are prone to nest in such places, in spite of the noise and rapidly moving air. Some solutions are shown in Figure 5.14. One is to fit a 'Chinaman's

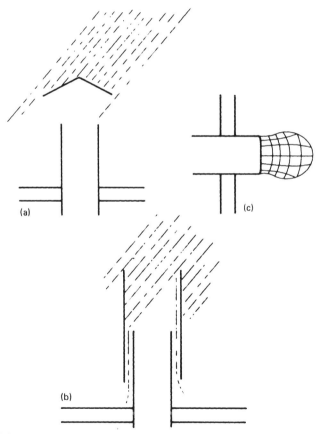

Figure 5.14 Fittings for discharge terminals. (a) Cowl, known in the building trade as a 'Chinaman's hat' which prevents rain from entering the trunking. (b) Annulus device (Darlow, personal communication) is effective because rain rarely falls vertically. (c) Wire cage which prevents birds nesting, known to builders as 'balloons'

hat' cowl to vertical or horizontal outlets, but when this is done the airflow at the cabinet face should be monitored. Sometimes fitting a cowl reduces airflow. The annulus device (Darlow, personal communication) protects against rain, which rarely falls vertically. The wire 'balloons' (spherical wire cages) are standard builders' goods, used to prevent birds and rats entering soil and drain pipes. They do not seem to impede airflow.

Trunking

It is generally agreed among cabinet manufacturers and engineers that circular cross-section trunking gives better airflows than that with a rectangular cross-section. In the early days of British and American safety cabinets flexible trunking, of 100–150 mm diameter was used. This so-called 'elephant trunking' served its purpose and allowed considerable latitude in placing cabinets relative to exhaust fans. This trunking still has much to commend it in awkward sites, but as it is corrugated it impedes airflow, so it should not be used for long runs. Another drawback, in some varieties, is that the lining sometimes becomes detached, especially where the trunking is fitted on to the cabinet exhaust or fan spigots. Again, this restricts airflow.

Some designers, but not cabinet manufacturers, have favoured trunking consisting of metal cylinders, about the size of baked bean or canned fruit cans, soldered or welded together. Such trunking (called 'bean-can' trunking in earlier editions) is expensive, cumbersome and prone to leak if it is knocked or disturbed. It has nothing to commend it.

Undoubtedly, the best and most favoured forms of trunking are the polypropylene (or similar plastic) tubes and fittings used by builders. Lengths up to about 4 m are available, as is a range of bends and offsets. The various components can be cut and assembled on site and fitted together on O-rings (they may also be cemented, but this is rarely necessary). The tubing can be connected to the cabinet and fan with rubber sleeves or if the spigots fit inside, with PTFE tape. Such an assembly does not leak, is rigid, but not so much that it splits or leaks when knocked or disturbed. The smooth lumen does not impede airflow.

It is very important that trunking is neither long nor tortuous. Long runs of trunking, even if the inner surfaces are smooth, reduce airflow. One right-angled bend can reduce it by as much as 20%. In a well-designed laboratory it is possible to duct cabinet air to atmosphere, through the wall or top of the window, or through the roof using only 2 or 3 m and not more than two bends. All bends should be 'easy', i.e. of large radius. These cause less reduction in airflow than sharp or abrupt bends.

Simple duct work is more efficient and therefore safer than complicated installations. It is also much cheaper. We have seen several examples of very expensive ducting of almost Möbian topology, which, of course, failed to remove enough, if any, air from safety cabinets. BS 5726 (1992) gives sound advice on trunking.

Blowback

If a very high wind blows directly into an unprotected exhaust air outlet it may create a high pressure in the trunking and dislodge material from the roughing filter into the cabinet. It is unlikely that this would happen while the fan is working, and when it isn't the front closure of the cabinet should be in place. This effectively seals the cabinet. To guard against the possibility of contamination of the floor and inside of the cabinet, BS 5726 (1992) specifies that an anti-blowback device must be fitted. Most manufacturers of cabinets fit these immediately above the cabinet plenum. Usually the device consists of hinged metal plates which are counterbalanced to close off the ducting unless air is being pulled through the system by the fan. In some cabinets they are balanced so that their position indicates the rate of flow to the operators, who can see them through perspex windows.

Testing microbiological safety cabinets

Performance tests for Class I and II cabinets

The UK *Control of Substances Hazardous to Health 1994* (COSHH) regulations include microbiological safety cabinets as 'local exhaust ventilation' and require that they are thoroughly examined and tested every 14 months but although this applies to airflows and filter integrity it is not clear if it applies to performance tests.

Three tests are applied, one to Class I cabinets, and three to Class II cabinets. They are

(1) the containment test (Classes I and II cabinets);
(2) the external contamination test (Class II cabinets);
(3) the cross-contamination test (Class II cabinets).

None of these is a 'routine' test, applicable during the ordinary working life of a cabinet. They are used

(1) as type tests, by manufacturers when they design new models or modify existing ones;
(2) when a new cabinet is installed and commissioned;
(3) when a cabinet is moved to a new site in a laboratory, or modifications are made.

All three tests require expensive apparatus and considerable expertise. These tests, especially that which measures containment, have evolved over several years as a result of the work of Williams and Lidwell (1957), Darlow (1967), McDade *et al.* (1968), Staat and Beakley (1968), Barbeito and Taylor (1968) and more recently in the theses of Barkley (1972) and Newsom (1976a). They led to the tests prescribed in NSF 49 (NSF, 1988) and BS 5726 (1992). Only an outline of the tests can be given here. For full details the reader is referred to the official standards documents and the references cited.

Performance tests for Class III cabinets and flexible film isolators

BS 5726 (1992) specifies a pressure integrity test for Class III cabinets. The cabinet must hold an internal pressure of 250 Pa to within ±10% for not less than 30 min. This test can be applied to flexible film isolators provided after the envelope is raised to the test pressure 30 min are allowed for the plastic film to stretch. Thereafter, a test pressure of 250 Pa is re-established (ACDP, 1985) and has to be held at 10% of this pressure for 30 min for the test to be passed.

Flexible film isolators may be tested in much the same way as microbiological safety cabinets. They can be tested for leaks by adjusting the dampers and flow controls to give an internal pressure and applying the soap solution test to all seams and service entry cones. They can be challenged with aerosols released inside and sampled at the outlet filter or released by the inlet filter and sampled inside.

The containment or operator protection test

An 'artificial arm', in practice a stainless steel cylinder, is placed inside the cabinet to simulate the disturbance to airflow caused by working within it. A measured amount of an aerosol containing a known number of spores of *B. subtilis*, var. *globigii* (NCTC 10073) is released inside a safety cabinet while it is operating and sampling devices outside the cabinet are set to capture on culture media any spores that escape. The culture plates are incubated and colonies—which are yellow in colour—are counted.

As there may be objections to the release of viable microorganisms an alternative method uses a solution of potassium iodide which is dropped on a spinning disc (Foord and Lidwell, 1975; Clark and Goff, 1981). The particles are collected in air samplers on membrane filters which are then exposed to a solution of palladium chloride, when the particles become visible and may be counted.

In accordance with the requirements of BS 5726 (1992), the protection factor is calculated. This is broadly speaking the ratio of the number of spores generated in the cabinet to the number which escape from it. The formula is given as $(N.s)/(10n)$, where N is the number of spores released (the challenge dose), s is the sampling rate in m^3/min and n is the number of spores that escape and are captured by the sampler (i.e., the number of colonies on the culture plate). Alternatively if s is in dm^3/min, the formula is $(N.s)/(10^4 n)$. For example, if $N = 4.3 \times 10^8$, $s = 30$ dm^3/min and the number of colonies on the plate was 3, the protection factor would be 4.3×10^5. For a pass, BS 5726 (1992) requires a minimum protection factor of 1.0×10^5 in each individual test. This standard also specifies how the protection factor can be calculated using an aerosol of potassium iodide. Commercial test equipment is shown in Figures 5.15 and 5.16.

Matthews (1985) and Kennedy *et al.* (1988) used fluorescent materials (polystyrene microspheres and an optical brightener respectively) generated by the same kind of nebulizer as that used for spores. Their results suggest that these materials might be used instead of either spores or potassium iodide.

The external contamination test

This tests if the curtain of air descending at the front of a Class II cabinet prevents contamination of material in the cabinet by room air. The nebulizer is placed centrally outside the cabinet with its nozzle pointing into it and 100 mm in front of the top edge of the working face. The 'artificial arm' is placed as in the protection test. At least 12 petri dishes containing nutrient agar are distributed over the working surface. The lids of these are removed and 1 min

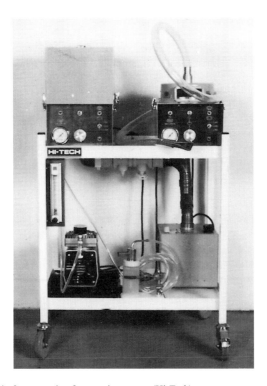

Figure 5.15 Test rig for protection factor using spores (Hi-Tech)

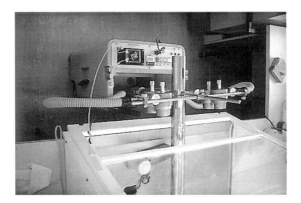

Figure 5.16 Test rig for protection factor using potassium iodide (Ki-Discus, Watson and Watkins)

later the nebulizer is operated. This should run for 4 min and produce a challenge dose of at least 3×10^6 spores. The test is repeated five times and a control test done with the cabinet fan switched off. The culture dishes are incubated overnight and the colonies counted. BS 5726 (1992) permits no more than five colonies per test (not per petri dish) with a control having more than 300 colonies.

The cross contamination test

This tests whether aerosols generated at one side of the cabinet will contaminate materials at the other side. BS 5726 (1992) requires that the 'artificial arm' is used and 12 petri dishes containing nutrient agar are placed at one end of the working surface to occupy not more than two-thirds of it. The nebulizer is placed at the other end and pointing towards them. The lids of the petri dishes are removed 1 min before spraying begins and the spray is run for at least 4 min to produce a challenge dose of at least 10^5 spores. Five tests are done and also a control test with the fans not working. The culture plates are incubated overnight and the colonies counted. The standard requires that there should be not more than five colonies per test.

Testing the filters *in situ*

This may be done as part of the commissioning tests or if leakage is suspected but until recently it was not usually done as a routine except in research laboratories which handle Hazard Group 4 agents. Any of the three challenge methods described on p. 123 may be used but the expense and portability of the equipment must be considered, as well as the availability of staff trained to do it. The challenge dose is released into the cabinet and measured with the fan running. A sample probe, connected to an impinger, a particle counter or a flame photometer is inserted through the sampling port, downstream of the filter.

The DOP test is widely used in the USA and the sodium flame test has been recommended for UK users (BS 3928:1963; HSE 1991). This test, however, could introduce an unacceptable hazard into diagnostic and similar laboratories because the flame photometers need hydrogen. The use of cylinders of this gas in laboratories is quite rightly discouraged by the Health and Safety Executive. The biological test is preferred, although it does not give the instantaneous result obtainable with the other tests. Lach and Wright (1981) compared the bacterial spore test with the sodium chloride method for *in situ* tests and found good agreement. The sodium chloride method gives almost immediate results (no delay for incubation) and does not contaminate the cabinet.

A 'good' filter should not pass more than three particles per 100 000 of the challenge dose. If, during a commissioning test, an unused filter does fail, it should be changed and tested on the rig described on p. 123. It may be possible to repair small leaks.

Other tests and requirements

Mainly for the benefit of manufacturers, BS 5726 (1992) specifies tests for leakage of cabinet carcase, resistance to overturning, distortion, deflection of the work surface and tipping and tests for chemical resistance and vibration resistance. Among other things, it specifies requirements for electrical safety (see below), lighting intensity and noise level.

Services

The earlier cabinets were illuminated by fluorescent tube lamps which were fitted on the ceiling of the enclosure. When such lamps were fitted in Class II cabinets they partially obstructed the airflow. It was also noted by several workers that the heat from them distorted the airflow. Current models of all three types of microbiological safety cabinets are illuminated from outside the front viewing panel. Failed lamps may be changed without decontaminating the inside of the cabinet.

It is often necessary to operate small electrical apparatus in these cabinets. Large apparatus, and equipment which generates heat should be avoided as both may compromise the airflow. It is more convenient to have electrical socket outlets inside cabinets than to trail electricity cable in through the front opening or through holes drilled in the walls. Such socket outlets should be waterproof or covered in such a way that no moisture can enter them when the cabinets are swabbed out with liquid disinfectant or when water condenses on the walls during decontamination with formaldehyde, which results in a high humidity. Switches for the outlets should be outside the cabinets but within reach of the operators as they sit or stand at work. Gas burners should be avoided in microbiological safety cabinets. The heat distorts the airflows, as described above, and if the flame goes out, as it may well do because of the air movements, gas may build up in the cabinet, plenum or ducting with risk of explosion. BS 5726 (1992) specifies that if there is a provision for a flammable gas supply to the inside of a cabinet this must be controlled by a solenoid valve that allows gas to pass only when the fan is switched on and which needs to be manually reset after any interruption of the electrical supply. It is spelt out in the standard that fittings for flammable gas must not be provided in Class III cabinets.

Choosing microbiological safety cabinets

While we are firmly of the opinion that selection of a microbiological safety cabinet should be the prerogative of the user, i.e. the person who will work at and with the cabinet and who is at risk, guidance should always be sought from a microbiological safety adviser (see Chapter 11) with reference to the guidance provided by BS 5726 (1992), Part 4 (see below). Much depends on the risk or hazard group of the microorganisms that will be handled and on the techniques used. Table 5.2 offers guidance to users.

It is essential that cabinets are purchased from and installed by reputable manufacturers and that they and their installation conform with the national standards, e.g. BS 5726 (1992); AS 2252 (1994); AS 2647 (1994) and NSF 49 (1983).

For work with Hazard Group 3 microorganisms the health and safety authorities in the UK have always favoured Class I, rather than Class II cabinets.

TABLE 5.2 Selection of safety cabinets

Hazard group	Class of cabinet	Degree of protection		Exhaust to
		Worker	Work[1]	
2, 3	I	++	cannot be relied on	Atmosphere
	II	++	+++	Preferably atmosphere
3, 4	III	+++	+++	Atmosphere

[1] e.g. tissue culture preparation.

This may have been the result of unsatisfactory reports of early cabinets. But as many of the current Class II cabinets offer the same worker protection as Class I cabinets, this view has been somewhat relaxed and the ACDP (1995) now gives guarded support for the use of Class II cabinets in appropriate circumstances. On the other hand Class II cabinets to the NSF 49 standard have been the norm in the USA and some other countries for many years, without any recorded incidents of associated infections.

All work with Hazard Group 4 pathogens requires a Class III safety cabinet except in those very specialized laboratories where the operators wear pressurized isolation suits.

There is no reason why Class III cabinets should not be used for less hazardous work and indeed some purists still insist that Class III cabinets are the only safety cabinets and that any work which merits a cabinet should be done in one of them. This is an extreme view which may be considered somewhat misguided in the light of Table 5.3 and practicalities must be considered. Work in a Class III cabinet is hampered by gloves and the procedures for transferring material into and out of the cabinet. For work with the less hazardous pathogens the inconvenience may not be justified. Nevertheless, if work with Hazard Group 3 or even Group 2 agents is likely to involve the deliberate production of aerosols a Class III cabinet should be considered. For some work with Hazard Group 4 agents the flexible film isolator (p. 114) should be considered. Cost, both of purchase and of maintenance, and protection of the work or product from contamination by room air needs consideration. Class I cabinets are less expensive and they require less maintenance than Class II cabinets. While it has been reported (Newsom, 1979a) that Class I cabinets can offer some protection to the work, as far as we are aware no manufacturer makes such a claim and work protection cannot be relied on.

The larger working area provided by Class II cabinets, makes them particularly useful for tissue culture work. So-called sterile tissue cultures may be contaminated with viruses and other agents without showing any signs and it is inadvisable for operators to inhale aerosols dispersed during dispensing, quite apart from the problems or external contamination.

Open-fronted cabinets (Class I and II) and enclosed cabinets (Class III and flexible film isolators) are limited in the degree of protection that is offered to the worker. Table 5.3 illustrates this with reference to portals of entry for infection.

TABLE 5.3 Worker protection: limitations of microbiological safety cabinets

Portal of entry	Class I and II types (open-fronted)	Class III types (enclosed)
Respiratory	yes	yes
Alimentary	no[1]	yes
Eye	possible[2]	yes
Mucous membrane	possible[3]	yes
Hand contact	yes[4]	no
Percutaneous	no	no[5]

[1] Partial barrier, mouth pipetting possible.
[2] Partial barrier, droplets in eye possible.
[3] Partial barrier, droplets in nose possible.
[4] Partial barrier, contact between contaminated hand and face and environmental surfaces possible.
[5] Possibility of transmission of infection by needle-stick following glove penetration.
Based on Kennedy (1995).

While it can be seen that Class III-type cabinets offer more protection because, being enclosed, they put a barrier between the worker and the material being worked on, nevertheless this barrier can be penetrated by a contaminated sharp object, such as a hypodermic needle, thereby presenting a risk of percutaneous transmission of infection. It is recalled that a case of laboratory-acquired Ebola fever reported by Emond *et al.* (1977) occurred in this way (p. 81). The limitations of microbiological safety cabinets need to be borne in mind when risk assessment is being undertaken (see Chapter 11).

Figures 5.17–5.19 are illustrative examples of microbiological safety cabinets. Figure 5.20 shows flexible film isolators.

Working in safety cabinets

It is most important that those who work at cabinets are comfortable. Discomfort and stress predispose accidents. Staff should be able to sit (or stand) so that the arms are in a natural position for working at the cabinet floor level and they should be able to reach all parts of it without contortions. They should be able to see through the front viewing screen—not under it, which negates the protection afforded—and vision should not be obscured by the front glazing bar. No work should be done in a Class I cabinet with the viewing screen raised. This

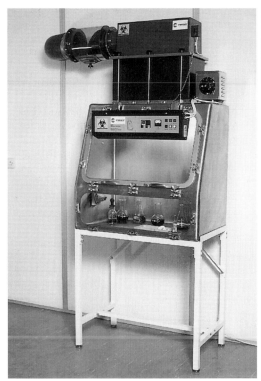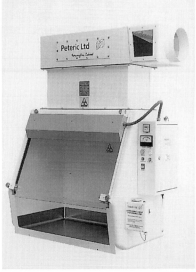

Figure 5.17 Class I safety cabinets. Envair (left) and Foramaflow (right)

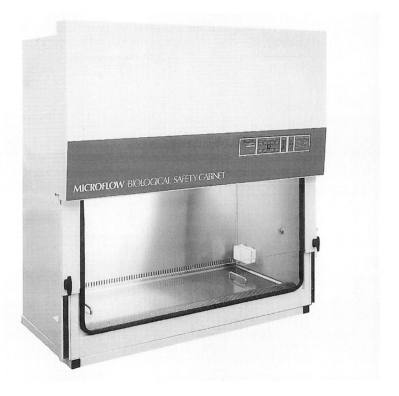

Figure 5.18 Class II safety cabinet (Microflow)

reduces the airflow to an unsafe level. Centrifuges should never be operated within open-fronted cabinets (see p. 90).

The operator should remember that the cabinet is intended to prevent the inhalation of aerosols. Open-fronted cabinets will not protect them from spillage and other accidents that release microorganisms. When working in Class I and II cabinets, the hands and arms will probably become contaminated. Operators should therefore be encouraged to wear protective gloves; certainly so if they have any cuts, scratches or other lesions on their hands. Appropriate protective clothing (p. 187) should always be worn.

The cabinet should be loaded with the materials necessary for the operation and not otherwise cluttered. Too much apparatus interferes with airflow. After switching on the motor the operator should wait about 30 s to allow the airflow to settle down and then check the airflow indicator to ensure that it is safe for him to proceed. The operator should work with hands well inside a Class I or Class II cabinet, not near to the front edge, and should avoid moving arms in and out like pistons or contaminated air may be pumped out out with them. The arms should not be entirely withdrawn from the cabinet until a set of operations is complete. The operator should then wait for about 1 min to allow any aerosols to be carried into the filter and for any larger particles to settle before removing arms and hands. The work can then be unloaded, hands washed and the cabinet reloaded.

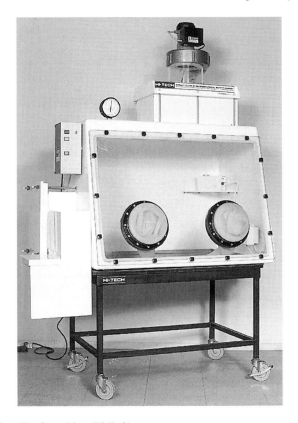

Figure 5.19 Class III safety cabinet (Hi-Tech)

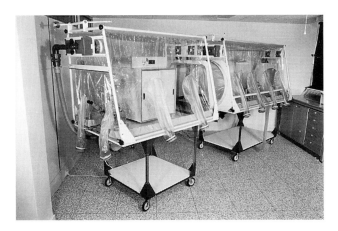

Figure 5.20 Flexible film isolator

It is advisable to use short graduated pipettes, plastic pasteur pipettes and plastic inoculating loops and needles for work in safety cabinets. Sharp objects should be avoided, especially in Class III cabinets where some tactile sensitivity may be lost through the wearing of gloves, and the risks of self-inoculation are greater are greater. When all work in a cabinet is finished and the work removed the cabinet fan should be allowed to run for a few minutes before switching off the motor and fitting the front closure.

Decontamination of safety cabinets

As safety cabinets are used to contain infectious aerosols which may be released during work, and spattering and spillage may occur, the inside surfaces and the filters will become contaminated. The working surface and the walls may be decontaminated on a day-to-day basis by swabbing them with disinfectant. Glutaraldehyde is probably the best disinfectant for this purpose as phenolics may leave sticky residues and hypochlorites may, in time, corrode the metal. For thorough decontamination, however, after large spillages, before maintenance, filter changing and testing (except for routine airflow tests (p. 117)) fumigation is necessary. This may be done with formalin (Darlow, 1967; Newsom and Walsingham, 1974) although vaporized glutaraldehyde was preferred by Evans and Harris-Smith (1970). Both of these aldehydes are toxic (see Chapter 7) and precautions should be taken before using them.

The installation should be checked to ensure that none of the gas can escape to the room or elsewhere. The front closure (night door) of the cabinet should seal properly onto the carcase, or masking tape should be available to seal it. Any service holes in the carcase should be sealed and the HEPA filter seating examined to ensure that there are no leaks. If the filters are to be changed and the primary or roughing filter is accessible from inside the cabinet it should be removed and left inside the working area of the cabinet. The supply filter on a Class III cabinet should be sealed with plastic film. Cabinets which recirculate air to the room cannot be decontaminated with formaldehyde without special precautions (see below).

Formaldehyde is generated by:

(1) boiling formalin which is a 40% solution of the gas in water;
(2) heating paraformaldehyde, which is its solid polymer.

Flexible film isolators may be wiped out with liquid disinfectant and decontaminated with formaldehyde. The capacity is given in the manufacturer's specification and the amount of formalin required may be calculated as described above. Care should be taken to ensure that the flexible exhaust hose is led through a window and well away from other, opened windows.

Boiling formalin

The volume used is important. Too little will be ineffective; too much leads to deposits of the polymer, which is persistent and which may contribute to the normal blocking of the filters in use. BS 5726 (1992) specifies a concentration of 0.05 g/m^3 which is approximately that obtained by Newsom and Walsingham (1974) when they boiled away 25 ml of neat formalin in a Class I cabinet with a capacity of 0.34 m. Their experiments showed that boiling away this proportion, which is 2 ml of neat formalin per 0.028 m^3 of cabinet space killed *Mycobacterium phlei* and the spores of *B. subtilis*, var. *globigii* on strips of aluminium foil in 2 hours, but if the formalin was diluted with equal parts of water even 8 hours' exposure was not always successful.

It has often been assumed that as formaldehyde requires a 70% humidity to kill bacteria (see chapter 7) it was necessary to add water when boiling formalin to decontaminate safety cabinets, but Taylor *et al.* (1969) and Newsom and Walsingham (1974) have shown that even dry gas is a good disinfectant. Boiling diluted formalin will result in a very wet cabinet. Formalin may be boiled in cabinets in several ways. When Darlow (1967) designed his Class III cabinets he incorporated an electric hot plate on a bracket on the wall. Formalin is dropped slowly on to this from a funnel fitted with a tap which passes through the roof of the cabinet. Some cabinet manufacturers supply and/or fit such devices. Evans *et al.* (1972) used a coffee percolator with an automatic thermal cut out, and Collins (1974) a flask (bolthead) heated on an electric Thermomantle. If the latter is used it should be connected to a timing device so that it is switched off when the formalin has almost boiled away. After checking the cabinet as described above the aldehyde is placed in the generator in the cabinet and the front closure sealed. A clear notice is placed on the front of the cabinet indicating that it is being decontaminated. BS 5726 (1992) recommends that 60 ml of formalin for each m^3 cabinet volume. HSE (1991) gives 25 ml for a cabinet with an internal volume of 0.38 m^3.

The heater is then switched on. When about half of the formalin has been boiled away the fan is run for about 15 s to bring formaldehyde into the filters.

Heating paraformaldehyde

Tablets (1 g) of paraformaldehyde are available from chemical manufacturers but the powdered or flake material may be used. Newsom and Walsingham (1974) found that heating four tablets for 2 hours killed the organisms dried on aluminium foil and exposure for 22 hours killed them if they were coated with serum.

There are two ways of heating the tablets. Taylor *et al.* (1969) used an electric frying pan; this is best connected with a 1-hour timing switch (NIH, 1978). Newsom and Walsingham (1974) used an electric hair dryer. The hot air dryers used by biochemists for chromatography are probably better and should be connected to a timing device. The Australian Standard (AS 2647:1983) recommends 10 g of paraformaldehyde for each m^3 of cabinet volume. This is mixed with high-temperature silicone oil to give a depth of 10 mm in a deep-fat fryer. This is heated at 200°C until it ceases to bubble, when all the formaldehyde has been driven off. The fan is run as with formaldehyde to decontaminate the filter.

One of us (DAK) has reported an explosion in a microbiological safety cabinet that was being decontaminated. Formalin was being boiled over a microbunsen and the cabinet was sealed. Eventually, when the oxygen was used up the burner went out. This was not noticed at the time and a concentration of flammable gas built up. There was an explosion when an attempt was made to relight the burner (Kennedy, 1988).

Exposure time

It is convenient to start decontamination in the late afternoon and let the gas act overnight. In the morning the fan should be switched on and the front closure 'cracked' open very slightly to allow air to enter and purge the cabinet. Some cabinets have a hole in the front closure, fitted with a stopper which can be removed for this purpose. With Class III cabinets the plastic film is taken off the supply filter to allow air to enter the cabinet and purge it of formaldehyde. After several minutes the front closure may be removed. The fan is then allowed to run for about 30 min which should remove all formaldehyde.

Decontamination of cabinets which recirculate room air

The problem of safely decontaminating cabinets which recirculate air to the room has already been mentioned (p. 126). If the air outlet is blocked off and the methods described above are used then there is no way of purging the cabinet and filter of formaldehyde. It is very unwise—even dangerous—to remove the front closure without first clearing the cabinet of gas. There are two solutions, neither of which is particularly satisfactory.

The first is used in the USA and Australia for Class II cabinets which return air to the room. A special fitting is made to cover the air outlet and this has a spigot so that a length of flexible trunking can be attached. The other end of the trunking is taken out of the nearest window. In buildings which have no openable windows this presents more problems!

The alternative is to decontaminate the room as well as the cabinet. This entails the provision of respirators, training in their use, handling concentrated ammonia to absorb formaldehyde and having the cabinet and room out of action for 24–28 hours (see Chapter 7).

Summary of decontamination procedure using formalin

The pre-filter should be removed from inside the cabinet (where possible) and placed inside the cabinet on the working surface. It is usually pushed or clipped into place and is easily removed, but as it is likely to be contaminated gloves should be worn. Formalin, 60 ml/cm^3 cabinet volume, is placed in its container on the heater in the cabinet or in the reservoir. The front closure is then put in place and sealed if necessary. Then the heater is switched on and the formalin boiled away. After switching off the heater the cabinet is left closed overnight. The next morning the cabinet fan is switched on and then the front closure is opened very slightly to allow air to pass in and purge the cabinet of formaldehyde. After several minutes the front closure is removed and the cabinet fan allowed to run for about 30 min. Any obvious moisture remaining on the cabinet walls and floor may then be wiped away.

Warning: Formaldehyde has hazardous properties. Work with formalin and exposure to formaldehyde causes irritation of skin, eyes and mucous membranes. It may cause sensitization in some workers and is a suspect carcinogen. In the UK, its occupational exposure limit is set at 2.0 ppm. Formaldehyde vapour is explosive at 7.75% (v/v) in dry air; its ignition point is 430°C. Every effort should be made to minimise exposure. Protective gloves and eyewear should always be worn (see Chapter 8).

Glutaraldehyde is also a hazardous substance; its exposure limit is now set at 0.5 ppm (HSE, 1998b). See Chapter 7.

Changing the filters and maintenance

Microbiological safety cabinets are clearly reservoirs of infection, especially the filters. Cabinets must be decontaminated before filters are changed and any work is done on the motor and fans. If these are to be done by an outside contractor, e.g. by the manufacturer's service engineer, the front closure should be sealed on again after the initial purging of the gas and a notice: 'Cabinet decontaminated but not to be used' placed on it awaiting the engineer's arrival. The engineer will also require a certificate stating that the cabinet has been decontaminated.

The primary, or prefilters should be changed when the cabinet airflow approaches its agreed local minimum (see Table 5.1). Used filters should be placed in plastic or tough paper bags, which are then sealed and burned. If the airflow is not restored to at least the middle of the range then arrangements should be made to replace the HEPA filter. This is usually done by the service engineer, but may be done by laboratory staff if they have received instruction. Unskilled operators often place the new filter in upside down or fail to set it securely and evenly in its place. Used filters should be placed in plastic bags, which are then sealed for disposal. They are not combustible. Some manufacturers accept used filters and recover the cases, but this is not usually a commercial practice and no refund is given. When manufacturers replace HEPA filters they may offer a testing service.

Physical hazards of microbiological safety cabinets

One of us (DAK) notes that there have been reports of a front glass viewing panel dropping out onto the user's hands, spontaneous shattering of glass panels and a case of conjunctivitis and erythema around the eyelids in a worker who was exposed to ultraviolet (UV) light when sitting at a Class II cabinet (Kennedy, 1988b). BS 5726 (1992) addresses such hazards by requiring that the viewing panel be made of safety glass or safety plastic and notes that while UV radiation is not recommended for use in safety cabinets, if it is required, electrical interlocking should be provided to prevent the operator being directly exposed to UV radiation when working at the cabinet. In addition, we are aware of an electric shock that was sustained when a cabinet was being tested and a case where a finger was lacerated by a very sharp edge of the perforated floor of a Class II cabinet.

Among other electrical safety requirements, the standard specifies that motors and other electrical equipment shall comply with the International Electrotechnical Commission's electrical safety standard IEC 1010:Part 1 (published in the UK as BS EN 61010-1,1993). BS 5726 (1992) specifies that the floor and any structures exposed when the floor is removed shall be free of sharp edges.

Management of microbiological safety cabinets

BS 5726 (1992) has four parts. They are:
Part 1. Specification for design, construction and performance before installation,

Part 2. Recommendations for information to be exchanged between purchaser, vendor and installer and recommendations for installation,

Part 3. Specification for performance after installation,

Part 4. Recommendations for selection use and maintenance.

Together these documents provide an ideal management system framework for microbiological safety cabinets because all the most important safety and use dimensions are addressed. It is to be noted that Parts 1 and 3 contain mandatory provisions, while the other parts contain recommendations. In particular, Part 3 specifies commissioning tests and Part 4 makes recommendations for routine maintenance. These are summarized in Tables 5.4 and 5.5 respectively. The advantage of this approach is that a workable standard, offering a high level of operator and environmental protection, is set for management that can be evaluated objectively by workers and regulatory authorities with reference to the written word. In a nutshell, it can be claimed realistically that compliance with all four parts of BS 5726 (1992) results in a well-chosen and well-made cabinet being properly installed and commissioned, well maintained and well used.

Commissioning tests for microbiological safety cabinets are shown in Table 5.4.

Mention was made earlier of a draft European standard, prEN 12469 (CEN, 1998) that addresses performance criteria for microbiological safety cabinets. This document is essentially a standard for manufacturers with emphasis on type testing, although it does make recommendations about installation testing and routine maintenance testing and recommendations about decontamination, cleaning and fumigation. If this draft European Standard is accepted, all four parts of BS 5726:1992 will, under European Union law, have to be withdrawn and the benefits of the management system outlined above will be lost. Clark (1997) has stated that this will be a retrograde and dangerous step because a recent survey of test results from an independent UK test house showed that 37 Class II cabinets (all with adequate type test certification and including 18 new installations failed to meet the operator protection factor requirements of BS 5726 (1992)). In all cases where containment failed, problems of the cabinet or the environment were identified and remedial action was taken. Without on-site operator protection factor tests—which are mandatory commissioning and routine maintenance tests in the BS 5726 system—potentially dangerous equipment would have been in service. Professor Clark is of the opinion that '. . . it is vital that, in the context of the proposed safety cabinet standard, testing for

TABLE 5.4 Commissioning tests for microbiological safety cabinets

Test	Class I	Class II	Class III
Pressure integrity (carcase[1], front sealable panel, exhaust duct and associated seals, tests of seals and gaskets)	+	+	+
Airflow velocity	+	+	+[2]
Airflow direction	+	+	
Operator protection factor	+[2]	+	

[1] If cabinet has to be dismantled and put together on site.
[2] Through glove port with glove removed.
Adapted from BS 5726, Part 3 (1992).

TABLE 5.5 Routine maintenance tests that should be carried out at least annually

Class 1 cabinets:
1. Visual examination of all internal surfaces and extraction duct system for defects, cracks and other damage.
2. Functional tests of anti-blowback valve and airflow indicator.
3. Measurement of inflow air velocity and flow visualization tests.
4. Test of filters and seal integrity.
5. Operator protection factor tests.

Class II cabinets
As for Class I cabinets, tests 1, 2, 4 and 5.
Measurement of downflow and inflow velocity and flow visualization tests.

Class III cabinets
As for Class I cabinets, tests 1 and 4.
Functional tests of anti-blowback valve, manometer and air pressure indicator.
Measurement of airflow through each open glove port.
Measurement of airflow through inlet filter.
Measurement of working pressure in cabinet.

All cabinets
Electrical safety tests.

Based on BS 5726 (1992) Part 4. If shortcomings are found, remedial work will be necessary.

containment both at commissioning and during routine maintenance remains a fundamental requirement' (Clark, 1997). We entirely agree with Professor Clark.

Hazards of home-made microbiological safety cabinets

Collins and Johns (1998) point out that when faced with the high cost of purchasing, maintaining and periodical testing of commercial microbiological safety cabinets, several attempts have been made in developing countries to design inexpensive home-made cabinets. While it may be possible to construct an inexpensive cabinet carcase that will approximate to the aerodynamic and other specifications to be found in the various national standards, no protection will be afforded to the operator unless the exhaust fan and associated system is capable of producing containment that meets the specifications that have been determined by the long and detailed investigations that have been outlined above. A reliable source of electrical power will be required. Any deviations from the standards that have been arrived at over many years by engineers, physicists and microbiologists will result in 'safety cabinets' that are not 'safe' and that may well be described as 'danger boxes' (Collins and Johns, 1998).

Chapter 6

Collection, transport and receipt of infectious materials

Large numbers of specimens of blood, faeces, urine, sputum and other material of unknown or unsuspected microbial content are collected from sick people every day and consigned to laboratories for investigation. During collection the outer surfaces of the containers may be contaminated. In some circumstances, e.g. taking blood samples, the hands or person of the operator may also be contaminated or some of the material may be introduced into his body by needle pricks or through cuts and abrasions (see Chapter 12 on blood-borne infections). Incorrect packaging, and damage in transit may lead to the escape of pathogens and the spread of infection.

Collection of pathological specimens

Containers

In most laboratories plastic, disposable, screw-capped 25-ml bottles have replaced glass containers. Unfortunately, a bewildering array of plastic containers confronts the laboratory worker and there is very little to guide the purchasing officer. Specimen containers must be sufficiently robust to withstand the stresses they are likely to meet and must be leakproof. There are British, European and international standards for some specimen containers (e.g. BS 5213, 1989; BS 4851, 1982a; BS EN 829, 1997; ISO, 1994) and a draft European standard is currently under review. Tests are prescribed for leakage and spontaneous discharge. Lewis and Wardle (1978) described a simple method. In principle the fluorescein-dextran solution (25 g fluorescein in 60 g/l dextran in 0.15 molar saline) is pipetted carefully into the containers to cover the capped part when it is inverted. After capping firmly the containers are inverted for 2 hours and then, still inverted, immersed in tubes of water for a further 2 hours. After removal of the test containers the water is examined under UV light for evidence of leaked fluorescein. Cook (1972) and Lewis and Wardle (1978) found a number of commercial containers which failed the leakage test, but reputable manufacturers are continually improving their products. Unfortunately, no action on the part of manufacturers or official bodies can ensure that the person who collects the specimen will cap the container securely. The screw caps of large containers, e.g. wider than 4 cm, are easily cross-threaded, and then will allow the contents to leak. Nor can one guarantee that press-on or snap-on caps will not allow leakage.

From time to time containers of other materials such as aluminium and waxed card have appeared on the market. Their popularity was short-lived, however; aluminium became too expensive, and many of the waxed card pots leaked.

Reusable (e.g. glass) containers must remain leakproof during their lifetime. They should be inspected before reassembly. Containers with chipped mouths, and caps and liners that are damaged, should be discarded.

Further comments on containers for particular kinds of specimens are made below.

Collection of blood

The obvious hazard here is the possible presence of hepatitis B and the human immunodeficiency viruses (HIV) but it should be remembered that other pathogens, such as *Salmonella typhi*, *Brucella* spp. and viruses may be present (see Chapter 12). Traditionally blood is collected with hypodermic syringes and needles and the hazards of using these have already been described (p. 80). A wide variety of plastic containers, with an assortment of anticoagulants and preservatives is in daily use. The stoppers of some of these leave much to be desired. Carstairs and Coates (1974) criticized plug-in stoppers and Lewis and Wardle (1978) found external contamination with a number of screw-in, push-on and plug-in stoppers. Screw-capped containers are claimed to be safer, but opening these is not without hazard (see p. 96).

Expelling the blood from the syringe into the container, especially a very small one, frequently results in contamination of the fingers and the outside of the container. It is not very easy to hold a syringe full of blood in one hand and to hold and uncap the container with the other. Fingers, either of the operator or an assistant who holds the container, are very easily pricked during the operation, especially if the container is held close to its mouth. Wearing gloves will protect the fingers from contamination but will not reduce the risk of finger pricks or of getting blood on the outside of the container.

Vacuum collection tubes minimize several of the hazards and problems of taking blood and disposing safely of the syringe and needle. These containers are robust, do not leak and the outside cannot become contaminated in the same way as traditional collecting tubes. Sometimes a small drop of blood is left in the well of the stopper after the needle is withdrawn although skilled operators seem to avoid this. It is easily mopped up with disinfectant.

Lach *et al.* (1983) did not detect local surface contamination by droplets or contamination of the needle holders, outsides of the specimen containers or the operators' hands. Holton and Prince (1986) noted more environmental contamination (hands of operator and benches) with the needle and syringe method than with the vacuum tube collection method. Some makes of vacuum collection tubes have screw caps (but see above). Some others, with plug-in stoppers, have plastic overcaps which prevent potential dispersion of droplets when the stopper is removed. A method for opening others safely is described on p. 95. Blood collection, phlebotomy, is discussed by Jagger and Bentley (1997) and Bouvet (1997).

There is now a US standard for work with blood that includes collection of specimens (OSHA, 1991).

Specimens other than blood

Faeces are probably the most hazardous of these because of their varied content of pathogens, not only of bacteria and viruses but also of protozoa and helminths. In addition, the specimens are usually collected by the patient, who is rarely properly instructed or who does not read the label on the container (if one is provided). Patients tend to fill the containers with faeces. Fermentation, with considerable gas production, may occur during transit. The pressure can cause leakage or even force the cap off the bottle or tube. When such a container is opened faeces may be broadcast with some violence. There is also the probability that the outside of the container will be contaminated. Patients should be told, preferably by including a printed slip with the collection outfit, to defaecate on a pile of toilet paper in the lavatory pan and to remove a portion the size of a pea with the spoon provided, to insert it carefully into the container and then to screw the cap on tightly.

Sputum specimens also present problems. Contamination of the outside of the container is not uncommon (Allen and Darrell, 1983). Unfortunately no really satisfactory sputum specimen container has been devised. It is difficult for patients to expectorate into the containers normally used for urine and faeces specimens without contaminating the outside and, as noted above, wider mouthed jars are prone to leakage. The best compromise is the 50 ml glass jar with aluminium cap and a rubber liner, but less satisfactory jars, e.g. plastic pots with plastic caps, may be justified if the specimen can be delivered in an upright position and has no great distance to travel, e.g. in a hospital.

The risks from urine are minimal in normal hospital practice, although a small proportion of patients may excrete *S. typhi*, leptospires, hepatitis and other viruses. It is debatable, therefore, whether any elaborate or expensive precautions need be taken in the collection of urine specimens, except in infectious diseases hospitals, and from patients with diseases where it is known that the agent is likely to appear in the urine. The problem is getting the urine into the container and not on the outside. This is easier for the male. There is a strong case for collecting urine from females in large jars (jam jars), which have been boiled in the ward or clinic sterilizer, and then transferring some into the laboratory container. In one hospital known to us half-pint enamelled iron jugs are used in this way.

Most other specimens, such as pus and aspirated fluids are collected by professional staff and although the microbial content is varied the method of collection minimizes external contamination.

Labelling specimen containers

Labels and stickers that identify various kinds of specimens should be self-adhesive for obvious reasons.

There was much controversy about 'Danger of Infection' and 'High Risk' labels. These are still used for specimens where there is a special risk, e.g. those that may contain hepatitis B virus (HBV), HIV or Hazard Group 3 organisms (HSE, 1991a), but the implication that there are two broad categories of specimens those that offer a high risk and others—a 'two-tier' system—was challenged by Whale (1986) who pointed out that although we know that about one in 800 people carry the hepatitis B antigen, the pool of people infected with HIV is not known.

We may add here that apart from HBV, which is a risk, and HIV, which is a lesser one, there is typhoid fever. Most specimens containing typhoid bacilli are sent to the laboratory before a diagnosis is made and will not be labelled 'Danger of Infection' or 'High Risk'. It is not reasonable to label all specimens. Fallon (1986) agreed that there will always be specimens that arrive without these labels, but thinks that abandoning the labels where there is a known risk would be unhelpful. In a survey conducted by Handsfield *et al.* (1987), 564 blood specimens were tested for HBV and HIV antibodies. There was not a great difference in the findings of unlabelled and 'High Risk' labelled specimens. This suggested that such labelling is likely to give a false sense of security to laboratory staff.

These problems have been largely overcome by the adoption of 'Universal or Standard) Precautions' which avoid the two-tier system (see Chapter 12).

Plastic bags for specimen containers

It is good practice to place specimens in self-sealing plastic bags. Pins and staples should not be used as they may prick the hands of anyone handling the bags. Request forms should be separate, not in the same bag and not stapled to the bag. Bags with two compartments, one for the specimen and one for the form, are available.

Transport

Many of these specimens, and also cultures and suspensions of microorganisms and research material, are moved about in public places on their way between patients and laboratories and between laboratories. They travel by hand, by public and private transport, by surface and air mail and by air freight. During transit the containers or the packages enclosing them may be handled by many people. The containers may be involved in accidents and be damaged or broken when the material may leak out and be dispersed; they may also be lost or stolen and opened by unauthorized people. Although there are no reports of illnesses attributable to such incidents it follows that any infectious material that is being transported from place to place could present a hazard to the health of any person who is in contact with it. Collection, packaging, transport and unpacking should therefore be strictly regulated.

Transport within hospitals and institutions

Leak-proof trays or boxes should be provided for the transport of diagnostic specimens from wards to the laboratory. These should be able to withstand autoclaving or overnight exposure to disinfectant. Suitable trays and boxes are readily available. Some are known as kitchen 'tidies' or tidy-boxes, and are sold cheaply by chain stores, hardware and tool shops for cutlery, kitchen utensils, shoe-cleaning equipment and handyman's tools. Ordinary hospital ward or surgical trays are also widely used. Some purpose-made containers are made of stainless steel, others of propylene ethylene copolymer. They should be deep enough for specimens to be carried upright to avoid leakage and spillage.

These trays and boxes should not be used for any other purposes. Organs in glass jars or plastic buckets, and 24-hour urines in 2-litre screw-capped bottles or the standard plastic carboys should be placed in disposable plastic (or paper) bags for transport for both hygienic and aesthetic reasons.

Some attention should be given to the staff who carry specimens. They should wear overalls. They should be warned about the possible hazards of handling the material they transport, although if collection is properly organized they need handle only the trays or boxes into which the specimens are placed. Frequent hand washing should be recommended, and taking specimens into canteens or through kitchens—both regrettably common practices—should be forbidden.

Surface transport between and to hospitals

Diagnostic specimens are frequently conveyed from one hospital to another because of the centralization of laboratory services. The usual means of transport is by hospital van or hospital car, i.e. the vehicle is under the control of the hospital authorities. Similarly, specimens are transported from local authority offices or clinics to laboratories by the authorities' own vehicles. Rarely, such material may be carried by taxicabs or by messengers on public service vehicles.

In the UK the Health Services Advisory Committee (HSE, 1991a) recommends that 'special' secure transport boxes with secure lids ('special' is not explained). These must be capable of withstanding autoclaving and prolonged exposure to disinfectants. Such boxes are in common use among food inspectors for conveying food, milk and water samples to public analysts and public health laboratories. Suitable boxes, used by some laboratories, included those which can be fitted to the carriers of motor cycles and scooters, and the plastic 'coolkeepers' or 'chilly bins' used by motorists for picnics. The boxes should be marked quite clearly with the name and address of the laboratory which owns them. In case they are lost or the vehicle is involved in an accident they should also carry warning labels 'Danger of infection, do not open' as well as the international biohazard sign, the meaning of which is rarely clear to lay people. The labels should request the finder to call the nearest hospital or police station. The boxes should be inspected daily for evidence of spillage and should be decontaminated and then washed out at least weekly. Again, the drivers or messengers should be warned that the material in the boxes may be infectious. If the boxes are suitable for the job and are packed with care the hazards are minimal and there should be no need for an 'emergency decontamination kit' (see p. 180) to be carried.

Some authorities send specimens to laboratories by hand on public service vehicles. The same type of boxes should be used but it may be advisable to label them less explicitly or transport employees and other passengers may be alarmed. A great deal of care is needed as some of these specimens, sent by local health authorities, may have been collected from typhoid carriers or contacts, or patients with salmonellosis or dysentery.

By inland post

Most of the material concerned here consists of diagnostic specimens, but there is also a considerable traffic in cultures, which qualify as infectious substances, and are sent to reference laboratories for further investigation.

Some research and quality control materials are also distributed by larger institutions. Local regulations must apply, but in the UK the regulations printed in the Post Office Guide (1986) apply. These are quite clearly written and are obtainable from UK Postal Headquarters or Crown Post offices. The only restriction on the nature of the infectious material sent through the post concerns agents in Hazard Groups 3 and 4 (see below). These must not be posted. If the sender knows the nature of the material, e.g. if it is a culture of typhoid bacilli or some other microorganism in Hazard Group 3 there must be a 'Danger of Infection' label on the container (but NOT on the outside of the box in which it will travel). In principle the container, i.e. the bottle or tube containing the culture, etc., must be robust and securely closed. It must be cocooned in enough absorbent packing material to retain the contents, should they leak or the container is broken. This should be absorbent cotton wool (not that which is used for plugging test tubes and pipettes), or cellulose wadding. Expanded polystyrene will not do. Although not specified by the Post Office it is wise to place the container, before cocooning, or the cocoon itself, in a self-sealing plastic bag. There should be enough packing material to wedge the cocooned container firmly in the container in which it will travel. Post Office approved outer containers are:

(1) a polypropylene clip-down container;
(2) a cylindrical light-metal container;
(3) a strong cardboard box with full-depth lid;
(4) the appropriate groove in a two-piece polystyrene box. Any empty spaces must be filled with absorbent material. The two parts of the box must then be firmly held together by self-adhesive plastic tape.

The UK Post Office does approve some boxes or outer containers submitted to it for specific purposes, but when approval is given it is for those purposes or types of specimen only and they must not be used for others. In spite of the readiness with which the generally approved boxes may be obtained and the ease with which they can be used, however, a great deal of ingenuity is displayed in some laboratories in selecting unsuitable boxes or cartons or in purchasing expensive and frequently unsatisfactory substitutes.

Packaging of diagnostic specimens, and even infectious substances, is some-times left to uninitiated members of the staff. It is not uncommon for a complaint about poor and unsafe packing to be answered by the apology that there was a new person in the office. That excuse is really an indication of poor laboratory management. It is certainly incumbent on the recipient to chide the sender when improperly packed infectious material is sent through the post. The Post Office has the power to prosecute offenders.

Some pathological specimens are posted by general medical practitioners and these sometimes give cause for concern. For example, an incident was described by Simpson and Zuckerman (1975) as 'Lassa by Letter' in which a tube of blood from a patient with suspected viral haemorrhagic fever was sent to them, unprotected and by ordinary letter post.

When the material, properly packed, is taken to a UK Post Office it is officially described as a 'package' not a parcel, and it must be sent by first class mail. It is an offence to send pathological specimens and cultures by second class or parcel post.

Restrictions on consignments

In the UK certain agents may not be sent by post. Indeed they must not be moved without notification to the Health and Safety Executive. These are:

- all agents in Hazard Group 4;
- rabies virus;
- simian herpes B virus;
- Venezuelan equine encephalitis virus;
- tick-borne encephalitis viruses in Group 3;
- monkeypox virus;
- Mopeia virus.

By airmail (overseas post)

Although considerably fewer packages containing infectious substances are sent by air than by inland post, it is probable that those sent by air are more hazardous, as they are more likely to contain highly infectious material for urgent diagnosis, or research. At one time it was feared that a large amount of potentially hazardous recombinant DNA material would be involved. Airline staff were made deeply aware of potential dangers of carrying such material by popular science and newspaper articles about 'doom viruses' and 'satan bugs'. This led to a stricter application of the rules for the transport of such materials. e.g. by the International Air Transport Association (IATA, 1994). If an accident occurs, and infections of humans, animals or plants result, the carrier might be held responsible.

Descriptions

Unfortunately, a number of different international, as well as national, organizations have been involved in describing the materials to be transported by whatever means, often with conflicting results. The materials concerned have variously been known as biological products; biological specimens; biological substances; cultures; aetiological agents; diagnostic specimens; genetically-modified organisms and microorganisms; infectious perishable biological substances; infectious substances; non-infectious biological substances; medical specimens; pathogens. Any or all of these may also figure in regulations as 'Dangerous Goods' and/or 'Hazardous Materials'

To add to this confusion some of these terms are synonymous; e.g. 'aetiological agent' and 'infectious materials/substance' (CDC/NIH, 1993); 'pathological specimen' and 'diagnostic specimen' (ACDP, 1995); and in the European standard (CEN, 1994) 'medical and biological specimens' are 'materials derived from man, animal or plant, destined by the sender for examination', i.e. 'diagnostic specimens'. Regulations that appear to lump together all these kinds of biological materials and to require specific packaging and restrictions on amounts clearly create many difficulties: there is a great deal of difference between diagnostic reagents which are harmless but nevertheless biological substances and samples for laboratory investigation and identification, which may be infectious.

Fortunately common sense has prevailed about the materials with which this book is concerned. The United Nations International Committee of Experts on the Transport of Dangerous Goods, advised by the World Health Organization, has formulated regulations (UN, 1996) taken aboard by the various other transport authorities with respect to (a) infectious substances and (b) diagnostic specimens. The WHO (1997b) has published very useful guidelines for the safe transport of infectious substances and diagnostic specimens.

(The transport of other biological material is not considered here; reference should be made to the recommendations of the United Nations Committee of Experts on Transport of Dangerous Goods (UN, 1996)).

Infectious substances—definition

These are substances containing viable microorganisms, such as bacteria, viruses, rickettsias, parasites and fungi that are known or reasonably believed to cause disease in humans or animals.

Diagnostic specimens—definition

These are any human or animal material including but not limited to excreta, blood and its components, tissue and tissue fluids collected for the purpose of diagnosis but excluding live animals.

Diagnostic specimens resulting from medical practice and research are considered to be a negligible threat to the public health on the grounds that they may contain only a limited amount of an infectious agent. This may be questioned as it is known that, e.g. 1 ml of blood from a patient with hepatitis B in the viraemic stage may have up to 10^8 infectious particles and 1 ml of blood from a positive HIV patient as many as 10^3 (Lanphear, 1994). This point should be considered when deciding if the material is a diagnostic specimen or a biological agent.

Preliminary arrangements

Before any material is sent to another country by airmail the sender and consignee must ascertain that it is acceptable to the authorities of that country. For medical and economic reasons some governments have banned the importation of some biological agents. This ban may extend to their air space. The consignee must notify the sender that the package has arrived.

Containers and packing

The internationally agreed 'triple packaging system' must be used. This must meet the requirements of the UN Class 2 specifications and packaging instruction PI(602) (UN, 1996) which impose strict tests, including surviving, undamaged, a 9 m drop on to a hard surface, and puncture tests.

(1) The material is placed in a watertight, leakproof receptacle—the 'primary container'. This is wrapped in enough absorbent material to absorb all fluid in case of breakage;

(2) The primary container is then packed in a watertight 'secondary container' with enough absorbent material to cushion the primary container.
(3) The secondary container is placed in an outer shipping package which protects its contents from damage during transit.

An example of a triple package that satisfies the requirements of the UN packaging instruction is shown in Figure 6.1.

The packaging and documentation requirements for infectious substances and diagnostic specimens differ and the sender may have problems in determining which applies to his material. For example, the definition of an infectious substance includes 'sample(s) from a patient with a serious disease of unknown cause'. Physicians not infrequently do not know the cause or may make an incorrect diagnosis. Clinical microbiologists often isolate quite unexpected agents from specimens when the request was for the presence of others. It may not be clear whether the material is an 'Infectious Substance' or 'Diagnostic Material'!

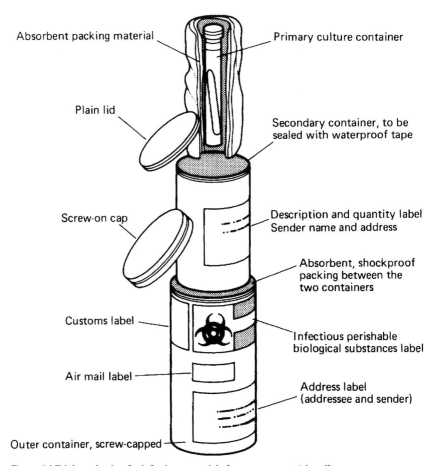

Figure 6.1 Triple packaging for infectious materials for overseas post (airmail)

INFECTIOUS SUBSTANCES

There are limits to the amounts of infectious substances which may be carried by aircraft. For passenger aircraft the limit per package is 50 ml or 50 g. For cargo aircraft the limit per package is 4 litres or 4 kg.

The outer package must be labelled with:

- the UN Packaging Specification Marking (Figure 6.2a), obtainable from the carriers or the appropriate national authority;
- the International Infectious Substances label (Figure 6.2b);
- the receiver's name, address and telephone number;
- the sender's name, address and telephone number;
- the UN shipping name, e.g. Infectious Substances Affecting Humans (or Animals) and the scientific name of the substance;
- the UN number (UN2814 for human and UN2900 for animal material);
- the temperature storage requirements if applicable.

Shipping documents, as supplied by the carrier, must be fixed to the outer package:

- the shipper's 'Declaration of Dangerous Goods' (Figure 6.2c)
- a packing list including the receiver's address, details of contents, weight, value (usually 'no commercial ...');
- an airway bill;
- an import/export permit/declation if applicable.

If the package is to be sent by cargo aircraft (see above) it must also be labelled 'THIS SIDE UP' or 'THIS END UP', with the international package orientation symbol (black or red arrows: Figure 6.2d).

DIAGNOSTIC SPECIMENS

The outer packaged must be labelled as follows:

- consignee's name, address and telephone number;
- sender's name, address and telephone number;
- the statement 'Diagnostic Specimen, Not Restricted, Packed in Compliance with Packing Instructions 650'.

Shipping documents, available from the carrier (Figure 6.2c) must be fixed to the outer package:

- packing list which includes consignee's address, details of contents, weight, value (usually 'no commercial');
- airway bill.

An 'Infectious Substance' label and UN 'Packaging Specification' label are not required for diagnostic specimens.

USE OF ICE OR DRY ICE

It may be necessary to use ice or dry ice (solid carbon dioxide) to preserve some materials. Wet ice should be placed in a leak-proof container and the outer package must also be leak-proof.

Dry ice must not be placed inside the primary or secondary container (risk of explosion) but in a properly designed outer package which is ventilated to allow the escape of the gas. UN Packing Instruction 904 applies.

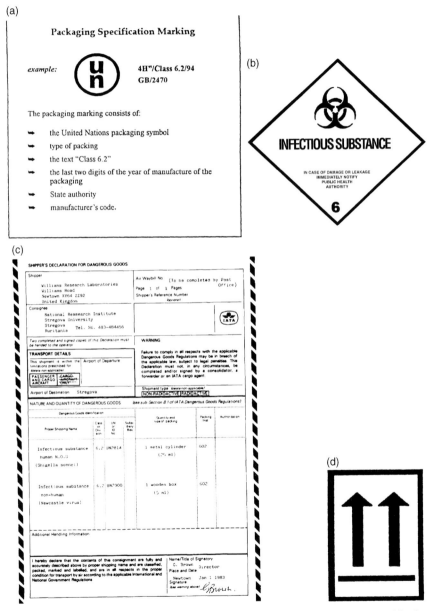

Figure 6.2 Documents for air transport of infectious substances. (a) The UN Packaging Specification Marking. (b) The International Infections Substances. (c) The shipper's Declaration of Dangerous Goods. (d) The International package orientation symbol

GENETICALLY-MODIFIED MICROORGANISMS

Genetically-modified microorganisms which meet the UN (1996) and the European Commission (EC, 1990, 1994) definitions of infectious substances (see above) should be classified as such. In effect, if the host or insert is in Hazard Group 2 or above it should be classed as infectious.

Air freight

This is normally used only for those packages which are too large to be sent by airmail, but the regulations are so complex and the whole procedure so fraught with difficulties that it is best avoided in favour of splitting the consignment into several separate packages and sending them by airmail. If it is unavoidable advice should be obtained from any large institution that has the necessary experience, as well as from a shipping company that has sent such packages before.

Transport-associated accidents

All institutions that consign or receive infectious substances and/or diagnostic specimens should have a well-organised procedure for dealing with emergencies arising from accidents to such materials that may happen outside their own premises.

The WHO (1980) offers guidelines for dealing with such accidents (Figure 6.3).

As these procedures involve decontamination and disinfection they, and other relevant emergency actions, are discussed in Chapters 7 and 11. See also WHO (1980).

Receipt of infectious material

There is clearly a difference between the hazards posed by specimens received by clinical and diagnostic laboratories and those received by specialist or reference laboratories.

Clinical and diagnostic specimens

It must be remembered that laboratories do not have any control over the microbial contents of specimens they receive.

For many years it has been normal practice for clinical specimens to be received and documented in the 'laboratory office' by clerical and secretarial staff. Office staff normally take their coffee and tea breaks, and eat their sandwiches at their desks. It was not unusual, therefore, to see food and drink being consumed close to, or even among, specimens of faeces, blood, urine and sputum, and even while the office worker was unpacking, sorting and documenting them. The disturbingly large number of untrained or ancillary staff who acquire infections in the laboratory (p. 36) undoubtedly includes members of clerical and reception staff. Although most specimens are probably harmless there is, properly, concern about the numbers of specimens that arrive in a

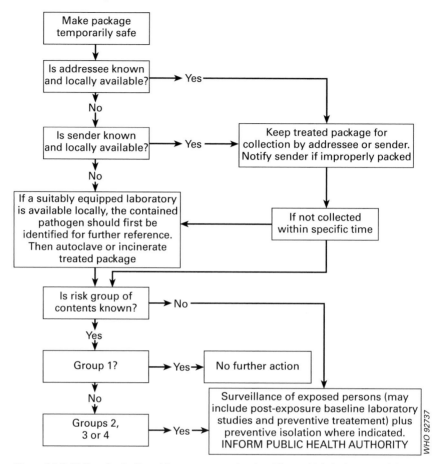

Figure 6.3 Guidelines for dealing with transport-associated accidents with infectious materials. (From WHO, 1993a, reproduced with permission of the World Health Organization)

leaking condition and those that have visible external contamination. In two separate surveys (unpublished) carried out on behalf of CHC, 17% of 103 blood samples had blood on the label, and 6% of 105 stool specimens had faeces on the outside of the container. The reception staff of another laboratory reported that between 4% and 5% of request forms that accompanied blood for biochemical and haematological tests were visibly blood-stained (see also p. 148).

It is obviously difficult to assess the extent of the risks of infection to laboratory clerical and reception staff, but it is clearly undesirable that they should suffer any more exposure than any other clerical workers. Unfortunately many laboratories rely on agency and temporary clerical assistance, much of which is very temporary indeed. Admittedly, a great deal of initial training is not necessary, but in this context training includes experience. The simple 'model rules' for reception staff and clerical staff have been updated by HSE (1991a). Most of these are simple hygiene rules and are considered in Chapter 8, but the important issues which must be considered here concern immediate contact with specimens.

Any specimen in a plastic bag which carries a 'Danger of Infection' or similar label should not be removed from that bag. The accession number can be put on the outside of the bag. Leaking or broken specimens should not be touched, nor should any others in the same box or tray. Provision should be made for a member of the technical or professional staff to deal with them. Children and visitors, which includes people from other departments, should not be allowed to touch anything on the specimen reception bench. These specimens should not be allowed to stray to other parts of the room. Accommodation for the reception of specimens is discussed in Chapter 10.

Accidents, and procedures for dealing with them, are considered in Chapter 7.

Specialist and reference laboratories

Packages received by these laboratories are likely to contain cultures or concentrates of infectious agents the identify of which may not be known to the sender and may therefore be more hazardous than expected. An example is the *Brucella melitensis* incident reported by Batchelor *et al*. (1992).

It is advisable, therefore, that cultures and such specialized materials are unpacked in the laboratories by professional staff and in a microbiological safety cabinet. Apart from the hazards inherent in the contents, there are risks in the unpacking. It is often necessary to use knives and other sharp instruments and it is not uncommon for operators to cut themselves while trying to open a particularly well-sealed package. The only solutions to this problem are great personal care and attempts to educate the clients in safe, but easily unpackable, packaging.

Importation of pathogens

Many states ban the importation of exotic pathogens or permit it only under licence to specified laboratories or individuals. In the UK, Hazard Group 4 agents may not be imported without approval from the Health and Safety Executive and with the knowledge of the Advisory Committee on Dangerous Pathogens. Importation of certain animal pathogens requires a licence from the Ministry of Agriculture, Fisheries and Foods under the *Importation of Animal Pathogens Order, 1980*. The USA places similar restrictions on importing some pathogens. The list of restricted animal pathogens, which contains a number of human pathogens, is too long to give here. It is included as an appendix by the ACDP (1995) and advice should be sought from the nearest government veterinary or plant pathology laboratory. The list of animal pathogens which may not be imported into the USA according to Department of Agriculture regulations is given in an appendix to the CDC/NIH (1993) book.

Anyone who receives unsolicited cultures or material containing pathogens which he believes may be restricted should inform the agriculture authorities (and in the UK the Health and Safety Executive) without delay. The package, whether opened or not, should be placed in a plastic bag, sealed, and refrigerated until collected or clearance is given.

Chapter 7

Decontamination

In the context of this book decontamination is the sterilization or disinfection of infected and potentially infected materials that are no longer required (i.e. waste), reusable equipment, surfaces and spaces in order to protect the staff, the public and the environment from infection and contamination.

Sterilization implies the complete destruction of all microorganisms, including spores.

Disinfection implies the destruction of vegetative microorganisms which might cause disease. Disinfection does not necessarily kill spores.

It is the moral responsibility of the microbiologist and, in addition, the duty of the staff to see that this contamination does not breach the barriers that are intended to protect the laboratory workers and the general public from infection.

Contaminated laboratory waste

'It is a cardinal rule that no infected material shall leave the laboratory.' (Collins, 1974.)

This simple precept offers no problems to properly-equipped and well-managed laboratories. Unfortunately not all laboratories have the necessary equipment and knowledge to fulfil the requirement. Some have been, and others still are, content to leave disposal to other organizations or individuals. In the UK, where infected laboratory waste is included in 'clinical waste' (HSE, 1992a), there is a requirement that 'All infected waste arising from work in laboratories should be made safe to handle, *ideally by autoclaving. If it is not reasonably practical to autoclave waste it should be disposed of by incineration*' (our italics). This indicates that the infected waste *can* leave the laboratory, although HSE stipulates that it is secured in 'strong, leak-proof containers and transported directly to the incinerator.' As few hospitals and institutions now have, on site, incinerators that satisfy the requirements of the *Environmental Protection Act 1990*, clinical waste, including that from laboratories (including large numbers of cultures of pathogens), can travel on the public highway, often for long distances because of the relatively small numbers of legally acceptable incinerators. There is clearly a hazard here: if the vehicle carrying such waste is involved in an accident cultures of pathogens could be widely distributed offering a risk to emergency personnel and the general public (Collins and Kennedy, 1993; Collins, 1994).

160

Transport accidents (see below) are not the only cause for concern. Within the past 10 years there have been several reports of laboratories that have handed over their infected waste to other organizations in the hope and expectation that it will be incinerated. A number of examples of public exposure of laboratory waste, e.g. on rubbish tips and beaches, are cited by Collins and Kennedy (1987, 1993). We have in our possession photographs, taken on a landfill site in 1989, of readily-identifiable used pathology specimen containers and cultures that had manifestly not been autoclaved or disinfected.

Now, the ACDP (1995) *recommends* that such waste should be autoclaved before incineration. As all competent (i.e. accredited) laboratories have, or should have, properly serviced and efficiently monitored autoclaves there would appear to be no reason why all waste that contains or might contain viable pathogens should not be made safe *before* it leaves the laboratory. The only possible exception to this would be when the waste is incinerated under the direct supervision of a member of the laboratory staff. Unfortunately, placing this responsibility firmly on the laboratory management may not solve the problem.

Regrettably, in some establishments there are very sketchy ideas on freeing material from living organisms. There is a touching faith in the ability of disinfectants at varying concentrations and indefinite ages to kill microbes submerged in or even placed near to them (see also p. 171). There is also a firm belief that any autoclave that gets hot and registers a certain pressure or temperature on its gauges will destroy any bacteria or viruses that have been placed in it.

A quite alarming practice that we have observed in several laboratories is the disposal or washing of specimen containers (usually for blood) and cultures that have been reported 'negative' for whatever tests had been requested without any previous decontamination.

The descriptions of laboratory waste given in several official publications, both in Europe and the USA, are not sufficiently itemized. Table 7.1 (Collins and Kennedy, 1993), which itself is not necessarily complete, may fill this void.

TABLE 7.1 Contaminated laboratory waste

Specimens or their remains (in their containers) submitted for tests: containing blood, faeces, sputum, urine, secretions, exudates, transudates, other normal or morbid fluids but not tissues.
All cultures made from these specimens, directly or indirectly.
All other stocks of microorganisms that are no longer required. Used diagnostic kits.
Used disposable transfer loops, rods, plastic pasteur pipettes.
Disposable cuvettes and containers used in chemical analyses.
Biologicals, standards and quality control materials.
Food samples submitted for examination in outbreaks of food poisoning.
Paper towels and tissues used to wipe benches and equipment and to dry hands.
Disposable gloves and gowns.
Hypodermic needles (with syringes attached if custom so requires).
Disposable knives, scalpels, blades, scissors, forceps, probes.
Glass pasteur pipettes; slides and cover glasses.
Broken glass, ampoules and vials.
Tissues and animal carcasses.
Bedding from animal cages.

Adapted from Collins and Kennedy (1993).

Segregation and identification of contaminated waste

Laboratory waste should be segregated into colour-coded containers. Recommended colours in the UK (HSE, 1992a, DE, 1993) are these:

Yellow—for incineration.

Light blue or transparent with blue inscription—for autoclaving (but may subsequently be incinerated).

Black—normal household waste: local authority refuse collection.

White or clear plastic—soiled linen (e.g. laboratory overalls).

Other colour codes encountered in UK hospitals, but not normally affecting laboratories, include red or red band on white for foul or infected linen. Yellow bags with black bands, intended for waste that, exceptionally, may be landfilled, have no place in laboratories. In the USA and some other countries, red, instead of yellow, colours are used.

There is a growing trend, especially in Europe, to use more robust and rigid disposable containers than plastic bags.

Methods and choice of treatment

There are three practical methods of treating contaminated laboratory waste. They are sterilization by autoclaving, chemical disinfection and incineration. The first two are laboratory processes; incineration involves off-site transport of the material.

While sterilization is the optimum, disinfection is useful as an immediate measure in the laboratory to reduce the numbers of organisms and make the material safe to handle pending further treatment. For the final treatment of infected material before it leaves the laboratory autoclaving is the method of choice. Although incineration, which not only kills microorganisms but reduces all organic material to ash, is permitted in some circumstances there are valid objections to its use as a primary method (see p. 186).

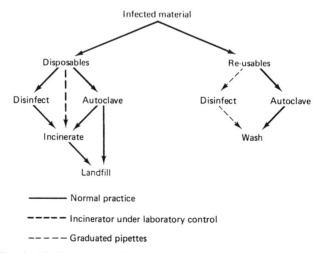

Figure 7.1 Flow chart for the treatment of infected materials

The choice of method may be determined by the nature of the material to be treated, i.e., if it is disposable, is adversely affected by heat, or heat treatment is impossible. With certain exceptions no methods are mutually exclusive and Figure 7.1 shows the options. It will be seen that disinfection should be followed by autoclaving or incineration, and autoclaving by incineration and/or land-filling. The exceptions, where reliance must be placed on disinfection alone, are certain types of graduated pipettes, surfaces, rooms and large equipment.

Autoclaving

Autoclaving involves the timed exposure of materials to steam above atmospheric pressure and hence at temperatures above 100°C.

The autoclave, in its guise as domestic pressure cooker or 'digester', was introduced into bacteriology by Pasteur around 1876. Similar instruments are still in use in some laboratories today. There is ample evidence that these 'old-fashioned' autoclaves achieved their purpose. They were used to sterilize culture media prepared empirically from a variety of natural and usually contaminated materials, collected from slaughterhouses, dairies, kitchens and pharmacies. If they had not been successful the science of bacteriology could not have advanced very far beyond its nineteenth century level. Although these autoclaves were not used in all laboratories to decontaminate waste material and used cultures (the disinfectant bucket was still popular in the 1950s!) a search of the literature has not revealed a single laboratory-acquired infection attributable to their failure.

On the other hand there are reports, too numerous to list here, of serious even fatal, infections that have resulted from the misuse of hospital and pharmaceutical autoclaves, and consequent failure to sterilize intravenous infusion fluids and dressings (see, e.g., Report, 1972; Meers et al., 1973; Phillips et al., 1976). Yet it is precisely these types of autoclaves, designed for 'bottled fluids' or 'porous loads' that have been supplied to some microbiological laboratories during the last three decades. It is not surprising that their performance, in the hands of some laboratory workers who are unaccustomed to their complexity, has been questioned, and failures to sterilize their contents have been reported and investigated (Gillespie and Gibbons, 1975; PHLS, 1978, 1981).

Autoclaves operate at high pressures and high temperatures and their manufacture, installation and use are regulated. In the UK they are subject to the *Pressure Systems and Transportable Gas Containers Regulations 1989*, which requires regular inspection and maintenance and regular checks on the the effectiveness of the sterilization cycles. Recording devices are required.

'Traditional' versus 'new-style' autoclaves

In view of these problems and what might seem to be a retrograde step, it is important to give good reasons why the traditional laboratory autoclaves have been replaced by what are called 'new-style' models, although they have been in use in hospitals and the pharmaceutical industries for some time.

The volume of microbiological work has increased substantially in the past two decades and there is a general acceptance, in informed circles, of the principle of autoclaving, rather than disinfecting discarded cultures and other contaminated materials. The traditional vertical autoclave chamber is, for practical reasons, limited in size, the maximum being about 80 cm deep and 45 cm in diameter. There is also a limit to the number of these autoclaves that can be accommodated in the space available in most laboratories. The newer models are horizontal and much larger. A horizontal autoclave is easier to load, either by hand or with a trolley and pallet. Traditional gas- and electrically-heated autoclaves take a long time to heat up, but the newer models are engineered to fit on to hospital or industrial steam lines. This shortens the heating-up time considerably. These newer autoclaves have temperature sensors (although these are not always in the right place, see below) so a direct temperature reading is possible instead of a pressure-to-temperature conversion. In addition the new health safety regulations require that 'pressure vessels' (the legal term which includes autoclaves) have safety locks and devices that prevent the operator from opening the door until the pressure and temperature have fallen to a safe level. These devices are an integral part of modern autoclaves but are difficult to fit to most of the traditional laboratory models.

The best of the new laboratory autoclaves operate automatically. Once preset, all the operator has to do after closing the door is to press a switch. The autoclave goes through its cycle and then indicates that the door may be opened.

Problems with 'new-style' autoclaves

Given that these 'new-style' autoclaves are a fact of life it is necessary to examine the possible reasons for the less than satisfactory performances of some of them. There are three main reasons for failure—the wrong type of autoclave; omitting to monitor the temperature in the load; and incomplete removal of air from the load.

THE WRONG TYPE OF AUTOCLAVE—AND THE RIGHT

As indicated in Chapter 10 there is a marked ignorance among some designers about what happens in laboratories and a strong disinclination to ask someone who might know. This has resulted in some laboratories being provided with the wrong kind, such as bed-pan sterilizers, instrument sterilizers, and even low-temperature formaldehyde autoclaves.

That the laboratory autoclave is required to take a 'mixed load' of assorted-sized bottles, tubes and petri dishes which may be made of glass or plastic or both is seldom appreciated by sterilizer engineers. Sorting contaminated material into separate batches, according to size and shape, as suggested by some engineers, is neither safe nor practicable. The more complicated and sophisticated an autoclave the more likely it is to go wrong or be misused. An instrument which frequently and repeatedly needs the attention of an engineer is frustrating to laboratory staff and may force them to adopt unsatisfactory and even hazardous methods for the disposal of contaminated materials. The people who work in laboratory wash-up rooms are likely to misuse—and misunderstand—the more complicated autoclaves, sometimes with unfortunate results.

The 'right' kind of autoclave for decontaminating used equipment and waste need not be very complicated. It can be a downward displacement, single-cycle model, without a jacket but for convenience and speed it should be on a steam line. A more sophisticated instrument should have a means of extracting air rapidly before the sterilizing cycle but problems may arise if the old system of discharge into an open tundish is used. Barbeito and Brookey (1976) recovered *Bacillus subtilis* and other tracer organisms from the air around the vent pipes. All effluent should be trapped so that organisms released from the load under reduced pressure cannot be discharged into the room.

The ideal sterilizer for laboratory waste should have these properties:

(1) Rapid removal of air to ensure adequate steam penetration into 'mixed loads'.
(2) No possibility of escape of microorganisms during removal of air.
(3) Correct time and temperature achievable in the load and recorded or demonstrable.
(4) Rapid exhaustion of steam to facilitate early cooling and opening.

In the UK laboratory autoclaves should conform to BS 2646 (1988, 1990a), and in some circumstances to BS 3970 (1990b). See also PHLS (1981).

Operational temperatures

For most purposes the following time/temperature cycles will ensure sterilization of a properly packed load;

3 min at 134°C
10 min at 126°C
15 min at 121°C
25 min at 115°C

These are the holding times at temperature (HTAT). The usual HTAT in microbiological laboratories is 15 min at 121°C but for the agents of the spongiform encephalopathies (prions, see Chapter 14) 18 min or six consecutive 3-min cycles at 134°C are recommended (ACDP, 1990).

The timing begins when the load reaches that temperature.

TEMPERATURE IN THE LOAD

Some autoclaves are fitted with dial thermometers or temperature recorders. The sensors for these are frequently placed in the chamber drain through which a mixture of steam and air is expelled until all the air is removed from the chamber, when a near-to-steam trap operates and prevents further loss of steam. Theoretically this is the coolest place in the autoclave, and when it reaches the required temperature, it is often assumed that that is also the temperature in the load. Unfortunately this is not always so, depending on the size of the load and how it is packed in the chamber, and if the cycle is timed from the moment the drain thermometer reaches say 121°C then the load will not be sterilized (PHLS, 1978). In Figure 7.2 (our observations) it will be seen that the temperature in the load, measured with a thermocouple, has reached only 65°C when that in the drain is at 121°C. It took a further 35 min for the load temperature to reach the required level.

It has become increasingly obvious that it is necessary to ascertain the temperature in the load, rather than rely on that in the drain if autoclaving is to be a reliable method of sterilizing contaminated materials.

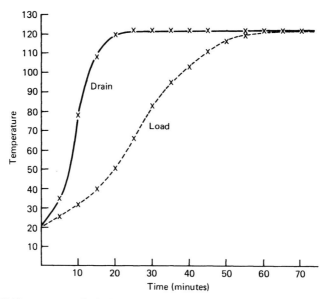

Figure 7.2 The temperature in the load compared with that in the drain of an autoclave

Monitoring temperatures

Temperatures may be monitored by thermocouples and this is preferred for modern autoclaves (HSE, 1991a). The probes may be distributed through the load and temperatures are recorded. Older instruments may not have integral thermocouples but independent monitors may be used as the probes are made of very thin wire and may be inserted between the door and its gasket without causing leakage of steam.

It is a salutary exercise to compare the temperature in the middle of a normal, mixed load with that of the chamber drain.

BIOLOGICAL AND CHEMICAL INDICATORS

The biological indicators may not be suitable for modern autoclaves. Those in common use consist of strips or discs of filter paper which have been soaked in suspensions of *Bacillus stearothermophilus* spores, then dried and packed in porous envelopes or sachets. These are placed in various positions in the load and after processing the strips or discs are removed from their packing and placed in nutrient broth which is incubated for 24–48 hours. Turbidity indicates failure to sterilize. The time and temperature combination at which all the spores are killed depends on several factors, such as the medium in which the organisms were grown and the incubation temperature. Commercial products, which have been subjected to rigorous quality control are therefore much more reliable than are locally made test strips. The results obtained with these strips are retrospective; one cannot wait for 24–48 hours before disposing of an autoclave load. They have their uses, however, as a periodic check that thermocouples and recording instruments are working.

There are at least three general kinds of chemical indicator. The well-known 'autoclave tapes' are used in many hospitals to show that a load of dressings, etc. have been processed. The ink of these tapes is steam-dependent, indicating that air has been removed, but the time and temperature relations are not critical. In the UK the Medical Devices Agency (MDA, 1998a) has issued a notice stating that indicator tape should no longer be used for the Bowie-Dick test for porous load autoclaves. Indicator sheets (BS EN 867, 1997) should be used instead.

There are also glass tubes containing pellets of a substance which melts at a given temperature, e.g. 121°C. Melting is independent of steam and partially dependent on time. The third kind of indicator is most commonly used in laboratories because it shows that steam was present and that the time and temperature combination was satisfactory. Again, there are three main varieties. One consists of a glass tube containing a liquid which changes colour from red to green if the cycle is satisfactory. Another is an indicator mounted on a paper strip which changes colour from yellow to mauve. The third is a blue, waxy substance which migrates along a tube in a foil and paper strip when it is heated in the presence of steam. The value and reliability of these chemical indicators may depend on correct storage and good technique. They are very useful for day-to-day monitoring, even in autoclaves which are fitted with thermocouples and automatic cycling.

REMOVAL OF AIR FROM THE LOAD

In a traditional vertical autoclave water is boiled vigorously by the external application of heat and the turbulence associated with the production of steam and its escape through a valve on top of the autoclave rapidly clears the chamber of air which would otherwise depress the temperature. Successful operation of any autoclave depends on the removal of all air and its replacement by steam so that when an internal pressure of 1.05 kg/cm^2 (15 lbf/in^2) is recorded on the gauge the temperature of the steam in the load is 121°C. This is sufficient to sterilize the contents in 15 min. It is obvious that with this system the larger the autoclave the less efficient it is likely to be in purging itself of steam. If all the air is not removed the time/temperature relation is altered and sterilization will not be achieved.

In the newer autoclaves steam enters the chamber under pressure from the hospital steam-line and displaces the (heavier) air downwards and through the valve in the chamber drain. Success in removing all air depends on the nature of the load, largely on the containers that hold it, and their distribution in the autoclave chamber.

CONTAINERS FOR AUTOCLAVING LABORATORY WASTE

It was the custom for many years to place materials for autoclaving in wire baskets. These, in turn, were placed in cylindrical buckets which stood in the chamber above the level of the water. A row of holes in the side of each bucket, 5–10 cm from the bottom, enabled steam to pass freely into the baskets and around their contents and retained some spillage. This may account for the success of traditional autoclaves.

As wire baskets do not retain leaks and spills from culture containers Collins (1974) proposed replacing baskets by shallow buckets, with straight sides,

5–10 cm less in diameter than the autoclave and guaranteed leak-proof. These buckets were made of copper or galvanized iron. Tests with chemical indicators and spore strips (thermocouples were not available) showed that the contents were sterilized (unpublished observations). The operative word was 'shallow' and Rubbo and Gardner (1965) stated that a depth of 25 cm should not be exceeded if all air was to be removed and sterilization achieved. Even so Gillespie and Gibbons (1975) showed that wire baskets were superior to what became known as 'solid-bottomed containers' for sterilizing bottled fluids.

Unfortunately, the containers adopted in some laboratories were frequently so tall that air was unlikely to be displaced and the articles at or near to their bottoms were not sterilized. Moreover, polypropylene replaced the much heavier and expensive copper and galvanized iron and eliminated the weight limit, so even larger buckets were used. Overlarge containers accounted for a high proportion of failures reported by the Public Health Laboratory Service (PHLS, 1978).

Containers with lids are another source of failure to remove air from the load. Such containers are often adopted as a safety measure in places where the autoclave is a long way from the laboratory; this may be inevitable in large research institutions or may be the result of bad planning of clinical laboratories. If lidded containers are used the lids should be removed when the containers have been placed in the autoclave. The lids should, of course, be autoclaved as well.

Thus, there has been a great deal of confusion about the choice of containers for autoclaving discarded cultures and other contaminated material. The conclusions reached by Everall and Morris (1976) are still sound. Such a container, they say 'should be reasonably cheap, resistant to corrosion, leak-proof and capable of allowing the passage of steam to all parts of its contents'. Polypropylene boxes, not more than 23 cm deep, which are leak-proof are available from a number of plastics manufacturers and laboratory suppliers. These may be used alone or as supports for autoclavable plastic bags.

The size of containers and their distribution in the autoclave are important. Tightly-fitting containers do not permit steam penetration. Nor do containers that are piled one above the other so that the bottom of one occludes the top of the one beneath it. Sterilizing-room staff should be instructed not to pack in as much as possible. This may save time but it will usually ensure failure.

Autoclavable plastic bags are now in general use. In the UK they should conform with BS 6642 (1985) and HSE (1992a). Those used for autoclaving waste should be permeable to steam. The plastic bags should be supported, e.g. in metal or plastic containers, to prevent environmental contamination if they burst or leak. They may be closed with wire ties after autoclaving and sent to the incinerator. The contents need not be seen or exposed.

It became the custom in many laboratories to close the bags before sending them to be autoclaved. The arguments for doing this were quite reasonable, being the same as those advanced for using lidded solid-bottomed containers. Unfortunately the bags were then usually autoclaved with their necks still closed, thus reducing steam penetration and the removal of air. The consequent failure to sterilize the contents was shown by Everall and Morris (1976). In our own (unpublished) experiments, as shown in Figure 7.3, the temperature in the middle of a closed bag containing small screw-capped bottles had reached 75°C when that in the middle of a similar load in a bag supported in a solid-bottomed container was 121°C. The temperature in the closed bag did not reach 121°C during the normal holding period. Everall and Morris pointed out that prolong-

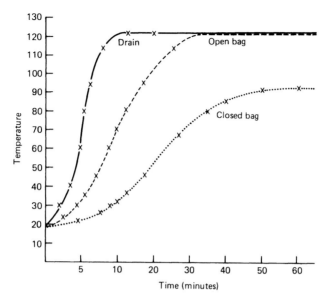

Figure 7.3 The temperatures in the loads in open and closed plastic disposal bags

ing the holding period is not likely to be effective: with no steam penetration the contents are receiving dry heat treatment, which, to be successful, needs a much higher temperature than is likely to be achieved, and much longer time than is practicable. In the report of the investigations by the Public Health Laboratory Service (PHLS, 1978) plastic bags impervious to steam are listed among the probable causes of a number of failures. The mouths of plastic bags must be turned back over the rim of the container to ensure maximum steam penetration. They should not be closed before autoclaving.

DISCHARGE OF INFECTED AIR

If infectious materials have been spilled into the waste containers or into the autoclave chamber aerosols containing them may be discharged in air which is removed from the chamber during the warming-up period. This potential hazard was recognized by Barbeito and Brookey (1976) and overcome by fitting a water-resistant microbial filter in the exhaust vent. This retained the test organisms (*B. subtilis* var. *niger*, *S. marcescens* and T1 coliphage). Oates *et al.* (1987) also fitted a filter in the chamber vent, and this, along with their 'concentric steam supply' (designed to overcome blockages in the drain caused by solidifying agar) successfully prevented discharge of microorganisms into the environment.

Testing and commissioning autoclaves

At commissioning, and at regular periods, autoclaves should be tested by the manufacturers' engineers. But laboratory staff should also test them from time to time.

Given that containers of the correct size and shape have been chosen, it is essential to test an autoclave to see if the correct temperature for sterilization can be achieved in the load itself within a reasonable time. The second requirement in the disposal of contaminated waste is important for economic reasons. If an autoclave takes too long to do its work, the waste will accumulate; this is undesirable as it is an additional hazard to the staff. Moreover, it is important if the autoclave is also used for sterilizing culture media; most of this will be spoiled by prolonged exposure.

Autoclaves should be tested under the 'worst-load' conditions. In most laboratories this would be a container full of 5 ml screw-capped bottles. This should be placed in the centre of the autoclave, and if space is available other loaded containers placed around it. A thermocouple should be placed in a bottle in the middle of this load. Other thermocouples may be distributed in other parts of the autoclave. The sterilization cycle is then started and timed. The time taken for the temperature in the chamber drain to reach 121°C is noted and then the time taken for the thermocouple in the load to register that temperature. This is when the sterilization time begins. After not less than 15 min the steam may be turned off when the cooling time begins. Thus, there are three periods:

(1) warming-up and steam penetration, until the recording thermometer indicates a temperature of, e.g., 121°C in the load;
(2) sterilization, during which the load is maintained at that temperature for the required time. This is the holding time at temperature (HTAT);
(3) cooling down time, until the temperature in the load falls to 80°C, when it may be removed.

If thermocouples are not available and reliance is placed on thermometers that record temperatures in the drain then the period of exposure after the temperature in the drain reaches 121°C is therefore (1) + (2) min. Automatic cycle autoclaves, which depend on the temperature in the drain should be modified accordingly.

In some autoclaves the door cannot be opened until the temperature in the drain falls to 80°C. This does not imply that the temperature in the load has also fallen to a safe level. The temperature in large, sealed bottles may still be over 100°C, when the contents will be at a high pressure. Sudden cooling may cause the bottles to explode. The autoclave should not be opened, therefore, until the temperature in the load has fallen to 80°C or below. This may take a very long time, and in some autoclaves there are locks which permit the door to be opened only fractionally to cool the load further before it is finally released. In others, complicated cooling arrangements with air blasts and cold water sprays are used but are unnecessary for discard material, although steam extraction facilities are desirable for larger laboratories.

Chemical disinfection

Many different chemicals may be used, collectively described as disinfectants or biocides. The former term is used in this book. Some are ordinary reagents, others are special formulations, marketed under trade names. Microbiologists and laboratory managers are often under pressure from salesmen to buy products for which extravagant claims are made. There are usually marked differences between the activity of some disinfectants when tested under optimal conditions by the Rideal-Walker or less discredited techniques and when they are used in practice. The effects of time, temperature, pH, and the chemical and physical nature of the article to be disinfected and of the organic matter present are often not fully appreciated. As long ago as 1961 Chatigny strongly recommended that the effectiveness of liquid disinfectants proposed for laboratory use should be evaluated for each agent and application. This counsel might well apply to new projects, e.g. in recombinant DNA work, but is hardly practicable for routine work.

It is our view that disinfection is a first line of defence, and for discarded bench equipment it is a temporary measure, to be followed, as soon as possible by autoclaving or incineration. Disinfectants should not be used as the sole method of treating bacterial cultures, even if they are completely submerged and all air bubbles are removed. This view was expressed by the late George Sykes who was a leading authority on disinfection and sterilization: 'It is not good enough to immerse them for a period in disinfectant and then simply wash and throw away' (Sykes, 1969). This is not a reflection on the quality of the products of reputable manufacturers but arises from the positive genius of poorly-trained laboratory workers for ignoring manufacturers' directions and for misusing disinfectants. It is fair to say, however, that as far as can be ascertained, improper use of disinfectants in laboratories has not resulted in any laboratory infections—although such infections might be among the 80% that have had no obvious cause (p. 40). This, unfortunately is not so with hospital practice, where misuse, leading to contamination and outbreaks of infection, has been reported (see Bassett, 1971).

Types and laboratory uses of disinfectants

There is a rough spectrum of susceptibility of microorganisms to disinfectants. The most susceptible are vegetative bacteria, fungi and lipid-containing viruses. Mycobacteria and non-lipid-containing viruses are less susceptible and spores are generally resistant.

The general properties of disinfectants used in microbiology are outlined in Table 7.2.

In the choice of disinfectants, consideration should be given to:

- spectrum of activity
- effective working concentration
- practicability of use
- stability
- compatibility with proteins and plastics, etc.
- health hazards to users
- other risks—fire, explosion, environmental.

Only those disinfectants that have a laboratory application are considered here. General information about the use of disinfectants, their chemistry and modes of action, is given by Gardner and Peel (1991) and Russell et al. (1992).

The most commonly used disinfectants in laboratory work are clear phenolics and hypochlorites. Aldehydes have a more limited application, and alcohol and alcohol mixtures are less popular but deserve greater attention. Iodophors and quaternary ammonium compounds (QACs) are more popular in the USA than in the UK, while mercurial compounds are the least used. The general properties of these disinfectants are summarized below (and in Table 7.2). Other

TABLE 7.2 Properties of some disinfectants

	Active against							Inactivated by					Toxicity		
	Fungi	Bacteria Gram+	Gram−	Myco-bacteria	Spores	Lipid viruses	Non-lipid viruses	Protein	Natural materials	Man-made materials	Hard water	Detergents	Skin	Eyes	Lungs
Phenolics	+++	+++	+++	++	−	+	v	+	++	++	+	C	++	++	−
Hypochlorites	+	+++	+++	++	++	+	+	+++	+	+	+	C	++	++	+
Alcohols	−	+++	+++	+++	−	+	v	+	+	+	+	−	−	++	−
Formaldehyde	+++	+++	+++	+++	+++[a]	+	+	+	+	+	−	+	++	++	+
Glutaraldehyde	+++	+++	+++	+++	+++[b]	+	+	NA	+	+	+	−	++	++	++
Iodophors	+++	+++	+++	+++	+	+	+	+++	+	+	+	A	++	++	+
QACs	+	+++	++	−	−	−	−	+++	+++	+++	+++	A(C)	++	−	−
Hydrogen peroxide	+++	+++	+++	++	+	+++	+++	−	−	−	−	+	+	−	−
Peracetic acid	+++	+++	+++	+++	++	+++	+++	+	+	−	−	+	+	+	−

+++, ++, +, −, indicate level of activity, inactivation and toxicity; v = depends on virus; C = cationic; A = anionic substances, such as ethylene oxide and propiolactone, are used commercially in the preparation of sterile equipment for hospital and laboratory use but are not used for decontaminating laboratory waste and the other activities mentioned above. They are therefore excluded from this discussion.

CLEAR PHENOLICS

These compounds are effective against vegetative bacteria (including mycobacteria), fungi, lipid-containing viruses (including Lassa and Marburg agents). They are inactive against spores and non-lipid-containing viruses. Most phenolics are active in the presence of considerable amounts of protein but are inactivated to some extent by rubber, wood and plastics. They are not compatible with cationic detergents.

Laboratory uses include discard jars and disinfection of surfaces. Clear phenolics should be used at the highest concentration recommended by the manufacturers for 'dirty situations', i.e. where they will encounter relatively large amounts of organic matter. This is usually 2–5%. Dilutions should be prepared daily and diluted phenolics should not be stored for laboratory use for more than 24 hours, although many diluted clear phenolics may be effective for more than 7 days.

Skin and eyes should be protected.

HYPOCHLORITES

The activity is due to chlorine, which is very effective against vegetative bacteria (including mycobacteria), spores, fungi and both lipid-containing and non-lipid-containing viruses. Hypochlorites are considerably inactivated by protein and to some extent by natural non-protein material and plastics and they are not compatible with cationic detergents. Their uses include discard jars and surface disinfection but as they corrode some metals care is necessary. They should not be used on the metal parts of centrifuges and other machines which are subjected to stress when in use.

Hypochlorites sold for laboratory and other use usually contain 100 000 ppm available chlorine (Av. Cl.). They should be diluted for use as follows:

Use	Dilution	Final conc Av.Cl.
Reasonably clean surfaces	1:100	1000 ppm
Pipette and discard jars	1:40	2500 ppm
Blood spillage	1:10	10 000 ppm

Some household hypochlorites (e.g. those used for babies' feeding bottles) contain 10 000 ppm and would be diluted 1:4 or used neat. Household 'bleaches' in the UK and USA contain 50 000 ppm available chlorine and dilutions of 1:20 and 1:5 are appropriate. Solid preparations such as sodium dichloroisocyanate (NaDCC), may have laboratory applications especially for spillages.

Diluted hypochlorites decay rapidly in use, although the products as supplied are stable. Diluted solutions should be replaced after 24 hours. The colouring matter added to some commercial hypochlorites is intended to identify them; it is not an indicator of activity.

Hypochlorites may cause irritation of skin, eyes and lungs.

ALDEHYDES

Formaldehyde (gas) and glutaraldehyde (liquid) are good disinfectants. They are active against vegetative bacterial (including mycobacteria), spores, fungi and both lipid- and non-lipid-containing viruses. They are active in the presence of protein and are not very much inactivated by natural or manmade materials, or detergents.

Formaldehyde is not very active at temperatures below 20°C and requires a relative humidity of at least 70%. It is not supplied as a gas, but as a solid polymer, paraformaldehyde, and a liquid, formalin, which contains 37–40% of formaldehyde. Both forms are heated to liberate the gas, which is used for disinfecting enclosed spaces such as safety cabinets and rooms. Formalin, diluted 1:10 to give a solution containing 4% formaldehyde, is used for disinfecting surfaces and, in some circumstances, cultures. Formaldehyde is used mainly for decontaminating safety cabinets (p. 140) and rooms (p. 184).

Glutaraldehyde is supplied as a 2% aqueous solution and may be used undiluted. It usually needs an activator, such as sodium bicarbonate, which is supplied with the bulk liquid. Most activators contain a dye so the user can be sure that the disinfectant has been activated. Effectiveness and stability after activation vary with product and the manufacturers' literature should be consulted.

Aldehydes are toxic. Formaldehyde is particularly unpleasant as it affects the eyes and causes respiratory distress, e.g. formaldehyde asthma. Special precautions are required (see below). The toxicity of formaldehyde is reviewed by HSE (1981), Smith (1992) and formaldehyde asthma by Newman Taylor (1997). The hazards of laboratory use are described by Cheney and Collins (1995). Glutaraldehyde is less harmful, but contact with skin and eyes should be avoided (DH, 1992a; HSE, 1998b). It may also be allergenic. Glutaraldehyde asthma in hospital workers exposed to it is discussed by Newman Taylor (1997).

ALCOHOL AND ALCOHOL MIXTURES

Ethanol and propanol, at concentrations of about 70–80% in water are effective, albeit slowly, against vegetative bacteria and lipid-containing viruses. They are not effective against spores, fungi and non-lipid-containing viruses. They are not especially activated by protein and other material or detergents.

Effectiveness is enhanced by the addition of formaldehyde, e.g. a mixture of 10% formalin in 70% alcohol or hypochlorite to give 2000 ppm of available chlorine (Coates and Death, 1975).

Alcohols and alcohol mixtures are useful for disinfecting surfaces (spraying with an 'atomiser').

Alcohols are relatively harmless to skin but may cause eye irritation.

PERACETIC ACID

This a comparatively new introduction to the battery of useful laboratory disinfectants. It is very active against bacteria, including spores, viruses and fungi.

It is a colourless liquid with a pungent odour and is supplied at 40%

concentration, containing 39% acetic acid, 5% hydrogen peroxide, 1% sulphur dioxide, 15% water, plus a detergent. It should be stored in a refrigerator in vented containers (oxygen is evolved) and contact of the concentrate with heavy metals should be avoided (violent decomposition, explosion).

Peracetic acid is used as a 2% dilution of this, freshly prepared daily, usually as an aerosol, e.g. for microbiological safety cabinets and other enclosures, but requires 80% humidity to be effective. There are no residues and it has the advantage of activity at subzero temperatures.

Much care is needed in its use and manufacturers' guidelines should be followed. It is an irritant. Eye protection, rubber gloves and an apron should be worn. Respiratory protection may be needed if it is used in any amount.

HYDROGEN PEROXIDE

This has quite a wide spectrum but although and its antibacterial and sporicidal activity has been known for many years (see Russel et al., 1992) its laboratory applications do not appear have not been investigated until 1990 (see below).

It is a colourless solution, generally available as '10 volume' or '20 volume' according to to the volume of oxygen liberated from 1 volume of the liquid. It is also commercially available as 90% concentration which is diluted for use to 3– 6%. It is useful as a spray disinfectant but apparatus has now been marketed which generates it as vapour for the disinfection of surfaces, e.g. in centrifuges, incubators, freeze dryers, etc. as well as enclosures such as safety cabinets and clean rooms (Klapes, 1990; Klapes and Vesley, 1990; Heckert et al., 1997).

The concentrated solution is corrosive, moderately irritant and toxic, and flammable but there are no hazardous residues whether it is used as a liquid or as a vapour (unlike, e.g. formaldehyde).

QUATERNARY AMMONIUM COMPOUNDS

These are cationic detergents known as QACs or quats, and are effective against vegetative bacteria and lipid-containing viruses and some fungi but not against mycobacteria, spores and non-lipid-containing viruses. They are inactivated by protein and by a variety of natural and plastic materials and by non-ionic detergents and soap. Their laboratory uses are therefore limited but they have the distinct advantages of being stable and of not corroding metals. They are usually employed at 1–2% dilution for cleaning surfaces, but are very popular in food hygiene laboratories because of their detergent nature.

QACs are not toxic and are harmless to the skin and eyes.

IODOPHORS

Like chlorine compounds these iodines are effective against vegetative bacteria (including mycobacteria), spores, fungi, and both lipid-containing and non-lipid-containing viruses. They are rapidly inactivated by protein, and to a certain extent by natural and plastic substances and are not compatible with anionic detergents. For use in discard jars and for disinfecting surfaces they should be diluted to give 75–150 ppm iodine, but for hand-washing or as a sporicide, dilution in 50% alcohol to give 1600 ppm iodine is required. As sold iodophors usually contain a detergent and they have a built-in indicator: they are active as long as they remain brown or yellow. They stain the skin and surfaces but stains may be removed with sodium thiosulphate solution.

Iodophors are relatively harmless to the skin but some eye irritation may be experienced.

MERCURIAL COMPOUNDS

Activity against vegetative bacteria is poor and mercurials are not effective against spores. They do have an action on viruses at concentrations of 1:500 to 1:1000 and a limited use as saturated solutions for safely making microscopic preparations of mycobacteria.

Their limited usefulness and highly poisonous nature make mercurials unsuitable for general laboratory use.

PRECAUTIONS IN THE USE OF DISINFECTANTS

As indicated above, some disinfectants have undesirable effects on the skin, eyes and respiratory tract. The maximum exposure limits (where available, and of the active ingredient) are as follows:

Formaldehyde	2.0 ppm
Glutaraldehyde	0.2 ppm (But HSE (1998) now recommend 0.05 ppm)
Phenol	10.0 ppm
Chlorine	3.0 ppm
Hydrogen peroxide	2.0 ppm
Ozone	0.3 ppm
Alcohol (ethanol)	100 ppm
Alcohol (propanol)	300 ppm

Disposable gloves and safety spectacles, goggles or a visor should be worn by anyone who is handling strong disinfectants, e.g. when preparing dilutions for use.

It is inadvisable to autoclave materials in disinfectants. The vapours may be discharged in the air which is removed from the autoclave before the sterilization cycle is commenced.

Full-face respirators, with the appropriate canister or compressed air supply should be worn when rooms are disinfected with formaldehyde (see pp. 184 and 190).

Testing disinfectants for laboratory use

Chatigny's (1961) counsel of perfection, that each disinfectant should be evaluated for each laboratory use, is no longer applicable for routine laboratory work now that there is much more information about the properties of the commonly used disinfectants. There is now a better understanding of the limitations of the 'standard' tests used essentially for marketing purposes. Much has been written about these tests which need not be reviewed here and the reader is referred to Gardner and Peel (1991) and Russell et al. (1992). There now seems to be no justification for doing any of them in the clinical or research microbiology laboratory. They are best left to the reference and other specialized establishments. Results of 'one-off' tests may not be reliable except in very skilled hands. Tests may be wrong in principle, when like is not compared with like (Croshaw, 1981), and—a common mistake—neutralization procedures may be inadequate or incorrectly applied (Russell, 1981).

THE IN-USE TEST

There is one test, however, which is useful and reassuring in laboratories where infectious materials are submerged in disinfectants for whatever purpose, notwithstanding subsequent heat treatment. This is the 'in-use test' devised for testing disinfectants in laboratory discard jars.

Full details of this test are given by Kelsey and Maurer (1966) and Gardner and Peel (1991). In principle, 1 ml of the disinfectant is removed from, e.g., a discard jar at the end of the day and added to 9 ml of diluent (quarter strength Ringer's solution for phenolic disinfectants and nutrient broth containing 0.5% sodium thiosulphate for hypochlorites). After mixing, 10 drops are placed on the surface of each of two nutrient agar plates (Figure 7.4). These are incubated for 72 hours, one at 37°C and the other at room temperature. There should be no growth on either plate. If there is, the management of the discard jars should be reviewed.

Discard jars

The jars or pots of disinfectant that sit on the laboratory bench and into which used slides, Pasteur pipettes and other rubbish are dumped have a long history of neglect and abuse (see Figure 4.7). In all too many laboratories these jars are filled infrequently with unknown dilutions of disinfectants, are overloaded with protein and articles that float, and are infrequently emptied. The contents, which certainly have not been disinfected, are then thrown away without further treatment (see Figure 4.8). Attention was drawn to the hazards of this kind of misuse, and firm recommendations made for the better management of discard

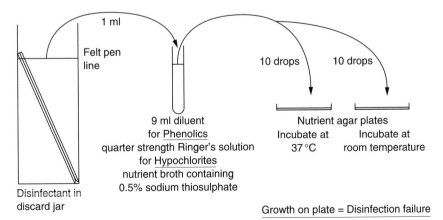

Figure 7.4 Maurer's 'in-use' test for the effectiveness of bench-use disinfectants. Growth on either plate culture indicates failure. (Reprinted from Maurer, 'The management of laboratory discard jars', p. 55. In *Safety in Microbiology* 1972, with permission of the publisher, Academic Press Ltd)

jars by Maurer (1972) and these were echoed by Collins (1974). They resolve themselves into (a) choice of container, (b) correct dilution of disinfectant (c) sensible use, (d) regular emptying, (e) sterilization of container before recharging, and (f) safe disposal of contents.

CHOICE OF CONTAINER

Old jam jars and instant coffee jars can no longer be regarded as suitable. Glass jars are easily broken and broken glass is an unnecessary laboratory hazard especially if it is likely to be contaminated. Discard jars should be robust and autoclavable and it is suggested here that the most serviceable articles are 1-litre polypropylene laboratory beakers or polypropylene jars. These are deep enough to hold submerged most of the things that are likely to be discarded, are quite unbreakable, and survive many autoclave cycles. They go dark brown in time, but this does not affect their use.

Wide-mouth screw-capped polypropylene bottles are better still. They are left open on the bench. At the end of a working session they are capped and inverted several times to ensure that all trapped air is removed from submerged objects so that they are in contact with the disinfectant (M. Scruton, personal communication).

CORRECT DILUTION

A 1-litre discard jar should hold 750 ml of diluted disinfectant and leave space for displacement without overflow or the risk of spillage when it is moved. A mark should be made at 750 ml on each jar, preferably with paint (grease pencil and felt-pen marks are less permanent). The correct volume of neat disinfectant to be added to water to make up this volume for 'dirty situations' can be calculated from the manufacturers' instructions. This volume is then marked on a small measuring jug, e.g. of enamelled iron, or a plastic dispenser is locked to deliver it from a bulk container. The disinfectant is added to the beaker and water added to the 750 ml mark.

SENSIBLE USE

Laboratory supervisors should ensure that inappropriate articles are not placed in discard jars. For example, a 30 cm pipette has no place in a 1-litre jar (see Figure 4.7). Apart from acting as a lever to tip over the jar, part of the pipette will not be disinfected. There is a reasonable limit to the amount of paper or tissues that such a jar will hold, and articles that float are unsuitable for disinfectant jars, unless these can be capped and inverted from time to time to wet *all* the contents.

Large volumes of liquids should never be added to dilute disinfectants. Discard jars, containing the usual volume of neat disinfectant can be provided for fluids such as centrifuge supernatant fluids, which should be poured in through a funnel that fits into the top of the beaker. This prevents splashing and aerosol dispersal (see p. 98). At the end of the day water can be added to the 750 ml mark and the mixture left overnight. Material containing large amounts of protein should not be added to disinfectants but should be autoclaved or incinerated.

REGULAR EMPTYING

No material should be left in disinfectant in discard jars for more than 24 hours, or surviving bacteria may grow. All discard jars should therefore be emptied once daily, but whether this is at the end of the day or the following morning is a matter for local choice. Even jars that have received little or nothing during the time should be emptied.

DISPOSAL OF CONTENTS

It is suggested above that the contents of discard jars should be autoclaved and/ or incinerated. This requires the separation of solid from liquid and Collins (1974) suggested pouring the contents of each jar through a colander, which, of course, should be of autoclavable material, into a bucket. The contents of the colander are then tipped into a bucket or bag for autoclaving or incineration. Stainless steel dairy sieves are probably better. The liquid waste is poured carefully down a sluice or deep sink without splashing.

RE-USABLE PIPETTES

These are a problem because they are an exception to the rule that disinfection is merely a temporary step before autoclaving and incineration. Safe methods for discarding these pipettes have already been described on p. 77. They should be completely immersed in the disinfectant so that no air bubbles remain to protect any part of the lumen from the action of the chemical. They should remain in the disinfectant for at least 18 hours and then removed with gloved hands and placed in several changes of hot (60°C) water before being washed and rinsed for recycling.

Accidents with infected materials

There is an immediate need for disinfection after spillage, breakage or other accidents involving infectious material. Local action will often suffice, but sometimes, e.g. after a massive release of aerosol, it may be desirable to treat a whole room or a vehicle.

Minor spills and breakage of contaminated material may be dealt with by the laboratory worker on the spot, but they must, of course, be reported to the safety adviser. Major events need his immediate attention. What constitute minor and major events must be determined by the safety adviser according to the nature or hazard group of the microorganisms concerned. He must also consider the risk from aerosols to people in the vicinity and whether such aerosols are likely to be spread around the building by the ventilation systems. Local knowledge should enable the safety officer to draw up protocols for decontamination procedures after such incidents as:

(1) leaking specimen containers and contaminated request forms;
(2) simple spills and those involving broken glass;
(4) spillage and breakage in safety cabinets;
(5) centrifuge accidents;
(6) transport-associated accidents.

Action to be taken will vary from simple mopping up with disinfectant to decontamination of large items of equipment or of whole rooms. Appropriate equipment should be available for all such emergencies.

Emergency equipment

Accidents requiring immediate action may occur outside (e.g. during the transport of infectious materials) as well as inside the laboratory building. At suitable sites in the building there should be an 'emergency kit' preferably on a trolley, ready to be taken to the site of an accident.

The kit should include the following:

(1) A supply of appropriate disinfectant at the correct dilution as specified by the manufacturer for 'dirty situations'. If hypochlorites are the disinfectant of choice, the small retail packs of bleach or domestic chlorine disinfectants are more economical for this purpose. These are usually not as concentrated as industrial packs supplied in large volumes, and may be used neat. Problems of stability after dilution do not arise. Alternatively one of the solid chlorine releasing compounds may be used. Activated glutaraldehyde (keeps at least 7 days) and 10% formalin in 70% alcohol are also recommended for this purpose. Gelling agents, supplied as a powder or as granules, may be sprinkled on a spill. Within a few seconds a stiff gel forms which is easily scooped up.
(2) Paper towels and swabs.
(2) Forceps for picking up glass, other debris, paper towels and swabs.
(3) Dustpans made of metal or polypropylene (autoclavable), a supply of heavy-duty polythene or paper sacks and polypropylene trays.
(4) Protective clothing, preferably of the disposable operating theatre type, disposable and heavy-duty gloves, rubber boots or disposable overshoes.
(5) Face masks and (where applicable) a full-face respirator with appropriate replaceable filters, e.g. submicron particle filters for aerosols and formaldehyde filters for disinfection work.

Leakage of specimens

This is of particular concern when it happens in reception rooms where the staff have neither scientific nor technical training. Saving the specimen, which may not be repeatable, and the request form, if only to determine its provenance, may be considered as important as protecting the staff from possible infection.

When a leakage is observed the reception staff should immediately request assistance from the safety officer, or a member of the laboratory staff. The person who deals with the leakage should don disposable gloves and then transfer the offending container and any others that are or may be contaminated to a tray which is then placed inside a large plastic bag and removed to a laboratory, preferably to a safety cabinet. The surface on which the leakage occurred should then be covered with paper towels over which the appropriate disinfectant is then poured. This should be left for at least 30 min before the towels are removed with gloved hands to a discard bag or bin. The area should then be swabbed with fresh disinfectant and left for a further 30 min before it is dried and restored to use.

In the laboratory or safety cabinet the tray should be removed from the bag. Material remaining in the specimen container may then be transferred to another one, using a pasteur pipette or spatula. If the request form is contaminated but legible the information on it can then be dictated to another worker. If no-one else is available the form should be placed flat in a plastic bag which is then sealed and labelled and stored until it can be copied. Containers that have not leaked but the outsides of which have been contaminated may be dealt with in the same way. The tray and its contents should then be flooded with disinfectant and left for several hours before the liquid is poured down the sluice and the solid debris autoclaved or incinerated.

Leakage into transport boxes should be treated in the same way except that the box can be autoclaved, with or without its contents.

Spillage and breakage

In general the following procedure should be adopted to deal with the simpler kinds of spillage of infectious material, and of blood, e.g. on the bench:

(1) Wear gloves and protective clothing, including face and eye protection if indicated;
(2) cover the spill with paper absorbent towels to contain it;
(3) pour disinfectant, e.g. hypochlorite (see above) over the paper towel and the area immediately around it;
(4) after 5–10 min use a piece of stiff cardboard to sweep the paper and any broken glass or other debris into an autoclavable or disposable dustpan;
(5) place the dustpan and its contents into a receptacle for autoclaving (not a plastic bag if the debris includes glass);
(6) pour more disinfectant over the area of the spillage and leave for 15–20 min before mopping up with absorbent paper towels; dispose of the towels into a container for autoclaving.

Modifications of this method include (a) covering the spill with a granular chlorine compound instead of paper towels; (b) sprinkling a gelling agent (see below) over the spillage before covering it with paper towels. Procedures for dealing specifically with blood spillages are given by Hoffman and Kennedy (1997).

Accidents in microbiological safety cabinets

If material is spilt in a safety cabinet, the fan should be kept running while the spill is dealt with. Some safety cabinets have perforated work surfaces and spilt material may go through into the catchment tray beneath. Enough disinfectant should be poured into this tray to dilute the spillage 10-fold. When work is finished the tray can be emptied through the drain cock and cleaned. After a spillage safety cabinets should always be disinfected with formaldehyde. The technique for this is described on p. 140.

Centrifuge accidents

Breakage of tubes in a centrifuge can disperse large amounts of aerosols unless the precautions described in Chapter 4 are observed. In a well-managed laboratory, where sealed buckets are used for all Hazard Group 3 agents, the consequences of centrifuge accidents are likely to be minimal, especially now that cultures of haemolytic streptococci and *Staphylococcus aureus* are not centrifuged as routine measures. There is usually a change in the noise a centrifuge makes when a tube breaks and this serves as a warning to the occupants of the room. The action to be taken is much the same as that for the breakage of a culture, as described above. After the room is considered safe to enter the centrifuge buckets and rotor can be removed and autoclaved and the bowl disinfected.

Major incidents

The most serious incident of this kind is when cultures, either liquid or solid, are dropped on the floor and break. There is much splashing and a considerable amount of aerosol is dispersed. Laboratory workers must be taught not to follow their natural instinct and bend down to inspect the damage. This brings the face into the aerosol cloud. All people in the room should hold their breath and leave. If anyone suspects or knows that his clothing has been splashed he should remove it. Laboratory overalls offer little protection. They should be placed in the appropriate discard bags for autoclaving or hot-wash laundering. Shoes, trousers and skirts may exercise the ingenuity of the safety officer or supervisor who may have contingency plans (see above). It may be sufficient to sponge the contaminated areas with a disinfectant-detergent mixture, but the nature of the fabric should be considered. Hypochlorites bleach most things.

The door should be closed and locked and a warning sign posted on it. Telephones should be left to ring; it is presumed that there are other extensions. Thirty minutes is a reasonable time to leave the room unoccupied while larger aerosol particles settle and small ones are cleared by the natural or mechanical ventilation. The safety officer should by this time have ascertained the probable nature of the microorganisms involved. This will enable him to decide (a) what respiratory and other protection he requires (if any) to enter the room, (b) which disinfectant to use, and (c) the extent of room decontamination procedures—from mopping up with the emergency equipment to decontamination of the room as described below.

Guidelines for dealing with accidents involving microorganisms are the subject of a WHO memorandum (WHO, 1980). (See also Chapter 11.)

Decontamination of automated equipment

In clinical laboratories the main concern in decontaminating this kind of equipment relates to hepatitis B and HIV (see Chapter 12), but it is always possible that material containing other pathogens is passed through the apparatus.

The HSE (1991a) recommends that the effluent discharge tube be taken at least 25 cm into the laboratory waste plumbing system or that it is trapped in a bottle. The instrument is then flushed through with a disinfectant recommended by the manufacturer.

Investigations performed by Death *et al.* (1982) in collaboration with a manufacturer showed that formaldehyde can be used for external decontamination of some automated instruments and for the dialyser assembly of one particular machine without any adverse effects. For the decontamination of dialyser assemblies, etc. they recommend placing the cartridge inside a smaller, sealable container for treatment with formaldehyde.

Decontamination of equipment before servicing

Although spillages, etc., which occur inside some equipment, may be dealt with as described above it is desirable to have a regular procedure for decontaminating equipment that is to be serviced on site or returned to a manufacturer for any reason. Many companies and their staff require that the equipment has been reliably decontaminated.

The interiors of incubators, refrigerators and similar cupboard-like equipment should be swabbed thoroughly with glutaraldehyde or alcohol-formalin mixture, observing the safety precautions described above. Cryostats should be brought up to room temperature first, or the aldehyde will not be effective. The equipment should then be labelled and left overnight. It should then be washed out several times with clean water and dried. Smaller equipment may be sealed in large plastic bags, with formalin, and left overnight. After decontamination the equipment should be taped or otherwise secured so that it cannot be used and a label fixed to it stating how it has been treated and the date.

Alternatively a hydrogen peroxide vapour generator may be used (see above).

A certificate of decontamination and a declaration that, as far as is possible, the equipment is microbiologically safe should then be given to the manufacturer or his agent.

Decontamination of laboratory protective clothing

Gowns, overall and coats worn in microbiological laboratories may become contaminated by microorganisms deposited on benches and equipment as a result of spillage or deposit of airborne particles. Wong and Nye (1991) have recovered viable organisms from such clothing, especially from the cuffs. Earlier, Oliphant *et al.* (1949) reported possible transmission of the Q fever agent from laboratory clothing to laundry workers.

Laboratory protective clothing should therefore be autoclaved before it is sent for laundering or placed in 'hot-wash' bags which should not be opened in laundries until after they have been exposed to very hot water.

Transport-associated accidents

These may range from leakage of a pathological specimen in a hospital van to leakage or breakage of a culture in a public place, post office, public service vehicle or aircraft. Accidents in hospital vans can usually be dealt with by a member of the laboratory professional staff armed with the emergency equipment described above. In principle, all the other accidents can be treated as described above for decontaminating surfaces and rooms, but the potential for the spread of infection is so great, particularly if the nature of the package or specimen is not known, that it is essential to inform both the senior medical microbiologist and the medical officer for environmental health at once. Protocols for dealing with these emergencies have been worked out by most health departments. A good example has been published by the World Health Organization (WHO, 1993) and is shown in Figure 6.3 (p. 158).

Space disinfection

It may be necessary to disinfect a room after a spillage of infectious material, before a change of use or before building alterations or redecoration. Two methods may be used—wet disinfection and 'fumigation' with a gaseous disinfectant.

Wet disinfection

This can be used only if the floors do not allow liquids to leak into the rooms below and if any equipment and furniture remaining in the room are not likely to be damaged by the disinfectant. Wet-mopping is useful only for floors but the usual practice, with a used mop-head and a single bucket of disinfectant, is unlikely to achieve much. Mop-heads are usually so dirty that they begin inactivating the disinfectant at once, and returning disinfectant from the floor to the bucket completes the process. A freshly laundered mop-head is required with two buckets, each fitted with a foot-operated wringer. One bucket contains the appropriate disinfectant, which may be mixed with a compatible detergent. The mop is dipped into this bucket, surplus fluid removed with the wringer and an area of floor is mopped. The mop-head is then wrung out into the other bucket, recharged from the first bucket and another area mopped. The floor should be left wet for at least 30 min when it may be dried with the mop and bucket or with a wet-vacuum cleaner fitted with a HEPA filter. Spent disinfectant in the bucket may be poured down a drain, but the bucket should then be treated with new disinfectant or autoclaved. The mop-head should be laundered.

If it is necessary to wet-disinfect the whole room a sprayer, e.g. a horticultural knapsack sprayer, should be used. This should have a lance that is long enough and angled so that crevices and corners can be sprayed. The operator should wear eye and face protection; if formalin is used respiratory protective equipment (RPE) should be worn. As RPE is not within the scope of this book, please see Harrington et al. (1998).

Fumigation

Formaldehyde fumigation is not now generally recommended as it poses problems and health threats. Fumigation is still practised, however, so the method is given here.

The room must be sealed. Windows, ventilators, pipe runs and cracks, and any aperture that might permit the gas to escape into other rooms should be sealed with masking tape. As a sensible safety precaution the 'two-man rule' should apply to this operation, and both individuals should have full-face respirators with appropriate canisters for formaldehyde, or breathing apparatus. One man should generate the formaldehyde while the other stands outside the door. The amount of formalin or paraformaldehyde needed depends on the volume of the room. For formaldehyde fumigation 100 ml of formalin plus 900 ml of water are required for each 30 m³ of space. The mixture is boiled away in an electrically heated pan fitted with a timing device. If paraformaldehyde is used 0.3 g/ft³ (10.5 g/m³) is heated in the same way.

The operator should leave the room immediately after starting the reaction, whichever method is used. The door should then be locked and sealed with masking tape. A warning notice should be posted and the room left for 24 hours. It is then opened by the operators, both of whom should be wearing respirators: one then enters the room and opens the windows. After he has left the room it should be locked again to allow clearance of formaldehyde, which may take one to several hours. If a Class I safety cabinet, exhausting to atmosphere, is in the room it should be switched on to assist in ventilation. Problems arise in those ill-designed premises that have no windows—or no openable windows. Clearance of formaldehyde may be hastened by exposing dishes of strong ammonia, or sheets of blotting paper soaked with it in the room but this offers another respiratory hazard. Respirator canisters that are effective against formaldehyde do not usually afford protection against ammonia.

For information and comment on formaldehyde disinfection of rooms see Cheney and Collins (1995) and Jones (1996).

There is now a safer alternative to formaldehyde fumigation. Machines which generate hydrogen peroxide vapour (see p. 175) are now available (from MDH, UK and AMSCO, Finland).

After a room has been decontaminated it may be necessary for a statement or certificate to be issued before work is resumed or building staff move in.

This certificate should be signed and dated by the safety officer or other designated person.

Disposal of contaminated liquid waste

Small amounts may be poured into disinfectant through a funnel as described above, but problems arise with large amounts, such as 24-hour urines, the effluents from automated equipment and sink and lavatory effluents from Level 4 laboratories.

The preservative normally put into 24-hour urine containers will prevent excessive multiplication of pathogens but urines in polythene containers cannot be autoclaved. It is safe to pour most specimens down a sluice or deep sink where they will join the large amounts of urine and faeces already in the public sewer. Sewage disposal plants deal quite effectively with most pathogens. The only hazard to the operator is from splashing and aerosol production while pouring, so this should be done with care. Afterwards or at the end of the day the sluice or sink should be flushed as gently as possible and enough disinfectant poured down it to fill the trap, which is then left undisturbed overnight. If it is known or suspected that the urine contains Hazard Group 3 pathogens, neat disinfectant (hypochlorite or phenolic) should be added to the urine to give the use dilution. After standing overnight the contents should be poured away as described above. Empty polythene containers should be autoclaved or incinerated, not washed and reused.

The effluents from automatic chemistry or haematology apparatus are unlikely to be very hazardous. Microorganisms and viruses in the original specimens will have encountered inimical chemicals on their way through the machines. Aerosols should be avoided, however, and the discharge pipes are best plumbed into the laboratory drainage system. The discharge tubes which lead directly to sinks from small machines should be made long enough to go right down the waste pipe or even round the bends of the traps.

The safe disposal of the various effluents from Containment Level 4 laboratories is a design consideration, not a matter for post-building or ad hoc decisions. The effluents are usually taken to one or more holding tanks where they are heated by steam for a predetermined time, then tested for the presence of the pathogens which were used (or suitable indicator organisms) before discharge into the sewers. Sometimes chemical treatment is preferred.

Incineration

The problems with this method of disposal are in ensuring that the waste actually reaches the incinerator and that if it does it is effectively sterilized: and that none escapes, either as unburned material or up the flue. Incinerators are rarely under the control of laboratory staff.

Sometimes they are not even under the control of the staff of the hospital or institution, but are some distance away and contaminated and infectious material has to be sent to them on the public highway. It may never arrive or may not be incinerated.

In recent years serious problems have arisen about ineffective and inadequate hospital incinerators that do not render material safe to handle and that contravene various control of pollution regulations. There is a trend towards larger, efficient and centralized incinerators which are well-engineered and operated under professional supervision (see Collins and Kennedy, 1993).

Laboratory waste will therefore have to be transported and such transportation is again covered by legislation. It is sensible, therefore, to make the waste safe by autoclaving it before it leaves the laboratory. Unfortunately current UK recommendations (ACDP, 1990; HSE, 1991a) still offer incineration as an alternative to prior autoclaving.

There is a British standard for incinerators for clinical waste (BS 3316, 1987).

Ultimate disposal of laboratory waste

The ash that remains after correct incineration is non-infectious and may be landfilled. In some areas landfilling of autoclaved (and therefore safe and generally unrecognizable) laboratory waste is permitted.

Chapter 8

The laboratory worker

In the first two decades of this century at least two bacteriologists (Eyre, 1913 and Fricke, 1919) stressed the necesssity of taking personal precautions against infection in the laboratory. Both authors recommended the wearing of protective clothing and gloves, the disinfection of hands after work with specimens and cultures, avoiding the licking of labels of placing anything in the mouth. Unfortunately these warnings were rarely repeated in later books until the 1950s and 1960s.

Even then in spite of attempts to inculcate good laboratory practices and the provision of the correct personal equipment, intended to protect the worker from the work, there seems to have been an ill-defined feeling among the staff of some laboratories that they were not getting the consideration they deserved. The areas of discontent are related to protective clothing, amenities, and medical supervision, which includes vaccination and immunization. Much of this concern has been alleviated by by the adoption (in some areas with poor grace!) of the official and other recommendations and codes of practice that stemmed from incidents that threatened the public health rather than that of the laboratory worker.

Protective clothing

It is now the accepted practice, and in some countries a legal requirement (in the UK the *Personal Protective Equipment at Work Regulations 1992*) to supply laboratory workers with protective clothing—coats, gowns, overalls or suits, depending on the nature of the work (Anon., 1981; HSE, 1991a; OSHA, 1991). Sufficient numbers of such garments per worker should ensure that there are at least two changes per week.

Over the years two kinds of protective clothing came into general use: gowns and front-buttoned white coats. The gowns, similar to but stronger and slightly shorter than those worn by operating theatre staff, protect the entire front of the workers' bodies. Their disadvantage is that they are fastened at the back by tape ties. Tying and untying tapes behind one's back requires contortions and tapes frequently become knotted so that the wearer requires assistance. It is very difficult to remove one of these gowns in an emergency. Another drawback is that tapes are often detached during laundering. Some gowns have large pockets like marsupial pouches at the front. These are much better than breast pockets: every time one bends down the contents of a breast pocket fall out.

It is argued that white coats which button at the front not only look better to the worker, especially as a status badge, but are more comfortable to wear. Certainly they are easier to remove than gowns. Unfortunately they were frequently worn unbuttoned and wide open (again as a status symbol), especially by younger members of the staff. They then afford no protection at all. Even when buttoned up these coats do not protect the neck and upper chest from splashes and contamination. The ends of the ties of male workers fall out onto the bench. Nor do the coats protect the thighs and knees as they gape open when the wearers sit down. The open cuffs allow the cuffs of shirts or blouses to project and pick up anything that has been spilled on the bench. It is also possible for aerosols and splashes to enter through the cuffs and contaminate the wrists and lower arms. Fricke (1919) noted these shortcomings nearly 70 years ago and recommended double-breasted coats with tight-fitting sleeves that covered shirt and dress cuffs and which could be tucked into gloves. The pockets are useful but the breast pockets are a nuisance, as with gowns.

Overalls that overcame all these objections, and met with the approval of many laboratory workers on aesthetic grounds, were introduced by Dowsett and Heggie (1972). They have high necks to protect the worker's front, wrap over and cannot gape at the knees, and have close fitting cuffs. The original versions had zip fasteners and later models have press-studs (poppers). The latter are easier to undo in a hurry. Some laundries seem to make a habit of wrecking zips and press studs. Velcro stands up to autoclaving and hot-washing, and if it fails to fasten because of accumulations of fluff it can be restored by brushing with stiff bristles. A distinct advantage of the position of the openings of these coats is that it is very uncomfortable to wear them unfastened.

Such coats, favoured by the HSE (1991a) have become popular with both sexes. They have almost entirely replaced the old style front button coats. They are made of a variety of fabrics, including cotton, polyester cotton, flame-resistant drill and nylon, and also in various colours. Styles, for men, women and unisex, vary slightly and intending purchasers would be well advised to obtain samples from the various suppliers and have members of the staff 'model' them before making a decision. In some laboratories one- or two-piece 'jump suits' are used for work at Levels 3 and 4. The workers change into these from their normal dress and discard them into the laundry bin at the end of the day. There are also one-piece suits, which may be worn over normal clothing. Some of these are disposable.

When re-usable protective clothing is removed it should be hung on the pegs provided inside or immediately outside the rooms in which it is worn and not in lockers in contact with street clothing. It should be removed before the wearer goes to the rest room or canteen. Some unthinking people object to this rule on the grounds that hospital doctors and nurses wear their overalls in the canteens. They need to be told that the laboratory environment is likely to be more heavily contaminated with microorganisms than are wards and patients and that, anyway, bad examples should not be followed.

There may be a case for colour-coding laboratory clothing—one colour for Level 2 and another for Level 3 work.

Plastic aprons

These are disposable and it is advisable to wear them over ordinary protective clothing when working with blood that might be infected, e.g. with HBV and HIV material. After a single use they should be discarded into a bag for autoclaving and/or incineration.

Gloves

There has always been some controversy about the wearing of gloves. The HSE (1991a) requires them for all Group 3 agents, HBV and where required by local rules. The ACDP (1995) specifies them for certain Group 2 and all Group 3 organisms. Too much reliance should not be placed on the integrity of gloves as there have been several reports of flawed and leaking products (see, for example, Palmer and Rickett, 1992). There is a British Standard (BS 4006, 1996c) for single-use medical gloves.

There is no doubt, however, that there is some loss of digital sensitivity, even with the best gloves and that this predisposes accidents. Some latitude seems desirable for all but work with agents in the highest category and when there are cuts and scratches on the hands.

Heavy-duty gloves should be provided in preparation rooms for handling hot materials and concentrated disinfectants, and in animal houses.

A wide variety of gloves is available and careful consideration is necessary in choosing them. Some individuals are allergic to certain materials, e.g. latex asthma (Newman Taylor, 1997). The allergens in the latex may be taken up in the glove powder, which is then inhaled. Latex sensitisation is reviewed by the Medical Devices Agency (MDA, 1996).

Eye and face protection

Several different kinds of goggles are available and those with side pieces are best. These may be worn over spectacles. It is also possible to obtain protective prescription spectacles. If these are used they should remain in the laboratory, not be taken home. There is a British standard (BS EN 168, 1996) for personal eye protection.

For some purposes, where there may be splashing of biological agents or chemicals and opening autoclaves, visors are preferred; the type that protects the throat is best.

Contact-lens wearers may be at risk from infection with *Pseudomonas* spp. and *Acanthamoeba*, either from these agents in the course of their work (manual transfer or splashes) or from contaminated eye wash bottles. Good hygiene is essential. (See Seal and Hay 1993 and Chapter 11.)

Masks and respiratory protective equipment

Hospital or surgeons' masks, made of cloth, may impede the passage of large droplets, but not of smaller particles, i.e. droplet nuclei (Andrewes, 1940; Jennison, 1942). These masks may offer protection, however, against the inhalation of the allergenic material in animal houses, where the particles are larger than those of droplet nuclei. A point has also been made that wearing any kind of mask will protect the mouth and nose from contact with infected fingers.

Better protection is afforded by the single-use submicron surgical masks, which are made of stiff, moulded fibre and can be pressed over the mouth and nose by light metal fittings. These permit a very good face seal. One such mask was tested by Chen *et al.* (1994) and found to be 97% efficient against particles averaging less than 1 μm aerodynamic diameter. See also Willeke *et al.* (1996) who tested the penetration of such masks by microorganisms.

The International Social Security Association (ISSA, 1998), which is concerned (among other things) with the control of risks in work with biological agents approves single-use masks of type FFP3 (EN, 149) and full-face or half-face masks fitted with high efficiency particulate air (HEPA) filters Class, British standard (BS 6016, 1993) type 203 or BS EN type FFO2 or FFP3 (BS 7355, 1990).

An alternative would be a HEPA respirator, which Chen *et al.* (1994) found to be 99.99% efficient in their tests. These are expensive and not very comfortable to wear, however, and their use may not be justifiable (Vesley, 1995).

Full respiratory protective equipment—self-contained breathing apparatus—may be necessary only in cases of major accidents with airborne pathogens and is beyond the scope of this book. Reference should be made to Croner (1997) and Harrington *et al.* (1998). There are British standards (BS 7355, 1990c, 1991d).

Official guidance is scanty. The Centers for Disease Control (CDC/NIH 1993) require for Level 3 work 'respiratory protection as needed; face protection (goggles, mask or face shield) for manipulations of infectious materials outside a biological safety cabinet' but do not specify the type of mask. Masks are not specifically mentioned by the HSE (1991a) nor the ACDP (1995). Respiratory protective equipment is not specifically approved by the Health and Safety Executive (ACDP, 1995: Appendix) for work involving exposure to infection; the responsibility for the choice of equipment is placed on the employer who must make a performance assessment.

Positive pressure suits are of interest although their details are outside the scope of this book. The operator is totally enclosed in a plastic suit and is supplied with air through a tube which he plugs into an outlet from a manifold. The suit is under positive pressure in relation to the room. Some Level 4 laboratories use this system in preference to Class III cabinet lines.

Footwear

It is rarely necessary for employers to issue protective footwear for microbiological laboratory work. The hazard comes from unsuitable shoes, e.g. flip-flops, loose sandals and very high heels which affect the stability of the wearer. Open-toed and fenestrated footwear should not be worn in laboratories. A number of accidents, involving spillage and breakage of toxic or infectious materials, have been attributed to the wearing of inherently unsafe footwear.

Disposable overshoes (foot-muffs) are a requirement in some institutions and are put on over the normal shoes at the laboratory door and discarded again on leaving the room.

Amenities

We are concerned here only with those amenities which might mitigate against microbiological hazards. These are mostly design features and are included in Chapter 10. In brief they are the provision of:

(1) hand basins in laboratories, in the very necessary interests of hygiene;
(2) lockers for staff clothing near to but not in laboratory rooms, and to protect street clothing from contamination;
(3) rest rooms for eating and drinking, again near to the laboratory rooms.

Health of staff

The Report of the Joint Committee on the Care of the Health of Hospital Staff ('The Tunbridge Report': Central Health Services Council, 1968) states that 'An employee's state of health must be consistent with the employment sought and unlikely to endanger the health of others.'

Pre-employment medical examinations

The HSE (1991a) does not consider that pre-employment medical examination is necessary. The only pre-employment medical tests which seem to be consistently observed in the UK, and then only recently, are a chest X-ray and a skin test for tuberculosis (or evidence of either or both). Thus, the very sensible recommendations of the Tunbridge Committee are too often ignored. This is in contrast with the requirements of the US Public Health Service which stipulates a pre-employment medical examination and specifies its nature (NIH, 1974, 1978). It includes a medical history, physical examination (including cervical smear for women), serology plus a serum specimen for the employee serum bank, selected biochemical tests, full blood count, urinalysis, immunization status, X-ray, electrocardiogram, visual and audiometric examinations. It would seem that this not only protects employers and employees but is regarded as good preventive medicine. The World Health Organization (WHO, 1993) also recommends such examinations.

For a more detailed discussion of these medical examinations see Wright (1985, 1987), the various guidance notes and guidelines of the HSE (1982) and of the Association of NHS Occupational Physicians (1986).

Medical monitoring

The most pressing need for this kind of health supervision is in those laboratories where especially hazardous agents are handled, i.e. in Levels 3 and 4 laboratories. The scope of the monitoring depends on the agent and is best determined on the advice of the medically qualified staff who are actually doing the work. Administrative decisions may miss the point.

In clinical or diagnostic laboratories, where there is usually a medically qualified microbiologist, monitoring is easier. He will know who is ill, and from the medical certificate provided by the employee's own doctor—or from that doctor personally—he can assess the likelihood of a laboratory-acquired infection, of any hazard the patient might be exposed to on his return to work and any risk to other employees. It is highly desirable that the names and addresses of all employees' family doctors are on record in the laboratory and that the list is kept up to date. Recommendations are offered by Wright (1985, 1987), HSE (1982) and WHO (1993). A good occupational health service is invaluable (Waldron, 1997).

Serological tests

The object of an employee serum bank is to enable a baseline titre to be determined if at some future date an employee becomes ill and further serological tests are required. Serum collected pre- or post-employment need not be tested unless the employee becomes ill. Comparison of titres might then establish the diagnosis or indicate that the antibody had always been present. Such a bank might well be mandatory in large research establishments but is hardly practical in clinical laboratories.

Another important serological investigation is for rubella antibody. This should be offered to all female staff of child-bearing age and if it is negative immunization should be considered.

Chest X-rays

Chest X-rays of apparently fit laboratory workers should be arranged only by medically-qualified staff in consultation with the radiologist. There may be contraindications. Staff who handle tuberculosis material should normally have an annual chest X-ray but for other staff a 3-year interval is thought to be adequate.

Pregnancy

Women who work with viruses should tell their supervisors as soon as they are, or think they are, pregnant because of the risks to the fetus, particularly in the first trimester (see Chapter 11). Their sera should be tested for antibodies to rubella. There should be an individual evaluation of the risks involved in continued employment. It may be necessary for them to change their work.

Limited information is available about laboratory exposure to cytomegalovirus.

Accident and incident reports

There should be a rule in all microbiological laboratories that all accidents causing personal injury, whether involving infectious agents or not, should be reported to the supervisor, safety officer or other designated person. In addition any incidents in which a worker is accidentally exposed to infectious material should be documented.

In the UK the *Reporting of Injuries, Diseases and Dangerous Occurrences Regulations 1985* (RIDDOR) requires that serious accidents and laboratory-acquired infections are reported to the Health and Safety Executive. Therefore, records must be kept of all injuries and accidents even if no injury has occurred, and of staff sicknesses.

Accidents that cause injuries, and 'dangerous occurrences' must be reported so that necessary investigations can be made in case of negligence and to ensure that action is taken to prevent recurrence. Whether such records are kept in the laboratory or in an occupational health department is immaterial so long as they are immediately available to the Health and Safety Executive officers. Accident records are particularly important for legal reasons, in case claims or litigation under any industrial injuries regulations ensue. Records must be kept for at least 3 years.

Infections must be reported in any case where a pathogen is knowingly handled as part of a work activity, e.g. in a clinical or research establishment, or where it is not intentionally handled it might be encountered in the course of the work.

The appropriate forms, (a) for reporting or dangerous occurrence, and (b) for reporting a case of disease, are available from the Health and Safety Executive, which also issues a guide to the regulations (HSE, 1986).

Medical contact cards

It was proposed by the UK health departments (DH, 1975, 1978) that each employee in a laboratory where pathogens were handled should carry a card and show it to his family doctor when he is ill. This informs the doctor that his patient may have contracted a serious infectious disease as a result of his work, which may require his isolation, and requests the doctor to contact the laboratory director. This seemed to be a sensible enough requirement, particularly as the symptoms of laboratory-acquired infections may not be the same as those of the naturally-acquired disease. There was a great deal of opposition, however, to what some people regarded as regimentation and interfering with individual rights. But as Howie and Collins (1980) pointed out, it does not seem to worry those who habitually carry such cards along with credit cards, bankers cards, kidney donor cards, corneal donor cards, allergy cards, driving and other licences and club membership cards.

The WHO (1993) and the HSE (1991a) endorse this requirement. The card should carry the following information:

(1) the employee's name, address and telephone number;
(2) the work address, nature of employment and brief statement of the hazards involved;
(3) the contact telephone number and/or address of
    (a) the employee's general medical practitioner;
    (b) the appropriate supervisor at work (laboratory director/consultant or manager at work;
    (c) the occupational health service (if any).

Copies of these cards should be kept at the place of employment.

Laboratory first aid

The word laboratory is used to qualify first aid here because some of the accidents that may happen in laboratories are outside the scope of ordinary first aid training. The subject is too large to be discussed here in detail and the reader is referred to e.g. Gunthorpe (1987), Edlich (1995), WHO (1997b). In the UK the *Health and Safety (First Aid) Regulations 1981* and its Revised Code of Practice (HSE, 1990) should be consulted.

It is highly desirable to have a qualified first-aider in the laboratory, but he should receive additional training in dealing with exposure to and ingestion of infectious, toxic and corrosive chemicals. Medically-qualified staff with adequate experience may not always be available, and many hospitals do not now have casualty departments. All staff should know who to contact if an accident occurs and where to send the patient.

The standard first aid kit for minor injuries should be in a prominent position and well signposted. Care should be taken with eye irrigation. The bottles of 'sterile' water, often growing algae and frequently contaminated with pseudomonads, should be scrapped and replaced by single-use packs (see Chapter 11).

Vaccination and immunization

These two terms are not synonymous. As Darlow (1972) has pointed out vaccination does not necessarily confer immunity. Serological evidence may be necessary to demonstrate that it does. Even then, immunity may be short-lived. Moreover, any immunity conferred by the available vaccines will have been assessed in terms of the infective (challenge) dose that is usually involved in naturally-acquired disease and is also related to the usual portal of entry. Laboratory workers may be exposed to much larger doses which may enter the body through different portals.

In spite of epidemiological evidence that some vaccines have been, and are, quite efficient in conferring immunity it is regrettable that some authorities have not offered vaccines to their staff. This may be due to personal inertia, the feeling that it is someone else's responsibility (family doctor, occupational health service) or even a belief that some laboratory infections are inevitable, and, a recent view, that if people do become infected then antibiotic treatment is usually effective.

In the larger microbiological research laboratories, however, vaccination programmes, with appropriate serological monitoring, are well-developed. In clinical laboratories the enforcement, by legal means or moral pressures, of codes of practice has also changed attitudes to preventive inoculations and in the UK, for example, it would be unthinkable to find an individual engaged in tuberculosis bacteriology who has not had BCG or evidence of a positive skin test.

This is not the signal for mass vaccinations of all laboratory workers against all possible infectious agents. Vaccination must be regarded as a secondary barrier and not as a means of avoiding the cost and possible inconvenience of effective primary barriers. Vaccination is not an alternative to safe techniques at the bench.

Choice of vaccines and recipients

Given the constraints mentioned above that challenge doses and routes of infection in laboratories may differ from those in other environments, that any immunity conferred may not prevent an individual from becoming a passive carrier or having a subclinical infection, and that some vaccines may be quite ineffective, a laboratory director, or his medical adviser has to choose which vaccine to give to which laboratory worker.

The important considerations are:

(1) the frequency with which the organisms concerned are encountered in the laboratory;
(2) the known incidence of infection with those organisms;
(3) the severity of the disease they may cause;
(4) who handles them.

For example, staphylococci, streptococci, many enterobacteria and oxidative Gram-negative rods are cultured daily in most laboratories, but they do not often cause laboratory infections. When they do the disease is not usually serious. On the other hand one never knows, in a clinical laboratory, when one may culture typhoid bacilli or receive a sputum containing large numbers of tubercle bacilli. A laboratory bench worker or animal technician may be at risk and merit vaccination but an office worker or glassware cleaner in the same building may not.

There is a case for having a basic list of vaccines for all workers, while reserving others for individuals who are particularly at risk. The list in Table 8.1 has been compiled from various current sources. Some of the prophylactics are readily available and laboratory staff may have been vaccinated in childhood. Booster doses, however, may be indicated. Some of the others in the list are restricted and consultations with the health authorities will have to be made for their release.

TABLE 8.1 Vaccines available for laboratory staff

Bacterial vaccines	*Viral vaccines*
Anthrax	Venezuelan, Eastern and
Whooping cough	Western encephalitis
Botulism	Tick-borne encephalitis[1]
Tetanus	Omsk haemorrhagic fever[2]
Diphtheria	Rift Valley fever[2]
Q fever	Influenza
Tularaemia	Hepatitis A
Haemophilus influenza b	Hepatitis B
Tuberculosis (BCG)	Kyasanur Forest fever
Neisseria meningitis A and C	Monkeypox[2]
Typhoid fever	Mumps
Cholera	Measles
Plague	Rubella[3]
	Varicella[2] (herpes zoster)

[1] Covers Central European, Russian spring-summer and strains of Absetterov, Hanzalova and Hypr viruses.
[2] Not available commercially. Consult health authorities.
[3] Women who have no immunity to rubella may be given the vaccine because of risk of fetal malformation.
Sources: DH (1992), CDC/NIH (1993), ISSA (1997).

Notes on some vaccinations

Anthrax
There is no case for general vaccination and it should be restricted to those who are exposed to the disease or to cultures. There are no contraindications, except that reactions may occur in people who have had the natural disease.

Botulinus
Vaccination is desirable only for people who work with the organism under conditions when toxin is produced. Severe reactions may indicate no further toxoid or a reduced dose.

Cholera
Laboratory infections are rare and use should be restricted. The vaccine confers only a limited immunity (3–6 months). It seems inadvisable to vaccinate during pregnancy.

Diphtheria
In developed countries most children receive toxoid (along with tetanus toxoid) and laboratory use should be confined to Schick-positive individuals who work directly with the organism. Laboratory infections are rare.

Eastern equine encephalitis (EEE)
Although laboratory infections are rare and the efficacy of the vaccine is not known it seems advisable to vaccinate individuals who work with the virus. Care is necessary with people who are sensitive to egg materials.

Hepatitis B
The (recombinant) vaccine is now generally available. There is a strong argument in favour of giving it to all laboratory staff, especially those who come into contact with blood. A combined hepatitis A and B vaccine is now available.

Influenza
Risks in the influenza laboratory are not sufficiently high to merit routine vaccination but on general health principles (avoidance of disease contracted elsewhere) vaccination with strains currently known or forecast to be prevalent may be useful.

Measles
Vaccination of adults is rarely necessary as nearly all individuals are immune by the time they leave school. Susceptible people working directly with the virus, however, might be vaccinated, but not if pregnant.

Plague
Laboratory infections are rare and vaccination should be restricted.

Poliovirus
Most young adults received the oral vaccine when at school and vaccination may therefore be restricted to those who work with poliovirus.

Q fever
This is a common laboratory-acquired disease and the agent is known to escape from laboratories. Although it is usually a mild disease, vaccination with *Coxiella burnetii* is indicated wherever Q fever work is done but egg-sensitive individuals should not be vaccinated.

Rabies
There is no case for general vaccination. Only a relatively few laboratories handle rabies material and vaccination is appropriate in those places, which always have well-organized prevention programmes. New vaccines are being developed at present.

Rubella
Laboratory infections are rare and the virus is not highly infectious. Pregnancy alters an individual's susceptibility. In developed countries most young girls have been immunized. Women of child-bearing age should be tested for rubella antibodies and vaccinated if none are present.

Smallpox
As this disease is officially extinct and only very few laboratories maintain stocks under WHO surveillance vaccination is considered unnecessary except in those establishments.

Tetanus
Tetanus toxoid is usually given to young people (along with diphtheria toxoid) and there are strong arguments for active immunization of the whole population. There seems to be no special case for immunizing laboratory workers on account of their occupation

Tick-borne encephalitis
The vaccine, which also protects against Central European, Russian spring-summer and strains of Absetterov, Hanzalova and Hypr viruses, should be reserved for those who work with these agents.

Tuberculosis
Although most young people in developed countries receive BCG vaccine while at school, some do escape the net and some immigrants who have not been immunized find work in laboratories. It is advisable to do skin tests on all new members of staff or to require them to provide evidence of having a positive reaction. Those with negative skin tests should be given BCG. There are strong arguments for applying these conditions to all clinical laboratory workers, not just those who work in microbiological laboratories.

Tularaemia
The numbers of laboratories working with *Francisella tularensis* is now limited and there is no case for vaccination in other establishments.

Typhoid fever
Typhoid is high on the list of laboratory-acquired infections and no clinical laboratory knows when it may expect to receive infected material or to culture

the organism. Monovalent typhoid vaccine is known to be more effective than TABC and except in cases of massive exposure, may protect 70–90% of personnel who receive it. Typhoid vaccine should not be given to workers who are receiving steroids.

Venezuelan equine encephalitis (VEE)
Vaccination is recommended only for those who work with virulent exotic strains as natural illness caused by 'domestic' strains may be less severe than vaccine reactions.

Yellow fever (YF)
Vaccination is recommended for individuals who work with virulent YF strains or with the 17D vaccine strain if they are exposed to high mouse passage virus that has reverted to virulence. Egg sensitivity, pregnancy, administration of corticosteroids and immunosuppressive drugs are contraindications.

DOSAGE AND FOLLOW-UP

It would not be appropriate here to detail dosage, as this varies with product. Guidance and other information may be obtained from health authorities and from WHO offices.

PROBLEMS OF CONTRAINDICATIONS AND REFUSAL

Problems may arise with staff who cannot tolerate some vaccine for medical reasons or who refuse vaccination on grounds of religion or militancy. When there are medical contraindications discussions are usually fruitful and accommodations, such as changing to another job within the laboratory can be made. When new appointments are made vaccination requirements can be incorporated into the job description or conditions of service, but when existing staff refuse vaccination, when, for example, new investigations are started, and also exercise their 'rights' not to be transferred to other work serious difficulties may arise. How far one can allow an individual to expose himself to infection becomes a moral issue. If, by doing so, he places other people at risk there may be redress from the courts in those countries that have occupational health legislation. There is no simple answer.

Chapter 9

Instruction and training

In the United Kingdom there is a legal requirement, under the *Health and Safety at Work etc. Act 1974* and the *Management of Health and Safety at Work Regulations 1992* for employers to provide information, instruction and training for their employees '... such as to ensure that persons at work on premises do not endanger themselves or others through exposure to substances hazardous to health.' (*Control of Substances Hazardous to Health Regulations 1994*: COSHH).

In many laboratories the information consists of a written local safety code of practice which, although it tells employees what they should or should not do, very rarely tells them why or explains the rationale of the instruction. There may or may not be a safety officer, whose duties, again, may or may not include training or instruction.

The ACDP (1995) states that 'In some cases, formal courses may be necessary, followed by refresher courses and lectures and other forms of instruction to keep personnel up to date with any changes that may have an impact on health and safety, for example the introduction of new equipment, materials and methods. A variety of audiovisual aids is available and some colleges and health authorities offer comprehensive course on microbiological safety.'

Regrettably, we have been unable to find this variety of visual aids (but see below). Nor do we know of any comprehensive (or other) courses on microbiological safety held by colleges or other authorities. The subject is sometimes mentioned briefly in respect of the regulations in the very popular management courses.

A few short courses were developed as a result, firstly, of the stimulus applied by a group of private individuals during the late 1970s, and, secondly, by the 'Howie' Code (DH, 1978a), but all petered out in the 1980s.

The Howie Report (Howie and Collins, 1980; not be confused with the 'Howie Code of Practice', DH 1978a) recommended officially sponsored courses and that the training of safety officers should be on a national scale to a national standard. The health services circular on training safety officers (DH, 1979b) set out a less than optimal syllabus, in spite of the fact that information was available from those who had made a study of these courses, and who possessed the necessary visual aids. It is of interest that the pre-course reading list in this circular did not contain the titles of any of the books that were readily available and which provide the reasons for the microbiological, chemical and other safety measures given but not explained in the Howie Code. A hardly relevant treatise on radiation protection, however, was included!

Some local health authorities responded by organizing courses and invited appropriate speakers. Others considered, quite erroneously, that any medical microbiologist or chief medical laboratory scientific officer must necessarily know all about laboratory safety. A few authorities organized courses on a do-it-yourself basis. Both kinds of local courses were short-lived.

In North America, such courses are the norm and standard textbooks treat the subject seriously (Liberman and Gordon, 1989; National Research Council, 1989; Rayburn, 1990) as does the American Society for Microbiology (Songer, 1993; Gershon and Zirkin, 1993). Courses are also held in Australia. The International Association of Medical Laboratory Technology is in favour of training in laboratory safety and has published a syllabus (IAMLT, 1992).

Who requires instruction?

The WHO subscribes to the 'train the trainer' system, the trainer in this case being the safety officer. Although this is a good principle, it is better to instruct every worker who can be spared to attend. Being spared, of course, is another problem. Many senior staff feel that they are indispensable, that they do not require instruction, or that it would be beneath their dignity. Nothing is further from the truth than the belief that graduates, medical laboratory scientific officers and technicians are all familiar with and always exercise good and safe laboratory practices.

The incidence of infections among ancillary staff also indicates that sterilizer attendants, glassware cleaners, janitors and cleaning ladies, as well as reception and office staff also need instruction, although not, of course, at the same level as the scientists and technicians.

Laboratories, especially those in hospitals and teaching institutions, have to co-exist with their neighbours. They usually share the same administrative, engineering and works services. Activities of one group may threaten the health and safety of the other. Again, instruction, but at a different level, is indicated.

These are but three target groups. Within the first group not all workers will need the same instruction. Biochemists, haematologists and histopathologists, for example, will need to learn only about the microbiological hazards that are inherent in their specific trades.

How the needs may be met

There are six ways in which instruction or training may be given:

(1) personal tuition and example by senior staff;
(2) in-service training;
(3) seminars and symposia;
(4) distance learning projects;
(5) journal-based learning;
(6) formal courses.

Personal tuition and example

This is an improvement on 'sitting next to Charlie' but it makes two assumptions. One is that the senior staff are actually doing the work. The other is that they are prepared to arrange this work so that they can give the tuition and set the example. This system works well where it is possible to do it on a one-to-one basis—where the learner first watches and listens, and then is watched—and still listens. Unfortunately it is difficult to achieve in large laboratories where the junior staff greatly outnumber their senior colleagues. Experience suggests that in many laboratories new entrants, and existing junior staff, receive very little guidance in safe practices—and sometimes not much in microbiological techniques—from the senior staff. There is a tendency to believe that the newcomer has been trained elsewhere, or at college. The modern trend in 'laboratory management' moves senior staff away from the work bench and into offices where their remoteness and preoccupation with administration and committees very often keeps them behind the times in technical methods and safe practices, especially where the former introduce new hazards.

Familiarity with certain microorganisms on the part of an experienced worker may lead to a contempt for their potential hazards, and a false sense of security and pride in his own prowess, especially if he has managed, in his own estimation to avoid infection. Darlow (personal communication) found rising titres against various agents in the sera of laboratory workers who have had no overt symptoms. This suggests subclinical infections, and, although these may have been acquired in spite of good technique, they could also be the result of breaches in good practice.

Personal instruction by senior staff can be highly successful. It can also lead to a skill in the safe handling of one microorganism that would be hazardous if applied to another. It may even result in the inculcation of unsafe practices.

In-service training

This differs from personal tuition in that all members of the staff are instructed in the same principles, and in practices depending on their status. Thus, most institutions would have two levels, one for all scientific and technical staff; the other for all support or ancillary staff. It should be a continuous, not a once-for-all-time process, both for those who instruct and those who are instructed, and should include basic training, with revision, and take care of techniques, equipment and agents which are new to that laboratory.

This kind of training may be very successful in large institutions or organizations where there is a biosafety officer, especially if this appointment is fulltime and is held by a microbiologist who heads a laboratory which is intended to monitor the activities of other scientists and departments in the interests of the safety of the staff and surrounding population. Microbiologists whose responsibilities for safety are only part-time may or may not keep themselves informed of developments within and outside their institution, and conflicts of interests and commitments may in either case make it difficult for them to arrange and keep active a programme of in-service safety training, particularly if they are relatively junior in rank.

Seminars and symposia

These are essentially 'one-off' meetings for lectures and discussions and take several forms. They may be local, within one laboratory or institution; they may be less local in that they are organized by professional bodies; or they may be arranged by companies who organize symposia of all kinds.

Local or institutional seminars may be part or instead of in-service training and may or may not include outside speakers. It is best if there are external contributions as these may question whether all is well within the institution itself. This may be embarrassing to the management. One unfortunate aspect of local seminars, however, is the reluctance of senior staff and research workers to attend along with their laboratory superintendents and technicians.

Seminars and meetings organized by professional bodies may be quite good or quite awful depending on the choice of speakers. It is a pity, however, that attendance at them is usually restricted to members of the bodies that arrange them.

There are two unfortunate features of the commercial enterprises. One is the price: the company promoting a symposium must meet its running costs, including fees for expert speakers (usually nominal or nil for other kinds of meetings). It also expects to make some profit, although there is no evidence that this is other than modest. The other feature is the choice of topics. Within a given subject the range of topics must be wide. If it is too restricted only a limited number of people can be expected to attend and the symposium ceases to be a commercial proposition. Although the organizers of these meetings seem to tread a middle course, it may well be that any individual who attends them will find himself paying a large fee to attend five or six lectures only one or two of which are relevant to his needs. Although seminars and symposia often make valuable contributions to microbiological safety and good laboratory practice they are too infrequent to be counted as serious instruction within the context of this chapter.

The interest and concern about genetic manipulation has stimulated a number of courses in mainland Europe (Germany and the Netherlands in particular) and these do have a direct bearing on safety in traditional microbiology.

Distance learning projects

These were introduced into colleges a few years ago in the form of voice-tape and slide presentations, or slides with reading matter. Recently video-tapes, either of the continuous or single frame variety, have become popular. Their great advantage is that they can be used by single individuals or by groups of any size at almost any time and place. The tape-slide and the script-slide presentations need only equipment that is readily available, and the video equipment may be rented. The tapes and slides may be purchased, hired or otherwise circulated.

Unfortunately only a small amount of material relevant to microbiological safety is available in the UK, although much more is available in the USA. This useful method of instruction is mentioned here, however, to indicate its potential, and if more material can be made and distributed internationally it could be of great value. It could be used alone or to supplement other kinds of instruction.

Journal-based learning

This is a comparatively new development. Trainees are given lists of journals through which they are expected to sift and extract information about subjects specified by their mentors. Unfortunately, as indicated on p. 2, there are not many papers in current journals about safety in microbiology but many papers and references, going back several years, can now be found on the Internet.

Formal courses of instruction

It is obvious that none of the approaches discussed above is optimal, and they raise two further questions: who instructs the instructors and what can be done for the staff of places where these options are not possible or are demonstrably inadequate? The obvious solution is the formal course of instruction. Such courses have proved to be valuable and successful in the USA over a number of years and also by the WHO. But their organization is complex and a number of factors must be considered. These are:

(1) objectives of the course;
(2) identity and numbers of the target groups;
(3) existing courses which might be adapted or extended;
(4) which organization should administer them and bear the cost;
(5) course content or syllabus for each target group;
(6) selection of tutors and instructors;
(7) availability of training aids and facilities.

OBJECTIVES

Although these should be obvious it is necessary to define them for administrative reasons: someone has to justify the cost. It may be stated that the courses are intended to create an awareness of microbiological hazards that might endanger the health of the individual and community. It must be emphasized that a qualification in science, microbiology or technology does not imply or guarantee any knowledge of microbiological and other laboratory hazards. It is important to define these objectives to avoid the inclusion or imposition of irrelevancies. Courses of any kind are frequently regarded by educationalists and training officers as vehicles for propagating their pet subjects or theories such as 'management techniques' and 'communicative skills'. Apart from the waste of time and therefore the exclusion of more useful subjects, such deviations from the proper objectives are likely to discourage genuine participants.

TARGET GROUPS

The nature and frequency of courses of instruction will depend on the kind of work done by prospective participants and their numbers.

The largest group contains the professional laboratory workers who must be considered together as they all need the same kind of instruction. In this age of databanks, registration and membership of professional bodies it should be possible to determine how many people in this group are in employment and how many enter employment each year. From these figures it should be possible to calculate the numbers who would need instruction in, say, a 5-year period, as not all of the 'backlog' could, or would need to attend the first flush of courses.

The other groups, ancillary laboratory staff, and hospital or institution administrative and engineering staff would be numerically smaller and less of a problem because their instruction could become part of the courses or training already in existence.

EXISTING COURSES

As indicated above there are now no courses for professional laboratory staff in the UK. In the USA formal courses are arranged by the Centers for Disease Control and Prevention, the National Institutes of Health, the National Institute of Occupational Health and Safety, the National Cancer Institute and the American Association of Clinical Pathologists, as well as in certain universities. In Canada they are organized by the office of Biosafety of the Laboratory Centre for Disease Control, and in Australia by the Occupational Health and Training unit of the Australian National University.

The administrative, managerial and works service staff of hospitals and other institutions that have microbiology and pathology departments frequently attend what are known as 'management courses'. It should be possible to graft onto these one or two lectures illustrating laboratory hazards.

Induction and general information courses are not infrequently arranged for ancillary workers and instruction on laboratory hazards could be included in these.

ADMINISTRATIVE RESPONSIBILITY AND COST

There seems to be some disagreement about responsibility for instruction in microbiological and other aspects of laboratory safety: whether it is that of the health authorities or of the education departments. The arguments seem to be semantic and to revolve around the interpretations of the words education, teaching, training and instruction. In reality they relate to cost. It should be obvious, however, to anyone outside such controversies that (a) laboratory safety concerns the health of the individual and the community and is therefore part of preventive medicine, (b) education departments are very experienced at organiz-ing the communication of all forms of skill and knowledge, whichever term is used to describe it; oddly enough, most health authorities employ 'training officers'. It does not really matter which body accepts responsibility so long as artificial administrative boundaries do not affect adversely the quality of the instruction. Professional organizations should be involved as they could provide some of the lecturers (but see below). Caution is necessary, however, to avoid the intrusion of vested interests and irrelevancies.

COURSE CONTENTS

Three outlines of course contents, essentially as described by Collins (1980a) and WHO (1993), are given here. Table 9.1 is aimed at scientific and technical staff, Table 9.2 at ancillary workers, including laboratory clerical staff and Table 9.3 at administrative, management and engineering staff. It will be noted that each has a section devoted to non-microbiological hazards. Although these are outside the scope of this book they are nevertheless of considerable importance.

The detailed contents of Table 9.1 help to emphasize the necessity for keeping the objectives of these courses very much in mind. Practical and useful assistance must be given to the participants. Generalizations are seldom useful as time is limited and many specific questions are likely to be asked, although a good syllabus with appropriate lecturing expertise will ensure that the 'whys' are explained and understood.

Practical work is a problem. It is only possible if the number of students is small and large teaching laboratories are available. It is an ideal to be aimed at, but unlikely to be achieved until these courses become generally accepted and their value is understood by those who hold the purse strings.

The courses illustrated in Tables 9.2 and 9.3 are designed for small numbers of participants.

TABLE 9.1 Instruction in laboratory safety. Course content for professional staff

(1) Legal responsibilities of employer and employee.
(2) Planning safe laboratories. Architectural and engineering requirements v protection of staff and community. Basic and containment laboratories. Siting of hazardous operations and materials.
(3) Infectious hazards. Routes of infections. History of laboratory-acquired disease. Classification of infectious agents on the basis of hazard. Assessments of risk and levels of containment.
(4) Aerosols and infectious airborne particles. How released, techniques for measurement and methods of control.
(5) Design, installation, testing and use of microbiological safety cabinets.
(6) Microbiological hazards in laboratories engaged in other aspects of pathology.
(7) Transport of infectious material.
(8) Decontamination. Autoclaves and disinfectants. Emergency actions.
(9) Personal protection. Hygiene and protective clothing. Health and medical surveillance. Immunization.
(10) Chemical hazards. Toxic and carcinogenic substances. Gases and vapours, liquefied and compressed. Threshold limit values. Normal and emergency disposal of chemical wastes. Radiation hazards.
(11) Electrical and mechanical safety. Equipment-related hazards.
(12) Laboratory fires. Prevention and control.
(13) Laboratory first aid. Burns, scalds, cuts. Accidental ingestion or exposure to infectious or toxic materials. Resuscitation.
(14) Accidents and incidents. Reporting. Emergency actions.
(15) Laboratory security. Vandalism and aberrant behaviour. Access controls.
(16) Conducting safety audits.

TABLE 9.2 Instruction in laboratory safety. Course content for ancillary staff

(1) The work of different departments and sections of the laboratory.
(2) Workers' and employers' legal rights and duties. Necessity for reporting accidents and injuries.
(3) Personal hygiene and avoidance of infection. Protective clothing. Eating, drinking and smoking. Biohazard signs and restricted areas.
(4) Specimen reception and packaging.
(5) Use and limitations of disinfectants.
(6) Autoclave practice and waste disposal.
(7) The hazards inherent in particular pieces of laboratory equipment, particularly in unskilled hands.
(8) Chemical hazards. Limitations in use of chemicals.

TABLE 9.3 The laboratory and its environment. Course content for administrative and service staff

(1) Outline of work done in each laboratory department and section.
(2) Infectious and chemical hazards that may be generated in the laboratory and which threaten the health of any employee and the general public.
(3) Hazards to laboratory workers and others that may be generated by non-laboratory staff (e.g. by cutting services without warning; arbitrary actions).
(4) Potential hazards in the cleaning of laboratories and the maintenance of services and fabric.
(5) Disposal of hazardous and unpleasant waste.
(6) Security: flood, fire and vandalism.

A syllabus for training in laboratory safety has also been published by the International Association of Medical Laboratory Technology (IAMLT, 1992).

TUTORS AND LECTURERS

If the courses are to be credible and are to satisfy the stated objectives and the requirements of those attending them it is obvious that the tutors should be established, well known experts in their chosen subjects. They should also be able to teach. 'Instant experts' abound but should be avoided. Organizers should beware of the commonly held opinion that anyone who has achieved a senior office necessarily knows a great deal about laboratory safety. Good, knowledgeable specialists in this field are few in number at present, but they are available and their numbers are increasing. Care must also be taken to avoid duplication, e.g. by having two people to talk about the same subject. The courses illustrated in Tables 9.2 and 9.3 would each require only one tutor, but again he should experienced and well-informed. It is just as important to give correct instruction to these target groups as it is to professional laboratory staff.

TRAINING AIDS

These are usually slides, video-tapes and films. Experienced lecturers possess personal collections of these and may be relied upon to use them. A limited amount of such material is available commercially, from the US Public Health Service, London University and Memo Media Marketing organization, Utrecht, the Netherlands. A videotape has been produced by the HSE (1997) about working at Containment Level 3. It must be remembered, however, that these 'visual aids' are not substitutes for good lecturers and personal contact between the teacher and the taught; they well may be, if the distance learning material mentioned above becomes available.

Conclusions

Training in microbiological laboratory hazards and safety precautions needs to be carefully organized and may entail some financial outlay, but it could become 'cost-effective' in terms of individual and community health. It should be regarded as a branch of preventive medicine.

Chapter 10

The safe working environment

This chapter is concerned with those aspects of laboratory planning which may affect the exposure to infection of the individuals who work in them as well as those whose contacts with them are occasional or peripheral. It is not intended to discuss overall design. For architectural and engineering details the reader is referred to the Hospital Building Note No. 15: Hospital Pathology Department (DH, 1991), British Occupational Hygiene Society (BOHS, 1993), Lees (1993) and Crane and Richmond (1993).

As long ago as 1951 Smadel pointed out that architectural design could influence the hazards of working in laboratories. The effect of design on microbiological safety was considered in the study made by Phillips (1961) when he visited 102 laboratories in 18 countries. In his own words: 'Good design features for buildings and rooms can be valuable in containing and controlling infectious agents. If a building is not properly designed its features can complicate or limit efforts to minimize risks of infection and cross contamination.'

Elsewhere in his report Phillips describes some laboratory infections and epidemics caused by the spread of airborne microorganisms from one room to other parts of a building. He found a number of design faults in the ventilation systems of laboratories he visited.

Phillips tended to place the responsibilities for poor and therefore hazardous design of laboratories on lack of adequate financial provisions by the administrative organizations and the difficulties laboratory directors have in convincing administrators that, in effect, laboratories are likely to cost much more than offices. He also noted that laboratory directors did not necessarily have enough knowledge of infectious hazards, laboratory-acquired infections or developments in building design that would allow them to argue their case successfully.

Howie and Collins (1980) noted that some very serious hazards to health and safety had been built into some new laboratories, and pointed out that other, serious design faults had been observed that although not immediately hazardous could create stressful conditions and inconveniences that could lead to errors and accidents. Somewhat unfairly, they placed the responsibility for bad design of some laboratories on the failure of architects to consult the users at all stages of design and building and to accept the guidance of the appropriate building note published by the Department of Health (DH, 1991).

In fact, the architect is instructed by a 'design team' which represents the client authority. It is the design team that must bear the responsibility for bad

207

design and for failure to consult with the users. Of course, a design team may argue that it has a whole building to design and it cannot have a committee consisting of users from every department. As a result it is not only laboratories that are frequently poorly designed, but other departments as well.

It is sometimes argued that the time-scale in building mitigates against good, up-to-date design; that the user of 10 years ago (now retired) was consulted, and the laboratory is to his design. An even more specious argument is that the laboratory is a new one and the users cannot be consulted as they have not yet been appointed! These arguments completely ignore the considerable amount of expertise and information that is available nationally, from other users, from faulty design in other laboratories, from professional bodies and health department architects and engineers many of whom have encountered design problems in earlier buildings. Much of the information is not new; much, for example, that concerns microbiological safety cabinets and directional ventilation was available 30 years ago. Much better use could have been made in the UK of the building notes, especially Building Note 15. Although this note came in for some criticism it contained, for all its imperfections and anomalies (easily resolved by consultation with laboratory workers), enough useful guidance for the building of reasonably good and safe laboratories.

It is to be hoped that we have seen the last of the regrettable experiences of laboratory workers who have moved into new premises, the design of which they were not consulted about, and from which they were, for no good reason, excluded during the design and building stages. On several occasions such 'victims' have found that their old laboratory was safer and more convenient. Although some quite good laboratories have been completed, others still leave much to be desired. Discombe (1985) drew attention to architectural failures apart from those concerned with laboratory design. These include large windows which make rooms cold, flat roofs and poor heating arrangements which result in laboratories that are either too hot or too cold.

Another problem that arises in the construction of a new laboratory, which may have been gestating for several years, concerns the inevitability of the perpetuation of bad design. If an error is discovered, or new developments in laboratory work make a change in design desirable, it is always too late to make that change. One is told that the contracts have been made, the quantities have been surveyed and that alterations will have to wait until the building is handed over. By then it may be too late, and money may not be available. Alterations which would cost little during building become very expensive when building is complete. Reports of the cost of rectifying design faults have emphasized the necessity for proper consultation (Committee of Public Accounts, 1981–82; *Daily Telegraph*, 1982a,b).

In contrast with the problems arising in new buildings alterations to existing premises seem to be more successful. Phillips (1961) noted that some older structures which have been extensively renovated provided better safety features than some new buildings. This has also been our experience in the UK, not only with old buildings, but with some of the newer structures. The Code of Practice (DH, 1978) and the interest taken by the Health and Safety Inspectorate resulted in the upgrading of not a few unsatisfactory premises. When this is done no design team is involved. There is, instead, direct consultation between users and architects and engineers, and there is a clear set of rules for both to follow. The result has been some excellent improvements in safety, comfort and convenience.

The 'barrier system'

The principle of this system (Figure 10.1) is to place barriers that prevent, or at least minimise the escape of biological agents with attendant risks to workers, the general population and the the environment. *Primary* barriers are placed around the agent; *secondary* barriers around the workers to protect them and hence their contacts outside the laboratory, and *tertiary* barriers around the whole building as a safety net in case the other two barriers are breached.

Location of laboratories

There are three equally important considerations when it is proposed to build a new laboratory—the environment, the site and the views of the local people.

The environment

Laboratories cannot exist in isolation: they will always have some impact on the environment. For this reason some states and local authorities require a formal environmental statement and/or planning permission before a laboratory can be built.

The site

The site should be surveyed geologically and with respect to climate. An institute placed on unstable ground e.g. in earthquake-prone areas, may suffer considerable damage, including the escape of laboratory animals, as happened in Alaska (Feltz and McAllister, 1964), at Sendai in 1978 and Kobe in 1995 (Shibata, 1997). Laboratories in areas that are subject to flooding, tidal waves,

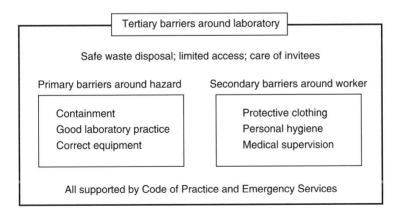

Figure 10.1 The 'barrier system'. (Reproduced from Collins (1988). *Safety in Clinical and Biomedical Laboratories* by permission of Chapman and Hall)

hurricanes, etc. may also received damage that leads to the escape of hazardous microorganisms.

Views of local residents

Consultations with the local residents and users of other facilities are essential. This will avoid objections to planning consents and possible public disaffection after the facility is built. The public needs to know what work will be done and if it is proposed to handle any microorganisms which they perceive to be a threat to their health. Bland assertions that all is safe will not suffice. Reports of escapes of pathogens from 'safe' laboratories into the community have been well documented in the news media. The World Health Organization (WHO, 1997a) recommends that 'high-level containment or high-risk laboratories should be located away from . . . public areas . . .'.

Position of laboratories in buildings

Unless a laboratory is to be a single purpose building—which is ideal, but does itself pose problems—it has to be fitted into a complex with many other departments. The ultimate site usually depends on the whims of the design team and the relative strengths of the heads of departments, if they are allowed to compete. The laboratory may therefore end up, to cite existing examples seen in recent years, in the basement, in the centre of a tower block, behind an ornate façade and therefore with a bizarre shape, or hurriedly added as an afterthought on whatever bit of ground was left over. When a site is to be allocated to a laboratory it is sensible to consider the impact it may have on surrounding departments.

There is no direct evidence that laboratories contribute to cross infection in hospitals, but Phillips (1961) gives examples of the spread of infections around buildings containing microbiological laboratories. As laboratories not only harbour infectious materials but also concentrate pathogens into large amounts it would be folly indeed to place them where infection can spread, e.g. near to intensive care units, open surgery areas and kitchens. Access of staff conveying specimens, and, if mortuaries are included, of cadavers, must be considered. Short cuts through wards, canteens and kitchens should be avoided.

Probably the worst site for any laboratory is at the core of a large, high building, where there are no windows. There is a curious belief among designers that laboratory workers do not need windows but that office staff must have them.

Most microbiological laboratories need microbiological safety cabinets and provision must be made for conducting the effluent to the atmosphere. The theory that it is safe to recirculate air from safety cabinets back into a room should be discounted (see p. 126) as none of the advocates of the procedure will accept this air into their own rooms. Ducting is therefore necessary to the appropriate exhaust point, and it is less than sensible (and also very expensive) to duct air through other parts of the building, where it may leak into other rooms. This problem is considered further under 'Heating, ventilation and lighting' (see below).

All these considerations lead to the conclusion that clinical microbiological laboratories are best sited on the top floors of hospital buildings, or in separate buildings some distance from the main blocks. Objections to such sites are frequently made on the grounds that they are too far removed from outpatient clinics. It is difficult to see why outpatients have to attend laboratories; inpatients do not and usually cannot. Specimen collecting facilities do not have to be in or attached to laboratories. Indeed it might be safer for the patients if they are elsewhere. Blood and other specimens are rarely collected nowadays by professional laboratory workers. Phlebotomists have taken over those duties. Rooms for taking blood and collecting other specimens can be near to clinics. They can be placed several floors below the laboratories and connected to them by small hoists (elevators) or 'dumb waiters'. Another possibility is the pneumatic tube system which has been introduced in some hospitals for the rapid distribution of drugs and the transfer specimens from phlebotomy rooms to laboratory reception areas.

Functions and shapes of rooms

Several rooms with different functions may be required to form a microbiology department. Industrial organizations may require only Containment Level 1 laboratories but hospitals and research establishments will probably require both Level 2 and Level 3 (but not Level 4) laboratories. The department may also require two preparation rooms, one for preparing culture media and reagents and the other for the treatment of used and contaminated materials and waste; a specimen reception room; one or more offices; a store; accommodation for staff clothing; a staff room; and lavatories. Built-in cold rooms and incubators may be added to the list.

Some designers divide laboratory areas according to function. Thus 'primary space' is said to be where the professional work is done; 'secondary space' is for support services, offices, etc.; and 'circulation' space means corridors and areas that will allow people to get from one room to another. It is difficult to see why any distinction is made between primary and secondary spaces and why this should involve calculations. Preparation and sterilizing rooms are just as important as laboratories. These predeterminations are often made without consultation and could lead to expensive alterations. One frequently hears complaints from occupiers of laboratories that the distribution of space is suboptimal or quite wrong.

Hazard zoning

This is a more sensible system. The principle is to designate zones ranging from 'safe' to 'highly hazardous' (WHO, 1997a).

This may be modified for microbiology departments, providing four zones—safety, low, medium and high hazard.

Safety zone: Here there would be the entrance and reception areas for visitors, offices, stores for non-hazardous materials, lavatories and cloakrooms, first aid and emergency control facility; specimens may be received in this area, but not unpacked.

Low hazard zone: In this zone materials that have been sterilized or disinfected are processed, culture media are prepared and chemicals are stored.

Medium hazard zone: This is where specimens are unpacked, work is done with microorganisms at Level 2 and infectious waste is autoclaved.

High hazard zone: This zone if for work with organisms at Level 3.

Table 10.1 suggests activities and equipment etc. suitable for each hazard zone.

Sensible planning requires that all rooms within each zone are interchangeable. This entails moveable partitions and 'flexibility'. Much good sense has been written about this kind of design, e.g. in Building Note 15 (DH, 1991), BOHS (1993) and by Lees (1993). Several systems have been developed by laboratory furnishing companies in Europe and America. The principle is that there are no, or few internal load-bearing walls so that the space may be divided into 'modules' by partitions which can be moved when occasion demands, subject to the vertical and horizontal distribution of services which are run in ducts or 'spines'. A laboratory room may consist of one or more modules and even half modules are possible. But very large laboratories, made up of a number of modules, are undesirable. The so-called 'open plan' laboratories, like 'open plan' offices seem to attract enthusiasm only from those individuals who are not required to work in them. Several separate laboratory rooms are safer

TABLE 10.1 Hazard zoning in microbiology laboratories

Activity	Zone	Equipment, etc.
Level 3 laboratory		
Processing and storage of Group 3 agents and materials. Decontamination of Group 3 agents and used materials.	HIGH HAZARD ZONE	Microbiological safety cabinets[1]. Dedicated[2] incubators, centrifuges, refrigerators and deep freezers. Dedicated[2] autoclave. Dedicated[2] handbasins
Level 2 laboratory		
Unpacking specimens. Processing and storage of Group 2 agents and materials. Decontamination of Group 2 agents and used materials.	MEDIUM HAZARD ZONE	Microbiological safety cabinet[1]. Incubators, refrigerators and deep freezers. Autoclave[3], handbasins
Technical services areas		
Media, etc. preparation. Washing and sterilization of decontaminated equipment. Disposal of decontaminated waste. Storage of non-flammable and non-volatile chemicals.	LOW HAZARD ZONE	Clean air cabinet. Autoclave.[4] Incubators, refrigerators and deep freezers.
Primary services		
Specimen reception[5]. Admin offices. Staff rest rooms. Cloakrooms and lavatories.	SAFETY ZONE	Entrance Normal office and leisure furniture. Lockers. Sanitary facilities

[1] Usually Class I, but Class II for cell/tissue culture work.
[2] Dedicated: For use only for activities in that zone.
[3] For decontaminating Group 2 infectious materials.
[4] For sterilizing reusable materials after decontamination and washing.
[5] But not unpacking.

than one very large one because they restrict hazards and the consequences of accidents to a smaller number of people. This was emphasized over 30 years ago (Frazer, 1972) and is, of course, the rationale of the containment laboratory principle for the handling of hazardous materials.

The standard module is the 'laboratory space unit' (LSU) and in Building Note 15 (DH, 1991) it is a rectangular room approximately 20 m² in area. It is claimed that a rectangular room is better than a square one as it gives a longer run of benching round the walls, approximately 14 m instead of 12 m for the same room area. While this is undoubtedly true it presupposes that the laboratory worker needs all that benching. In fact he needs floor space for free-standing equipment such as incubators, refrigerators and centrifuges. Some of this apparatus is quite deep, as much as 0.9 m. Microbiological safety cabinets to the British Standard (BS, 5726, 1992) are as wide, and Class II cabinets may be wider. There may be serious problems in accommodating such equipment in a narrow cell only about 3 m wide, while allowing some workers to sit at their benches and others to move around and possibly manoeuvre trolleys loaded with cultures. In addition, at least one worker in such a room needs somewhere to read and write and it is not good laboratory practice to have books and papers at a bench where they may be in contact with infectious materials (Figure 10.2).

There is space for a desk or writing table in the middle of a square room but not in a long, narrow one.

There is also the question of light. It has long been recognized that microbio-logical laboratories should be given a north light and that microbiologists like to work under a window during the hours of daylight. The narrow LSU allows fewer windows and less space to work under them. Long narrow rooms require more artificial light, which is a financial consideration (see also p. 218).

It has been argued that square rooms would make a building smaller or narrower. This need not be so; space between laboratory rooms and corridors

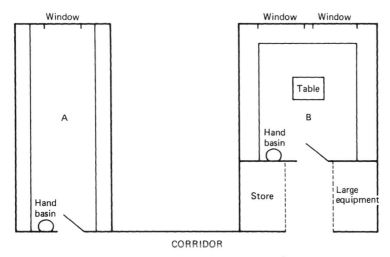

Figure 10.2 Two rooms which are the same size—approximately 20 m². Room A is long and narrow, gives approx. 12 m of narrow benching, has poor natural light, no space in the middle. Room B is square, also gives 12 m of benching, much more natural light and room for a writing table in the middle. There is space for storage and large equipment between room and corridor. This does not need natural light and saves storage space elsewhere

could be used for local storage. Store rooms do not need daylight. This is also shown in Figure 10.3 (p. 220).

Containment Levels 1 and 2 laboratories

Although Containment Levels 1 and 2 laboratories are considered to be adequate for work with microorganisms which offer minimal or low risk to the worker the potential is enough to merit design features additional to those of say, school science laboratories and offices. The features to be considered include:

(1) the size and shape of rooms;
(2) access by staff who do not work in them;
(3) materials of floors, walls and ceilings;
(4) heating, ventilation and lighting;
(5) benching and services;
(6) furniture and fittings.

Sizes of rooms; working space

A safe working environment implies, among other things, enough working space. The handling of hazardous material in crowded and confined conditions increases the likelihood of accidents, either directly or by placing the worker under stress.

When new laboratories are designed the area made available may be calculated according to the estimated workload. The latter will certainly increase annually and therefore any new laboratory that is designed to cope with the existing load is unlikely to be large enough within a year or two. Various formulas have been presented from time to time, which, it is alleged, will allow designers to predict the required area from the number of samples or specimens received or tests performed. These formulas cannot take into account changes in the nature of the work, new techniques and equipment and sudden changes in population and demand, none of which is predictable. An alternative approach is to relate the space required to the number of staff, allowing for a possible increase—never likely to be large, and excluding senior people who merit their own rooms. Although the average space per person (56.5 m^2) in Phillips's (1961) survey is almost the same as the official requirement of the US Army Biological Laboratories (Fort Detrick) at that time, over half of the laboratories seen by Phillips provided less space ($9.3–46.5 \text{ m}^2$).

Those laboratories where the more hazardous materials are handled should be allocated more space per worker, e.g. 18.6 m^2 per person according to Frazer (1972) and DH (1978).

Calculations and statements about the space required for laboratory work can be misleading. It is never quite clear whether the space per worker includes large pieces of equipment. The most important part of what designers call 'free space' is, in the context of safety, the length of bench, uncluttered by permanent apparatus, that is available to each worker. Little has been written about this. It is now generally accepted in the UK that each worker should be given 3-m run of benching, not more than half of which is occupied by permanent equipment, and 24 m of free air space (DH, 1991).

Access

Access to laboratory areas by people who do not work in them should be strictly limited. This is to protect such people against possible infection or other hazards, as well as to protect the laboratory workers against aberrant behaviour and unannounced interference with services (like switching off the electricity when safety cabinets are in use). Members of the general public, and especially children, should get no further than the reception areas or waiting rooms. It is more difficult to restrict the entry of the staff of other departments but some arrangements should be made between managements whereby authority to move about and perform service and maintenance work is given by the laboratory director or supervisor. Even authorized visitors should be encouraged to go first to the reception area or office.

Floors, walls and ceilings

Serious, as well as minor, accidents may occur in laboratories if people slip on floors, trip over irregularities in the surface, and drop hazardous materials. In the interests of safety, therefore, floors should be slip-resistant, seamless or have welded seams, be impermeable to liquids and resistant to most, if not all, chemicals that are normally used in the laboratories. There are no problems in meeting these requirements: the materials are available and are in use in many hospital, university and industrial buildings. Fanciful and artistic features should be resisted. These include concrete tiles, marble, wood blocks, linoleum and carpeting, all of which we have observed, either in use, or at the design stage. The junctions of floors and walls should be coved and doorway thresholds should be flat, not raised to create difficulties with the movements of trolleys.

The surfaces of walls and partitions might be splashed with infectious materials if there is an accident. They should therefore be smooth, impervious and easily cleaned, not rough and absorbent. Epoxy and polyurethane finishes are available. Bizarre colour schemes and 'murals' should be avoided. Far from being 'restful and interesting' as some designers claim, they are disturbing and likely to cause stress to people who are doing close and possibly hazardous work. Windows, which are essential for humanitarian and psychological reasons, should be sealable, but not necessarily sealed. Any window through which the sun can shine at any time of the working day should be fitted with external shades or internal blinds. If blinds are used they should be Venetian or semi-opaque. Those made of loosely woven or spun fibres, through which the sun's rays can shine or even be concentrated, are quite useless in laboratories. Doors should be fire-resistant (20 min) and fitted with vision panels ('wired Georgian') to avoid collisions when people are carrying infectious or hazardous materials (a common accident). This combination is possible in spite of the protestations of some designers.

Ceilings also need to be impermeable and should be coved to the walls. False or floating ceilings are generally undesirable, but if it is necessary to hide pipework they might be permitted providing that there is a proper ceiling above them and not a space running on over other rooms.

Openings in walls and ceilings for the entry of pipes, etc. should be sealed around such pipes. Designers should keep in mind the possibility that a room may need fumigation and this should be possible without placing the occupants of adjacent rooms in jeopardy from the fumigant.

Heating, ventilation and lighting

HEATING

Provided that a laboratory is adequately and sensibly heated (or in warm climates is cooled) to within the limits prescribed by most governments or their health and safety organizations, there are no microbiological hazards inherent in keeping a building warm. Unfortunately, there are some methods of space heating that make laboratories uncomfortable places in which to work. Discomfort causes stress and stress may lead to accidents. Most rooms can be heated by radiators or steam pipes around the walls and near to the floor. This system works well in laboratories and has the great advantage to the laboratory workers that it is under their control, i.e. they, and not a remote individual, controls the temperature of the laboratory. It also has the advantage to the engineer that it is relatively simple and commonplace and easy to maintain.

It has been argued that one cannot have wall radiators and wall benches. This is untrue. There are many laboratories that have both. Alternative heating systems include steam coils behind false ceilings and ducted warm air. As pointed out above, false ('floating') ceilings are undesirable in microbiological laboratories which may need fumigating, and are unacceptable in Containment Level 3 laboratories which must be capable of being sealed. In addition, ceiling heating, whatever is said in theory, usually heats the top part of a person but not his legs and feet, and this leads to discomfort and stress. Moreover, such heating is not under local control. We know of a serious accident that was caused by this form of heating. The laboratory workers, suffering from cold feet, were permitted to have an electric fire on the floor. A woman tripped over the fire cable while she was carrying some cultures and sustained serious cuts on a hand and arm, which became infected (from the broken cultures) despite prompt medical attention.

The success of heating by mechanical ventilation in some laboratories can best be judged by the caustic remarks of its victims and the proliferation of electric fires, bottled gas fires and paraffin heaters. While mechanical ventilation seems to work well in the USA its efficiency in the UK is proclaimed mostly by its advocates but rarely by those who suffer from it. It is, however, intimately connected, where it is used, to the ventilation of laboratories and the buildings in which they are sited, and even more serious problems may arise as a result.

VENTILATION: THE CLEAN-TO-DIRTY AIRFLOW PRINCIPLE

Since the end of the Second World War a great deal has been learnt about the generation and dispersion of aerosols and infected airborne particles during laboratory manipulations (Chapter 2). The association of these with ventilation becomes significant when one considers the proportion (some 80%) of all known laboratory infections that have probably been acquired by inhaling infected particles and the fact that not a few of the victims were some distance away from the site of aerosol formation even in other parts of the same building or in one case outside it. Some of these incidents are described in Chapter 2.

It is known that the infectious agents are moved around the buildings by air currents produced by natural or mechanical ventilation. In natural ventilation infectious particles may travel from one area to another on the random air currents caused by the movement of people and the opening and closing of doors and windows. With positive mechanical ventilation, where air is forced into rooms and left to find its own way out, such movement of particles may be accelerated. A total-loss extract system, where air is removed from each room and make-up air enters from wherever it can will probably remove any particles generated in that room, but may well attract into it particles released in a room where the extract is not as efficient. In view of the difficulty, if not the impossibility, of keeping each room at the same pressure there is not much to choose between these two systems.

The mechanical ventilation system that recirculates air offers further problems. Theoretically, air is removed from rooms and corridors through one set of ducts and after filtration and the addition of 'make-up' air from atmosphere and adjusting to the desired temperature and humidity (conditioning or tempering) it is returned to the rooms by another set of ducts. When it works to the satisfaction of the occupants (who often refer to it as canned air because it is far from fresh) it can save a great deal of energy and therefore money. But the filters may not be effective, and it offers an excellent means of distributing infectious airborne particles from any source to a wide area. In addition, such air-conditioning arrangements have undoubtedly been associated with the dispersal of infectious airborne material from rooms. Some of the 'sick building syndrome' incidents have been caused by the multiplication of the organisms in the water used in the humidifying systems (see Collins *et al.*, 1997).

Ventilation systems designed to prevent the distribution of infectious airborne particles were developed during and after the Second World War, especially at the US Army Biological Laboratories at Fort Detrick, Maryland and the Ministry of Defence Microbiological Research Establishment, Porton Down, England. The principle is simple: more air is extracted from the rooms where hazardous materials are handled than from any other area. Close-fitting doors and, if necessary, air locks are used. This gives a pressure gradient so that air always flows from clean to potentially contaminated areas, i.e. from corridors to laboratories and not in the opposite direction. The air extracted from the contaminated areas may be ducted directly to atmosphere, either through microbiological safety cabinets or filtered first, according to the hazard group of the agents handled. This 'clean-to-dirty' airflow principle should not offer any problems to a competent ventilation engineer who is involved in the design of new Level 2 or Level 3 laboratories (see below).

It is not always necessary to fit microbiological safety cabinets into Levels 1 and 2 laboratories, but if this is to be done then all the details of siting, ducting and airflows discussed in Chapter 5 must be considered.

In general, six air changes per hour are adequate for Level 2 laboratories but 10 changes per hour are desirable for Level 3.

LIGHTING

Microbiologists spend much of their time examining small objects like colonies of bacteria and the contents of small tubes, and in performing tests with minute amounts of materials. Such work requires good general and local light, the former when daylight has faded and the latter all the time. The light is required over the work bench. Poor lighting can lead to accidents such as spillage of cultures and self-inoculation. Lack of consultation and incorrect decisions by design teams frequently result in the placing of general (ceiling) lights above and behind the seated workers so that they cast a shadow over their work. It is expensive to correct this design fault.

There is also opposition from some designers to adjustable bench lamps. Their arguments against local lighting are that the general lighting provided is adequate for all purposes and that bench lamps waste electricity and that trailing electricity cables are unsafe. In fact the provision of an adequate number of socket outlets minimizes that hazard.

Although ceiling lighting does not influence safety so long as there is enough of it, some saving in energy could be achieved if the switching arrangements permitted the rear, and darker part of the room to be illuminated without lighting up the window end, which may not at that time need it. It seems that most banks of fluorescent lamps in LSUs are switched parallel with the long axis of the room instead of parallel with the short axis.

Benches and services

The heights and widths of benches are frequently bones of contention between users and planners. Critical and close work with small apparatus is done sitting down. Therefore microbiologists need benches at which they can sit comfortably. There is, unfortunately, a tradition based on the design of chemical and 'science' laboratories that most people stand up to work and that any one who wishes to sit simply uses a high stool. Many ergonomic studies have been done on office and factory workers. These have been concerned with comfort, and the avoidance of stress and fatigue which may predispose accidents or physical illnesses such as backache. There is no reason why the findings in these investigations should not be applied to microbiologists. Sitting comfortably, with adequate back support, requires one's feet to be on the floor, not on the rail of a chair. It should be possible to rest the elbows on the front edge of the bench. Anthropometric dimensions are well documented, and for most people a bench-top which is 700–750 mm high is ideal. In reception and preparation areas, however, where people stand more of the time and move up and down the length of their benches 850–900 mm is a comfortable height.

The depth of benches should depend on the reach of the individual. If benches are too deep the rear becomes a dead area or dump, out of reach of the sitter, and, unless the service outlets are well placed it may be necessary for the worker to rise from his seat to turn on the gas or switch on the electricity. Anthropometric studies have indicated that 600–850 mm is a convenient depth. In practice, 600 mm is not all that convenient for microbiological work for two good reasons. The first is that it is often necessary to have large numbers of cultures and stocks of media for immediate use readily available and to store them temporarily at the back of the bench. They are usually in baskets or racks and they reduce the working space considerably. An extra 100–200 mm is highly desirable, and still brings the articles within the reach of the average person. The second reason relates to the depth of large bench equipment such as incubators, ovens, bench centrifuges and microbiological safety cabinets. A bench only 600 mm deep will not accommodate them. They protrude over the front edge, which may lead to instability. This problem has already been mentioned in connection with the shape of laboratory rooms. It is not in the interests of flexibility to have purpose-made benches for particular pieces of equipment which may be changed every few years.

Bench surfaces should be impervious to liquids, and not easily corroded or stained by chemicals. The modern laminates are excellent, but problems may be encountered with joins. Some products can be moulded into shape and provide coved front and raised rear edges. Even hard, polished wood makes a good bench surface. Colour is important. White surfaces reflect too much light and pretty colours can be disturbing. Buff or brown seem to be acceptable to most workers.

Microbiologists need gas and electricity services to their benches. Water and waste plumbing are not universal requirements each worker may not need a sink, as staining is best done away from the work-bench and water is rarely required for other purposes. Staining and utility sinks, and handbasins may be placed at the rear of the room. This has the advantage of economy in plumbing. Gas and electricity services can be provided from ducts or spines above and at the rear of benches. This allows flexibility with benches and free-standing equipment. It is sometimes argued that the horizontal ducting cannot be carried round the window end of a room, particularly if it consists of several LSUs. This argument should be resisted as all that is required is good planning. Ducting can be taken up and over doorways.

Each worker should have two gas taps and at least two electrical socket outlets, one of which would be used for adjustable lighting. More gas and socket outlets should be provided between workers to avoid long, trailing flexible tubing and cables which can create both microbiological and fire hazards. Socket outlets should also be provided in non-benched areas for free-standing equipment. Microbiologists rarely need vacuum lines or special gas supplies to their personal work-benches. If they are required at all, e.g. for anaerobic work, they can be piped to utility areas at the rear of the laboratory.

Figure 10.3 shows good and suboptimal benching and service arrangements in microbiological laboratories.

Furniture, fittings and free-standing equipment

Most of these have been considered already, as incidental to other design features. They affect microbiological safety only if they cause inconvenience. For example, under-bench and over-bench cupboards are often a source of nuisance.

Under-bench units should be mobile, so that they may be moved easily when necessary. But they should not be so mobile that they move when someone opens a door or a drawer. Over-bench cupboards are frequently too large. If the cupboards are low enough for workers to reach the top shelf easily they are likely to bang their heads on the bottom when they rise from their seats or reach to the rear of the bench. If the cupboards are raised to avoid this workers may have to climb up to reach inside them.

Handbasins have been mentioned already. Every laboratory should have at least one, and if more than 10 people work in one room there should be two basins. Laboratory workers should not be expected to wash their hands in sinks used for staining and down which chemicals, disinfectants (or even urine) are poured. Paper towel dispensers should be provided; communal cloth towels, e.g.

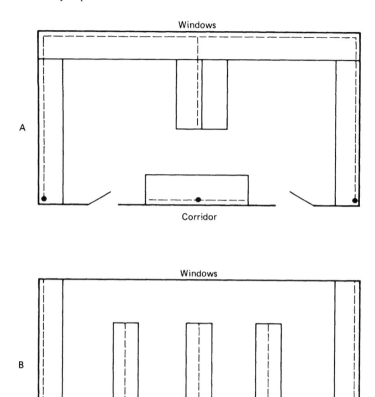

Figure 10.3 Good and poor bench arrangements in two rooms of the same size and shape. Room A allows good natural, lighting to the main work bench, easy escape in case of fire, simpler services and most benching. Room B gives poor natural lighting to any bench, escape from bays may be difficult, more services are required for less benching

roller towels, are considered to be unhygienic in offices, factories and food shops. They are even more so in microbiology laboratories. Towel machines are satisfactory if they are serviced so that they never run out but this ideal seems difficult to achieve. Pegs for protective clothing should be placed near to doorways.

Containment Level 3 laboratories

These rooms are intended for the safe handling of Hazard Group 3 biological agents. The object is to confine, or contain, the organisms so that only a minimum number of people are exposed to them. Hence the policy, hopefully proposed by some authorities, of designating a whole microbiology department as a Level 3 laboratory (to save the expense of providing one) is fatuous. A Level 3 laboratory, consisting of one LSU or its equivalent is suitable for one or two people only. If the amount of work merits more staff then additional, and separate Containment Level 3 laboratories should be provided.

All the design features advocated for Level 2 laboratories apply, with special emphasis on some of them. Although Level 3 laboratories may open off non-public corridors it is best if access is from other laboratories or though lobbies. If both are possible then the door to the corridor could be kept locked (key on the inside) or replaced by a breakthrough panel to allow emergency escape. There should be glass panels in the partitions or the doors so that the occupants of Containment Level 3 laboratories are visible to others, again a precaution in case of accidents. If parts of the laboratory cannot be seen through this panel mirrors, suspended from the ceiling, should make that area visible.

Microbiological safety cabinets are essential features of these laboratories. Care is needed in siting these in relation to airflows and staff movements, as explained in Chapter 5. They must be considered in conjunction with the clean-to-dirty airflow principle, whereby air flows from the corridor to the Level 2 laboratory and from there to the Level 3 laboratory (giving, ideally, 10 air changes per hour) and finally to atmosphere. One way of achieving this is to close off any mechanical ventilation inlets and outlets and to fit an extract fan in the window or external wall. This is likely to provide a better airflow into the room than the building ventilation system. The fan is linked electrically to the safety cabinet(s). Three switching positions are necessary:

(1) extract fan ON, cabinet exhaust OFF, when the room is occupied but the cabinet is not in use;
(2) extract fan OFF, cabinet exhaust ON, when the cabinet is in use;
(3) both OFF, for servicing, etc.

Transfer grilles must be fitted in or over the door to allow air to pass from the corridor to the Level 2 laboratory and from there to the Level 3 laboratory. These, like all pipe ducts, should be sealable so that rooms may be fumigated.

If space permits, a lobby could be provided between the two laboratories. Clothing can be changed there. An incubator room could open directly from a Level 3 laboratory and there should be enough storage space, e.g. for refrigerators and deep-freezers so that Hazard Group 3 organisms need not be kept elsewhere. The benching, services and equipment are otherwise similar to those in the Level 2 laboratory. A handbasin is essential, and should be near to the door, as should a bin for discarded overalls.

Access to Level 3 laboratories should be strictly limited and controlled and the doors should be kept locked when the rooms are not in use. The International Biohazard sign, with appropriate additional warning should be displayed on the outside of the door.

Suggested designs of Containment Level 3 laboratories are shown in Figure 10.4.

It is obvious that it is easy to convert any reasonably sited room into a Level 3 laboratory and that no great expense need be incurred. If suitable rooms are not available, it is probably better, and cheaper, to purchase factory-made structures that are delivered on site, completely fitted and engineered to a high standard.

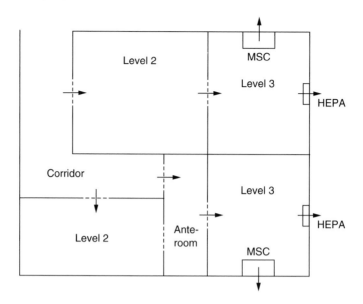

Figure 10.4 Designs for Level 3 laboratories. Arrows show direction of airflows

Connecting them to local services presents no problems. It is practicable to place these buildings alongside or on top of existing buildings.

Containment Level 4 laboratories

These laboratories are necessary for work with viruses which are particularly hazardous to laboratory workers and the general public (i.e. are in Hazard Group 4). As this work and the use of these agents is severely restricted in most countries by government regulations, a great deal of consultation is necessary, followed by close supervision in planning and building these laboratories. It is, of course, essential that individuals and organizations that have had experience in building and using these laboratories are involved in the design of any new facility. Useful information is given by van der Groen and Trexler (1982), ACDP (1995), CDC/NIH (1993) and WHO (1993).

The architectural and engineering features are highly sophisticated and can only be outlined here. The laboratory should be isolated or physically separated from other parts of the same building so that access is difficult and can be strictly controlled. It should be airtight, i.e. completely sealed, except for doorways, so that no infectious material can escape. Likewise, it should be vermin-proof. Ingress and egress should be through air-locks, changing rooms and showers. The ventilation system should be completely controlled with pressure gradients maintained at all times so that air flows via air-locks into the laboratories. Class III microbiological safety cabinets and (or) flexible film isolators should be maintained at a lower pressure than the rooms in which they are placed. All effluent air, from rooms and cabinets should be passed through double banks of HEPA filters before discharge to atmosphere. Provisions for positive pressure suits may be necessary, when special decontamination showers will also be required before exit. Pass-through facilities, with air-locks, to get specimens, etc., in the rooms while people are working should be one-way only and operated from the outside. A double-ended autoclave, with locking devices, is essential. This would usually open from a Class III cabinet line into a lobby outside the room and the devices ensure that nothing can pass out without being sterilized. All effluents from sinks, handbasins and laboratories are sterilized (see p. 113).

Specimen reception rooms

It has already been made clear in Chapter 6 that some of the outsides of some of the specimens which arrive at microbiology laboratories may be contaminated. A reception room is therefore a potentially infected area (medium hazard zone) and it should be designed as such. It should be separated from offices, and not treated as an office. The floors and surfaces may become contaminated with spilled material and need disinfecting. Carpeting and polished desk tops should therefore be avoided in favour of laboratory flooring and laminate-topped benches. It is best to regard a specimen reception room as a Level 2 laboratory without laboratory equipment other than racks and trays for specimens, and shelves for specimen containers. A handbasin is essential.

Access should be restricted to authorized people. A separate bench or table should be reserved for documentation.

Preparation or utility rooms

One or more of these rooms should be designated for the reception, treatment and disposal of contaminated waste. The design features should be those of a Level 2 laboratory equipped with autoclaves, a sluice, a waste disposal unit plumbed to the public sewer, deep sinks, glassware washing machines, drying ovens, sterilizing ovens and large benches.

These should be arranged to preclude any possible mixing of contaminated and decontaminated materials. The designers should therefore work to a flow, or critical pathway chart provided by a professional microbiologist.

Such a chart is shown in Figure 10.5. The contaminated materials arrive in colour-coded containers (p. 162) onto a bench or into an area designated and used for that purpose only. These are then sorted according to their colour codes and despatched to the incinerator or loaded into the autoclave. Nothing bypasses this area. After autoclaving the containers are taken to the sorting bench where the contents are separated into:

(1) waste for incineration, which is put into yellow colour-coded bags;
(2) waste for the rubbish tip, which is put into black colour-coded bags;
(3) waste suitable for the sluice or waste disposal unit;
(4) recoverable material which is passed to another room for washing and re-sterilizing.

The area which received the sterilized articles for reuse should have a separate autoclave. Contaminated waste and materials for re-use or re-issue should not be processed in the same autoclave.

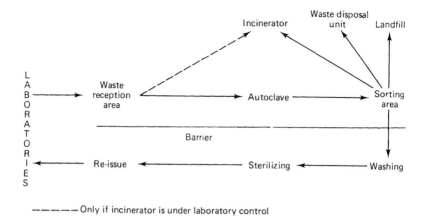

————— Only if incinerator is under laboratory control

Figure 10.5 Design of preparation (utility) rooms; a flow chart for the treatment and disposal of laboratory waste and for treatment of reusable materials

To avoid any possibility of cross contamination a separate room should be provided for the preparation of culture media and reagents. Otherwise this room offers no microbiological hazards (although some chemicals are suspect). This is the only room in the laboratory building that might require a laminar flow clean air cabinet for pouring and distributing culture media.

Walk-in incubators and refrigerators

The microbiological hazards associated with these concern, firstly, their distance from the laboratories and, secondly, raised thresholds. It should not be necessary for cultures to be carried, or trollies loaded with cultures to be pushed long distances or taken up and down stairs or elevators. Spillages and breakages of cultures in corridors are much more hazardous than in rooms.

Raised thresholds are sometimes fitted to incubator and refrigerator rooms to accommodate floor insulation. People trip over them and drop things; trolleys are difficult to manoeuvre over them, even if they are ramped, and cultures may fall or be shaken off. There is little need for floor insulation. The average concrete floor, covered with normal laboratory flooring material will not lose or gain enough heat to affect an incubator or cold room.

Chapter 11

Risk assessment

Risk assessment is an essential procedure in the control of laboratory-acquired infections, but before it is considered, it is necessary to say something about the interrelated notions of hazard and risk. The *hazard* presented by an article, substance, process or activity is its potential to cause harm in some way, e.g. to cause an infection. The *risk* from an article, substance, process or activity is the likelihood that it will cause harm in the circumstances under consideration, e.g. give rise to an infection in a microbiological laboratory worker. In terms of harm presented, a risk can be perceived qualitatively at one end of the spectrum as 'vanishingly small' and acceptable and at the other end as being so severe at to make it totally unacceptable. Deciding what is an acceptable risk is a management task; a risk that is acceptable in one set of circumstances may be unacceptable in another.

It should be borne in mind that where microbiological laboratories are situated in places where there is a high public perception of infection risk, or where there is a possibility that agents with a high risk profile (e.g. plague, Ebola fever, anthrax) will be handled, there may be differences of opinion between the laboratory and the public about the acceptability of risk. In such cases, we think that the onus is on the laboratory management to allay fear of infection by demonstrating that every possible containment measure is reliably in place and to provide all the supporting documentary evidence that is necessary (see below). It is worth noting here that the World Health Organization (WHO, 1997a) advises that wherever possible laboratories should be sited away from patient, residential and public areas and that high-level containment or high-risk laboratories should be located away from patient or public areas.

It is a reasonable assumption that for microbiological laboratories the higher the level of containment the more complicated will be the working procedures and the greater will be the capital and running costs. For most microbiological laboratories, especially those carrying out routine diagnostic work, it will not be economically possible, nor justified in terms of infection risk, always to work at Containment Level 4 or even at Level 3. Risk management involves the identification and evaluation of risk coupled with cost/benefit analysis of potential control measures.

In developed countries legislation will require that in workplaces hazards are identified, risks are assessed and measures are put in place to prevent or control exposures to the hazards. The law may even prohibit the use of certain substances hazardous to health for certain purposes. For example, in the UK, the *Control of Substances Hazardous to Health Regulations 1994* (COSHH), prohibit the manufacture and use for all purposes of benzidine, its salts and any substance containing it, in any other substance in a total concentration equal to or greater than 0.1% by mass.

In the general context of biomedical research laboratories, risk assessment has been defined as *'A systematic examination of the hazards associated with the work, an evaluation of the risks to health associated with the hazards and a judgement on the measures required to eliminate or control harmful exposure to the hazards'* (MRC, 1996). In microbiological laboratories, a range of hazards may be encountered intentionally or incidentally. They include biological agents, chemical agents, sources of ionising radiation, fire, electrical hazards and equipment-related hazards. Biological agents will be the main focus here, other hazards being generally outside the scope of the book. Those who need more information about such hazards in health-care laboratories should consult WHO (1997a). The basic elements of chemical risk assessment are dealt with by Moses (1997), and chemical safety in the microbiological laboratory is specifically addressed by Lisella and Thomaston (1995).

In the UK, risk assessment is a requirement of COSHH. A biological agent is defined as *'... any micro-organism, cell culture, or human endoparasite, including any that have been genetically modified, which may cause an infection, allergy, toxicity or otherwise create a risk to human health'*. Agents that fall within this definition include:

(1) any microorganisms in Hazard Groups 2, 3 and 4 that are held as stocks or which might arrive at the laboratory for investigation, and
(2) any microorganisms in Hazard Group 1 that might be allergenic or have toxic metabolites.

Risk assessment is a stepwise process that can be summarized conveniently as follows (HSE, 1993):

Step 1: Gathering information about the agents being handled, relevant laboratory practices and all people who may possibly be at risk of infection with the agents being handled.

Step 2: Evaluating the risks to health.

Step 3: Deciding what needs to be done to control or prevent exposures.

Step 4: Recording the assessment.

Step 5: Reviewing the assessment.

With reference to COSHH, approved codes of practice for control of biological agents, chemical and other substances hazardous to health and carcinogenic substances have been published (HSE, 1997).

Responsibility for risk assessment

Assuming that he or she will wish to delegate the task, the head of the laboratory will have to decide who should have responsibility for carrying out a risk assessment, either as a sole function or as a coordinator for a team approach. Whoever is given the responsibility for the assessment should be well-versed in microbiological safety and have a thorough understanding of relevant legal requirements. The responsible person should be (must be) given the necessary facilities and authority to do the work competently. He or she will need to have enough time and status to gather information, talk to the appropriate people, look at records to examine the workplace and, where necessary, seek the help of experts from outside the organisation (HSE, 1993).

Safety advisers

Whether or not there is a specific legal requirement for a specific appointment, it is our opinion that all laboratories need to have at least one person on the staff who is sufficiently experienced in safe practices and who is sufficiently competent to pass on his or her expertise to others. Large and multidisciplinary institutions may require several such people, each qualified in one particular field. Such individuals have variously been called safety officers, supervisors, managers or advisers and often there has been confusion about their duties and responsibilities. This person, whose title may vary from one institution to another, will be responsible to the head of the laboratory or organization and his or her detailed duties will vary. The term 'safety adviser' is used below because it seems the least controversial of titles.

SUGGESTED DUTIES OF A SAFETY ADVISER

(1) Advise management on the formulation of a safety policy (which is required by law in the UK) and in risk assessments.
(2) Assist scientific staff in drawing up standard operational procedures (SOPs) that incorporate safe working practices.
(3) Carry out safety audits and inspections and bring to the attention of individuals and management any infringements of SOPs.
(4) Investigate accidents and 'near misses' and ensure that they are reported and documented, as required by law where appropriate.
(5) Ensure that hazardous materials are correctly labelled and stored.
(6) Ensure that protective clothing and equipment is in good order and is kept so.
(7) Oversee routine decontamination procedures and carry out effective decontamination after an accident.
(8) Maintain a library of appropriate literature and disseminate information on safety matters.
(9) Liaise with emergency services.

In large organizations the various safety advisers, together with representatives of management and staff, may form a safety committee (which may be a legal requirement), or it may be useful to set up a full-time biosafety office.

Step 1: Gathering information

Information is needed about infection hazards, i.e. the biological agents that may possibly be encountered in the laboratory, and in particular to what hazard group they have been assigned. Information is also needed about possible routes of exposure to the biological agents, i.e. mechanisms whereby they can enter the human body and cause an infection. Information is required on work practices and people who could possibly be at risk from exposure to biological agents.

Infection hazards

Information on hazard categorization is available in authoritative official publications, e.g. those of the Advisory Committee on Dangerous Pathogens in the UK (ACDP, 1995) and of the World Health Organization (WHO, 1993).

Routes of infection were considered in Chapter 2 (see Figure 2.1, p. 41).

There are three problem areas which will receive attention below. These are agents that are:

(1) not listed in official or other authoritative publications;
(2) present in clinical specimens that in a microbiological laboratory have to be cultured and otherwise manipulated before they are identified, thereby to enable a hazard grouping to be assigned to them, or in other workplaces, e.g., clinical biochemistry laboratories and postmortem rooms, where manipulation of specimens containing pathogens in sufficient concentration presents an incidental risk of infection;
(3) pathogenic agents that have been incorrectly assigned to a low hazard group because of mis-identification.

UNLISTED BIOLOGICAL AGENTS

In the UK employers whose work involves keeping or handling biological agents not appearing in the ACDP's (1995) categorization are required (Schedule 9 of COSHH) to place it in one of the hazard groups (see Chapter 3). The decision about which hazard group is appropriate has to be based on all available information about the agent in question. If there is doubt about which of two hazard groups is appropriate, the higher of the two groups must be selected.

All viruses isolated from humans must be allocated to Hazard Group 2 as a minimum, unless there is clear evidence to show that they are not pathogenic. Where a provisional categorization results in an agent being placed in Hazard Group 3 or 4, there is a legal requirement to notify the Health and Safety Executive, which is the regulatory authority.

CLINICAL SPECIMENS

The type of specimen is indicative of the range of biological agents to which exposure is possible. The level of containment appropriate for handling the specimen can be assigned with reference to an agent or agents of the highest hazard group to which exposure is possible. Therefore, with reference to relevant publications, laboratory records and the experience of staff, there is a need to be aware of the range of agents likely to be encountered in different specimens. Examples are given below.

Sputum samples may contain a range of pathogens which are spread by the airborne route, including *Mycobacterium tuberculosis*, which is an agent in Hazard Group 3 (ACDP, 1995). For this reason, all sputum specimens must be handled in a microbiological safety cabinet during preparation for cytological or microbiological examination (HSE, 1991a; see Chapter 13).

Blood samples received by a haematology laboratory may contain a range of agents (Hunt, 1997a, Collins, 1997) including HBV and HIV which are spread by the parenteral route. For this reason, 'Universal Precautions' (Hunt, 1995b; Kibbler, 1997), including measures to prevent injury by blood-contaminated sharp objects, are required (Kennedy, 1997). In addition, patients with AIDS may have a *M. tuberculosis* bacteraemia (Salzman *et al.*, 1986). Blood cultures may contain a range of agents (Collins, 1997), including *Brucella* spp. (see below).

The country of origin, together with what clinical information is available, can be a useful indicator of the agents that may be present in a sample. For example, a blood specimen from Zaire with a diagnosis of haemorrhagic fever should send out a signal that viruses in Hazard Group 4 (ACDP, 1995) may be present, thus requiring Containment Level 4 conditions. Similarly, a culture from Russia with a diagnosis of severe sore throat should indicate that Hazard Group 3 organisms naturally disseminated by the airborne route might be present, thus necessitating the use of a microbiological safety cabinet (see below).

MATERIAL DISTRIBUTED BY EXTERNAL QUALITY ASSURANCE SCHEMES (EQAS)

It should not come as a surprise that materials distributed to test a participant laboratory's ability to isolate and to identify a pathogenic microorganism may actually contain viable pathogens (see Chapter 2). However, two reports illustrate that EQAS participants may lack proficiency in the safe handling of such samples.

Blaser *et al.* (1980) reported that of 24 cases of laboratory-acquired typhoid fever, 21 cases occurred when *Salmonella typhi* was introduced voluntarily into the laboratory for proficiency testing or for research purposes. On the basis of their data, they estimated that for three national proficiency testing programmes involving about 4600 laboratories, there was one case of laboratory-acquired typhoid per 655 laboratories (range 1:466–1:912) receiving *Salmonella typhi* material.

Chin (1998) reported that an experienced medical laboratory scientific officer became infected with a toxigenic strain of *Corynebacterium diphtheriae* while handling an EQAS sample. It is interesting to note that participants were informed that this came from a patient with a severe sore throat who had recently returned from Russia. Nevertheless, a heavy suspension of organisms was prepared on the open bench for biochemical testing.

MISIDENTIFICATION OF PATHOGENS

Reliable categorization of biological agents in hazard groups depends upon reliable identification. Misidentification can lead to increased risk of exposure because of misclassification. A report by Batchelor *et al.* (1992) illustrates this principle. *Brucella melitensis* isolated from clinical material was misidentified as *Moraxella phenylpyruvica*, on the basis of biochemical tests carried out with a commercial identification system. This is generally regarded as a harmless commensal organism that would normally be assigned to Hazard Group 1. Had the organism been correctly identified, it would probably have been assigned correctly to Hazard Group 3 (ACDP, 1995) and work done in a microbiological safety cabinet. Mis-identification led to the work being carried out on the open bench. This, in turn, led to infections with an organism that heads the list of the 'top ten' laboratory-acquired infections (see Chapter 1).

Laboratory practices

The people responsible for a risk assessment will need to know in exact detail every stage of every process in which biological agents may be encountered, including the collection and transport of specimens, laboratory manipulations involving biological agents, the treatment and disposal of liquid effluent and solid waste and the recycling of equipment and materials. They will also need to know how laboratory infections are acquired (see Chapter 2) and about the consequence, in terms of release of viable agents, of foreseeable accidents. It is important to involve employees in the assessment process. They have the most direct knowledge of the how work is carried out. Their information is vital in order to ensure a reliable assessment that reflects work as it actually happens, rather than how the management thinks that it should. The involvement of employees promotes their interest and commitment to precautions established by the assessment (ACDP, 1995).

People at risk

The range of people at risk from microbiological laboratory work will vary according to circumstances and detailed knowledge of procedures will be required for risk assessment purposes. Examples include:

- Phlebotomists and other laboratory personnel who collect or handle blood and other material from patients (see Chapter 4). The risk of becoming infected with tubercle bacilli during the collection of sputum specimens from patients is quite high because of the high level of exposure to airborne organisms. Laboratory workers who collect sputum specimens directly from patients are more likely to be exposed to tubercle bacilli than when preparing sputum smears on the open bench (Collins and Johns, 1998).
- Staff who transport samples to laboratories (e.g. nurses, porters, drivers, laboratory receptionists). These are at risk from blood-contaminated outer surfaces of the blood culture bottle, from leaking closures, from spillage of contents or from breakage in transit (Allen and Darrell, 1983; Garner and Masterton, 1990).
- Laboratory staff involved in the isolation and identification of agent
- Portering and domestic staff who may clean laboratories and handle waste. A laboratory porter contracted typhoid, which was fatal, after a container containing a culture toppled over and spilled on him (*Times*, 1977).
- Visiting contractors who may repair and maintain equipment within the laboratory, and other visitors.
- Those who handle equipment removed from the laboratory for repair, maintenance, etc., and who come into contact with such items, including transport drivers and repair staff in outside workshops.

- Those who remove and dispose of solid waste and effluent including waste disposal contractors, landfill site workers and sewage workers.
- Anyone who may breathe contaminated air exhausted from the laboratory (see Chapter 5).

Step 2: Evaluating the risks to health

The assignment of biological agents to one of the four hazard groups, has been done in the light of the answers to the following questions (ACDP, 1995):

(1) Is the agent pathogenic to humans?
(2) Is it a hazard to employees?
(3) Is it transmissible to the community?
(4) Is effective prophylaxis or treatment available?

The resultant categorisation does not, however, allow for the special factors, agent-specific and host-specific, that need to be taken into consideration in risk assessments. These factors are discussed below.

In a particular individual, risk of infection with a particular agent can be evaluated in the light of the following criteria:

- whether the viable agent is present in large enough numbers to enable infection;
- what is the lowest number of organisms required to initiate an infection, i.e., the minimum infective dose (MID) (ACDP, 1996, see also Chapter 2);
- is there a mechanism whereby the MID of the organism can gain access to a host through one or more of the portals of entry (mouth, skin, conjunctiva, other mucous membranes, lungs)? Examples of such mechanisms are production of a pathogenic aerosol that is inspired by the host, and a skin puncture with a sharp object that is contaminated with a blood-borne virus;
- whether the agent is able to survive natural defence mechanisms such as phagocytosis and low stomach pH (for a fuller coverage of this area, see Mims, 1982);
- whether the host is immune or especially susceptible to the particular infection. Some hosts are naturally immune or have conferred immunity to some infections. In come cases there are factors that predispose a host to particular infections (see below).

Reference to these criteria is a good introduction to the development of measures to prevent or to control exposures to biological agents (see below).

Agent-specific factors

These include increased virulence, antimicrobial drug resistance, robust organisms and working with organisms at high concentrations.

INCREASED VIRULENCE

Escherichia coli provides a good example of this problem. In general, this organism is assigned to Hazard Group 2, with the exception of non-pathogenic strains which would be assigned to Hazard Group 1 (ACDP, 1995). However, verotoxin-producing *E. coli* O157:H7 may cause severe human disease, may have an infective dose as low as 10 organisms and may cause laboratory-acquired infection. Accordingly it has recently been promoted to Group 3 (HSE, 1998).

ANTIMICROBIAL DRUG RESISTANCE

A laboratory-acquired infection with an agent that has multiple drug resistance is more difficult to treat and therefore the consequences are more serious for the affected person. Agents that cause particular concern are multiple-drug resistant strains of *Mycobacterium tuberculosis,* drug resistant *Plasmodium falciparum* and methicillin-resistant *Staphylococcus aureus*.

ROBUST ORGANISMS

A current cause for concern are prions—the transmissible spongiform encephalopathy agents. These are very robust and appear to be able to survive most of the usual sterilization procedures (see Chapter 19).

Pathogenic bacterial spores and protozoan cysts may be able to resist decontamination and disinfection by commonly-used agents.

AGENTS AT HIGH CONCENTRATION

Working with biological agents at high concentrations increases the risk of laboratory-acquired infection thus necessitating a higher level of containment. In three separate incidents laboratory workers became seriously ill with meningococcal infection following the preparation of a heavy suspension of *Neisseria meningitidis* on the open bench. The use of a heavy suspension of organisms was a requirement of a new protocol that was intended to increase the sensitivity of a commercial bacterial identification kit. Previously, a lighter suspension of organisms had been required and consequently the risk of exposure was lower. A hazard notice issued by the UK Department of Health (DH, 1993a) advised that a microbiological safety cabinet should be used when making and manipulating a heavy suspension of a culture which might be possibly be *Neisseria meningitidis.*

GENETICALLY-MODIFIED MICROORGANISMS

In the Brenner Scheme for quantitative microbiological risk assessment (ACDP, 1996), three factors are used. Each factor is assigned a value lying between 1 and 10^{-12} in increments of 10^{-3}. The *access* factor is a measure of the ability of the modified organism to colonize or otherwise persist in the human body, and to transfer genetic material to other organisms. *Expression* is a measure of the amount of protein expected to be produced by the insertion (a value of 1 being assigned when the expressing system is designed to produce at a maximum rate in the host). *Damage* is a measure of the likelihood of harm being caused by exposure to to the product of the inserted genetic material. Table 11.1 gives recommended values for *damage factors*.

The assigned values are then summed to provide a figure that is used to assign the level of containment required for working with the modified organism.

TABLE 11.1 Recommended values for damage factors

Damage factor	
1	A toxic substance or pathogenic determinant that is likely to have a significant biological effect.
10^{-3}	A biologically active substance which might have a deleterious effect if delivered to a target tissue, **or** a biologically inactive form of a toxic substance which, if active, might have a significant biological effect.
10^{-6}	A biologically active substance which is very unlikely to have a deleterious effect, or for example where it could not approach the normal body level (e.g., less than 10% of the normal body level).
10^{-9}	A gene sequence where any biological effect is considered highly unlikely either because of the known properties of the protein or because of the high levels encountered in nature.
10^{-12}	No foreseeable biological effect (e.g., non-coding DNA sequence).

Reproduced from ACGM (1993) by permission of the Health and Safety Executive.

Detailed guidelines on risk assessment of genetically-modified microorganisms have been prepared by the Advisory Committee on Genetic Modification (ACGM, 1993). The HSE (1997) has issued a compendium of guidance on genetic modification.

HOST-SPECIFIC RISK FACTORS

For convenience, these can be divided into two classes—intrinsic and extrinsic factors. Intrinsic factors include immunodeficiency, immunosuppression, pregnancy, atopy and old age. Extrinsic factors include habits such as nail biting, and pen chewing that increase the risk of infection through the mouth, and contact lens wearing that increases the risk of localised eye infection and systemic infection via the eye.

INTRINSIC FACTORS

The ACDP (1995) notes that their hazard categorisation does not allow for any additional risk for those people who may be more severely affected because of compromising factors, including pre-existing disease, compromised immunity, the effects of medication and pregnancy. Laboratory workers who are immunodeficient are likely to be at greater risk of occupational infection with pathogens and with agents not normally regarded as being pathogenic. This is evidenced by the secondary infection problems of patients with AIDS including extra-pulmonary mycobacterial infections (Shafer et al., 1991) and infections with bacterial opportunists such as pneumococci, and *Pseudomonas* (Shanson, 1989). Ridzon et al. (1997) reported that a phlebotomist with a nosocomially-acquired HIV infection developed tuberculosis after exposure to multidrug-resistant *M. tuberculosis*. They pointed out that health-care workers with immunosuppression are at increased risk of tuberculosis and if exposed should be considered for preventative therapy regardless of tuberculin skin test status.

Workers who are receiving cytotoxic immunosuppressive therapy, e.g., following a renal transplant, are also likely to be at greater risk of occupational infection. The *British National Formulary* (Anon., 1997) notes that susceptibility to, and severity of, infections may be increased when prednisolone, a steroid drug that is prescribed, among other things, for the suppression of inflammatory and allergic disorders, is taken. Clinical presentation of disease may be atypical and severe infections such as septicaemia and tuberculosis may be at an advanced stage before being recognized and there is an increased risk of severe chicken pox and measles when prednisolone is being taken (Anon., 1997). It is estimated that in the UK approximately 4 million prescriptions per annum are made out for prednisolone.

Knobloch and Demar (1997) reported that a laboratory technician under immunosuppressive therapy because of systematic lupus erythematosus developed cutaneous leishmaniasis after accidental percutaneous inoculation with amastigote culture forms of *Leishmania mexicana*. The authors recommend that the exposure of immunodeficient laboratory workers to *Leishmania* spp. should be avoided.

The ACDP outlines infections that, if they are contracted in pregnancy, present a risk to the fetus or newborn baby (ACDP, 1997c). The agents concerned are:

Chlamydia psittaci	*Listeria*
Cytomegalovirus	Parvovirus
Hepatitis A virus	Rubella virus
Hepatitis B virus	*Toxoplasma*
Human immunodeficiency virus	Varicella zoster virus

In addition, the ACDP advises that a wide range of microorganisms may infect pregnant women and may or may not have an adverse effect on the baby. These include:

Borrelia burgdorferi	*Mycobacterium tuberculosis*
Campylobacter	*Salmonella* spp.
Coxiella burnetii	*Treponema pallidum*
Lymphocytic choriomeningitis virus	

Furthermore, any severe infection, whatever the cause, may be detrimental to the health of the mother and child. Consequently, this should be taken into account when setting up control measures (see below) to tackle the risks of infections in the workplace (ACDP, 1997c). It is estimated that about one-third of the UK population is sensitized to common environmental sensitizers such as grass pollen, house dust mite and animal dusts. Such people are said to be atopic (HSE, 1994). Atopic individuals may be more susceptible to occupational allergies. Allergy to laboratory animals which may lead to the development of asthma is an occupational hazard among laboratory animal handlers especially those who are atopic and sensitized to domestic animals (see Chapter 17). It seems a reasonable presumption that atopic laboratory workers will be more at risk from biological agents that are respiratory sensitizers such as *Aspergillus fumigatus* and *Candida albicans*. Latex sensitisation is a problem for some workers (see below).

In the general population many protective immune responses are impaired in old age leading to an increased risk of infection (Venjatraman and Fernandes, 1997). Whether older laboratory workers are more at risk of occupational infection is unclear.

EXTRINSIC FACTORS

Hand-to-eye (see Chapter 2), hand-to-mouth and hand-to-nose contacts are commonly observed and may possibly be routes for transmission of occupational infection. Environmental surface contamination with blood may be the norm in clinical laboratories (Kennedy, 1997) and fingers in contact with contaminated surfaces help to spread contamination.

We are aware of a case of laboratory-acquired shigellosis in which the only definite risk factor that could be identified was that the individual concerned was a nail-biter. It is a feature of nail-biting that there are frequent involuntary contacts between the potentially contaminated finger tips and the lips and the teeth. It is easy to see how minute traces of material that could contain a minimum infective dose of *Shigella* spp. (see Chapter 2) could be transmitted in this way.

Another habit that could result in the transmission of infection in occupational settings is finger licking while page turning. Those who are familiar with Umberto Eco's book *The Name of the Rose* will recall that some monks with this affectation were poisoned with arsenic that they had picked up from the pages of forbidden books. Books and papers that are consulted in a laboratory may become contaminated with materials being handled. Blood contaminated computer cards may have been implicated in an outbreak of hepatitis in a laboratory (see Chapter 2).

Pen chewing is another habit, and a chewed pen may be kept in the top pocket of a laboratory coat. In one study of contamination in a clinical laboratory, blood was detected on ballpoint pens and felt-tipped markers (Kennedy, 1997).

Seal and Hay (1993) reported that approximately 1.3 million people in the UK wear contact lenses and a proportion develop microbial keratitis as a direct consequence of their use. *Pseudomonas aeruginosa* is the most important cause of acute necrotizing keratitis for the contact lens wearer and some wearers develop keratitis as a result of corneal infection with *Acanthamoeba*. While there are no published epidemiological data identifying contact lens-wearing laboratory personnel as being at greater risk than other contact lens wearers of acquiring microbial keratitis as a direct consequence of their work, nevertheless the microbiology laboratory does provide an environment with increased risk of exposure to biological agents with the potential to cause keratitis. Agents may gain access to the eye as a consequence of splashing or via direct transfer from contaminated fingers or microscope eyepieces (see Chapter 2) to the eyelid margin. Seal and Hay (1993) advise that extended-wear contact lenses are not recommended for staff working in microbiological laboratories and that contact lens wearers should avoid touching their eyelids or lenses when handling bacterial culture plates, especially those with *P. aeruginosa*. Other organisms recognized as potential pathogens of eye include *Serratia marcescens*, *E. coli*, *Klebsiella pneumoniae*, *Stenathrophomonas maltophilia*, *P. acidivorans* and *P. fluorescens* (Ready, 1998).

Because the eye is at risk from localized infection and is a portal of entry for biological agents that cause systemic infection, there is a very good case to be made always to require that protective spectacles be worn in a microbiological laboratory. Seal and Hay (1993) advise that goggles should always be worn for handling cultures of *Acanthamoeba* or for handling liquid cultures of other organisms, especially in large volumes. Work with large volume cultures should be done in a microbiological safety cabinet.

Step 3: Deciding what needs to be done to prevent or to control exposures

The classic approach in occupational hygiene, which underpins the COSHH legislation in the UK, is that for all hazardous substances in a workplace, the employer must give first priority to trying to prevent exposure. This might be achieved by: (a) changing the method of work so that the operation giving rise to the exposure is no longer necessary; (b) modifying the process to eliminate production of a hazardous by-product or waste product; or (c) where a hazardous substance is used intentionally, substitution by a new substance or different form of the same substance, which, in the circumstances of the work, presents no risk or less risk to health (HSE, 1988). Where prevention of exposure is not reasonably practicable, except in the of carcinogens (for which there are special legal provisions in the UK), adequate control of exposure should be achieved by measures other than personal protective equipment.

Prevention of exposure to biological agents

In the microbiological laboratory, especially the clinical laboratory, the scope for absolute prevention of exposure to a particular infection risk is often limited, because of the need generally to handle viable organisms. However, wherever possible, materials to be handled should be sterilized or otherwise pretreated to remove the infection hazard completely. To illustrate this point, we recall that in some clinical chemistry laboratories 6-day collections of faeces were autoclaved before fat determination, and more recently experiments have been carried out with heat treatment and with addition of β-propiolactone to inactivate pathogens in blood and serum (Kennedy, 1997). In the latter case, it should be borne in mind that there is a definite chemical risk attached to the use of this toxic agent which will have to be weighed against any infection risk. A method of decontaminating blood films is described in Chapter 12.

There is a case to be made for preventing workers with host-specific risk factors (see above) from exposure to biological agents that are more likely to cause infection to them, e.g., nail biters could be moved from tasks that expose them to agents that are normally transmitted by the faecal-oral route, and pregnant staff should be moved from tasks that would expose them to any of the agents listed above as likely to cause fetal damage.

A problem arises where immunosuppressed staff are involved, because they may be liable to become infected even with agents in Hazard Group 1. If a decision is taken by laboratory management specifically to prevent exposures to workers with host-specific risk factors, great sensitivity will have to be exercised, full agreement of staff will have to be obtained and the legal rights of affected workers will have to be safeguarded. In most cases, it is likely that measures to control exposures will be sufficient to protect such workers.

Control of exposure to biological agents

Where there is a definite need to work with viable agents, control of exposure to infection is necessary. For convenience, methods of controlling exposure can be grouped as follows: (a) engineering controls; (b) personal protection; (c) good

TABLE 11.2 Examples of engineering controls

Negative pressure laboratories
Microbiological safety cabinets
Sealed centrifuge rotors and buckets
Pipetting devices
Robust and leakproof specimen containers
Puncture-resistant 'sharps' containers
Biochemical and haematological analysers with features designed to minimize exposure to samples
Anti-needle-stick devices

laboratory practice; (d) decontamination. The risk assessment will need to take account of any hazard which is inherent in the use of a control measure (see below).

ENGINEERING CONTROLS

These include control of laboratory ventilation (Chapter 10), microbiological safety cabinets (Chapter 5), sealed centrifuge rotors and buckets and other devices designed to minimize exposure to infection (Chapter 4). Table 11.2 list these and others.

PERSONAL PROTECTION

This includes personal protective equipment (e.g., respirators, visors, laboratory coats and gloves) and occupational health services including vaccination and immunization (Chapter 8).

GOOD LABORATORY PRACTICE

This includes standard operating procedures that incorporate universal precautions (e.g., avoidance of 'sharps', rules prohibiting smoking, drinking, eating, application of cosmetics and requiring regular handwashing) designed to minimize exposure to infection, staff training programmes, procedures for dealing with accidents, in laboratories and involving transport of cultures and specimens, where there is a risk of release of biological agents and safety audits (Chapters 9, 12 and 13).

Decontamination
This is covered in detail in Chapter 7.

Step 4: Recording the assessment

A written record of the risk assessment should always be made. This should show why decisions about risks and precautions have been made and should reflect the detail with which the assessment has been carried out. The record should be meaningful to all those who need to know about it, both at the time that the assessment is done and in the future. In particular, there should be sufficient information available within the written record to enable the validity of the risk assessment to be considered by all who have a legitimate interest in the safety of the laboratory's activities, e.g., management, employees, inspectors from enforcement agencies, and representatives of the public in areas where there is a climate of high risk perception or when there is a need to handle agents that have a very high perceived risk profile (see above).

Step 5: Reviewing the assessment

The risk assessment should always be reviewed at regular intervals and should be reviewed immediately if there is any reason to suppose that the original assessment is no longer valid, or if any of the circumstances of the work should change significantly (HSE, 1993). Examples of changing circumstances necessitating review are receipt of samples from areas where Hazard Group 4 agents are endemic, pregnancy in staff handling agents listed, and when for any reason there is a need to scale up a process where viable agents are handled.

Emergency contingency plans

One or more SOPs should be drawn up for dealing with natural disasters (fire, flood, etc.) serious contamination of premises, accidental exposure of staff to infection, emergency medical treatment, inquiries into dangerous occurrences and epidemiological investigations. These should take note of the presence and location of Groups 3, and 4 pathogens and hazardous substances, location of high risk areas, personnel who are at risk, identification and whereabouts of emergency civil and medical services, sources of prophylactics and therapeutics sources and provision of safety and life-saving equipment. WHO guidelines provide a basis for local planning (WHO, 1980).

Hazards inherent in control measures

The chemical hazard associated with the use of β-propiolactone has already been mentioned. Other decontamination agents are likely to be toxic or have other hazardous properties. It should be borne in mind that no human activity is without risk and that the substitution of one practice for another may bring with it a new risk to consider.

An example of this is that when certain types of pipetting aids were introduced into some laboratories to prevent mouth pipetting, cut fingers resulted. This was because of the pipettes fitted tightly in the devices and considerable force had to be used to apply them. In some cases, the glass pipette broke cutting fingers.

Anglim et al. (1995) reported an outbreak of needle-stick injuries caused by discarded needles piercing sharps containers that were part of a contamination control programme. We have observed this in institutions where fibreboard (instead of heavy duty plastic) containers were used.

Latex sensitization is another example. An increase in the use of latex gloves by health-care workers as a control measure against infection has led, overall, to an increase in the reporting of adverse reactions to latex, residues of materials used in the manufacture of gloves and powder contained in gloves, including irritation, immediate hypersensitivity and delayed sensitivity. Atopic individuals are more at risk. The problem is reviewed and advice on management of sensitized workers is given in a publication by the UK's Medical Devices Agency (MDA, 1996).

An additional concern for all laboratory staff is contamination of emergency eyewash solutions with *Acanthamoeba*. Such contamination could result in amoebic keratitis following accidental injury to the cornea. Eyewash solutions, often depend on chlorine-based disinfectants which may be ineffective against *Acanthamoeba* cysts. Single-use eyewash sachets should be used (Seal and Hay, 1993). While there does not appear to be evidence to implicate it in transmission of laboratory-acquired infection, personal protective equipment that may be shared, such as gloves and goggles, may be a reservoir of infection. Accordingly, all such items should be regularly cleaned and decontaminated.

The inherent physical hazards of microbiological safety cabinets and the need for cabinets that offer adequate containment of pathogens are considered in Chapter 5.

Chapter 12

Blood-borne infections: universal precautions

Although the transmission of infection by blood-to-blood contact has a long history it has become a matter of great concern to laboratory workers (and, of course to other health-care staff) in the past two decades because of outbreaks of hepatitis B, followed by the onset of the AIDS epidemic. According to Hadler *et al.* (1985) and Jacobson *et al.* (1985) the occupational risk to laboratory workers is 10 times greater than that to the general public. The CDC (1992) reported that of 101 documented cases of occupationally-acquired human immunodeficiency viruses (HIV) 25 (24.8%) occurred in laboratory technicians. References to hepatitis B and HIV infections among laboratory workers will be found in Chapter 1.

Although the hepatitis B and HIV are currently the most important that may be acquired from percutaneous and mucocutaneous exposure laboratory workers are often unaware that other blood-borne agents, bacteria and endoparasites may pose a threat to their health.

Although some blood samples may contain relatively small numbers of some of these agents laboratory procedures may concentrate them into infectious doses, thus creating a hazard to workers. Thus we may distinguish between *primary* transmission, i.e. blood-to-blood, and *secondary* transmission, i.e. from aerosols and contaminated surfaces. This chapter is concerned with the former, as the latter may be controlled by the methods described elsewhere in this book. It should be remembered, however, that, any organism isolated from blood, e.g. by blood culture, has the potential for transmission to laboratory workers.

Concern about blood-to-blood exposure has now been extended to the hazards of exposure to other body fluids.

Agents of blood-borne infections

Table 12.1 lists the agents that have been documented as agents of occupational diseases associated with exposure to blood (Hunt, 1997, Collins, 1997). Although these are not necessarily all laboratory acquired (see Chapter 1) they indicate the potential for such infections.

Table 12.2 lists a wide variety of organisms that are isolated from blood cultures in the ordinary course of clinical investigations, all of which offer a potential for secondary transmission to laboratory workers.

TABLE 12.1 Agents incriminated in blood-borne infections

Viruses	Bacteria and protozoa
Colorado tick fever	Borrelia spp.
Crimea-Congo virus	Brucella spp.
Cytomegalovirus	Mycobacterium spp.
Ebola fever virus	Treponema pallidum
Hepatitis B virus	Rickettsia rickettsii
Human immunodeficiency virus	Leishmania spp.
Lassa fever virus	Plasmodium spp.
Marburg virus	Trypanosoma spp.
Parvovirus B19	

Adapted from Hunt (1997) and Collins (1997). References are given in Chapter 1.

TABLE 12.2 Bacteria that have been isolated from blood cultures in the UK: potential for blood-borne infection

Acinetobacter	Mycobacterium avium-
Bacillus	intracellulare
Bacteroides	Mycobacterium tuberculosis
Candida	Neisseria meningitidis
Clostridium	Pasteurella multocida
Corynebacterium	Proteus
Cryptococcus neoformans	Pseudomonas aeruginosa
Enterobacter	Salmonella typhi
Escherichia coli	Salmonella other species
Haemophilus influenzae	Shigella dysenteriae
Klebsiella	Staphylococcus aureus
Listeria	Streptococcus pyogenes
Morganella	Xanthomonas maltophila

Adapted from Hickey and Shanson (1993).

Routes of transmission

As indicated above, these are percutaneous and mucocutaneous. The most common form of percutaneous exposure is by needle-stick injury. Hollow-bore needles can retain enough hepatitis B virus (HBV) to initiate infection. In simulation experiments Napoli and McGowan (1987) found that 1.4 µl of blood was retained; Hoffman et al. (1989) a mean volume of 0.03 µl was left and Gaughwin et al. (1991) that up to 0.75 µl was transferred. Needle-stick injuries have been reviewed by Collins and Kennedy (1987) and more recently by the authors of several papers in Collins and Kennedy (1997).

In laboratories mucocutaneous exposure is most likely to arise from contact with blood spills and splashes (Kennedy and Collins, 1997), many of which may not be visible to the naked eye (Hoffman and Kennedy, 1997). According to Lanphear (1994) 1 ml of infected blood may contain 10^2-10^8 HBV, $10-10^6$ or $10-10^3$ HIV, although Satter and Springthorpe (1991) mention as many as 10^{13} HBV.

HBV may survive in dried plasma and remain infective for some time, as shown by Bond *et al.* (1981) and Bond (1984).

Inactivation of specimens

If possible specimens should be treated to render them non-infective before they are examined. Heat treatment is not thought to be useful, especially at the usual temperature and time—56°C for 30 min (ACDP, 1990; see Kennedy and Collins (1997). β-Propiolactone (BPL) would appear to be the only chemical disinfectant that does not interfere with biochemical tests (Ball and Griffiths, 1985, Ball and Bolton, 1985) but this is a toxic substance.

Universal precautions

The two-tier system, under which certain specimens, mainly blood from patients with or suspected to be suffering from, hepatitis B (but not others) were labelled 'High Risk' was questioned by many workers (see Chapter 4). The Centers for Disease Control (CDC, 1987b, 1989) proposed a set of guidelines for the prevention of the transmission of HBV and HIV. These were termed 'Universal Precautions' (UPs). These guidelines formed the basis of the US Occupational Safety and Health Administration's Standard (OSHA, 1991), expanded to all clinical settings.

Meanwhile and subsequently the CDC's UPs, with various modifications, were adopted by several other states. In the UK, after several organizations had published their recommendations (Royal College of Nursing, 1987; DH, 1990, 1993) they finally emerged as guidance by the ACDP (1995b), mainly concerned with the various HIVs (HIV-1, HIV-2, HTLV-1 and HTLV-2) and hepatitis viruses (HBV, HCV, HDV), which applied to any workplace where blood might be handled as well as giving specific advice on laboratory work with blood, body fluids and tissues. Apart from blood itself, the accepted list of body fluids includes:

- blood-stained fluids (urine, faeces, sputum);
- amniotic, cerebrospinal, pericardial and pleural fluids;
- semen;
- vaginal secretions;
- human tissues, e.g. placentas.

Quality control material is also a potential source of infection. Simmons *et al.* (1990) found that all five batches of immunoassay control sera of human origin tested gave anti-HCV results. A pregnant laboratory worker developed hepatitis B after suffering a cut while handling quality control material which was found to give a positive test result for HBV (Anon., 1989).

In the OSHA standard these are referred to as 'other potentially infectious materials' (OPIMs).

Reviews, with comments, have been made on UPs by Kibbler (1997b) and on the OSHA regulations by Hunt (1997b). Many of the precautions advocated or required are common to other laboratory procedures and are covered in other chapters of this book, but are summarised below with references to other parts in this book.

Precautions

Level 2 containment (p. 214) is acceptable for most work in diagnostic laboratories, e.g. with HIV, etc. and hepatitis viruses but concentration or culture of the viruses requires Level 3 (p. 220). Work on haemorrhagic fever viruses must be done at Level 4 (ACDP, 1995, 1997a). For bacterial and protozoal infections the containment level should be appropriate to the hazard group of the organism.

Although there is no evidence of transmission of either virus by inhalation it is possible to aerosolize blood, certainly if it is diluted, e.g. in saline. Microbiological safety cabinets, Class I or Class II (see Chapter 5), should therefore be available, and should always be used for the concentration and culture of the viruses.

Personal protection

Protective clothing as described in Chapter 8 should be worn at all times and augmented by plastic aprons. Good quality disposable gloves should be worn. If there is a possibility that the face might be splashed with blood or other material then visors or masks and goggles should be worn.

Hand inspection for cuts, scratches or other lesions should be encouraged, although this is best done by the worker himself or his peers rather than by the supervisor. Workers should be reminded that inapparent lesions are just as effective portals of entry for the virus as obvious cuts and abrasions (p. 48).

Collection and transport of specimens

Methods for the collection and transport of specimens should be reviewed (Chapter 6) to reduce as far as possible the number of operations that expose the operator and the possibility of leaking containers. For blood, the vacuum collection system seems to offer fewer of these hazards than the traditional methods.

Opening specimen containers

Blood may be splashed when containers are opened, and suitable precautions should be taken (p. 95).

Blood films

Care is necessary in making and handling blood films. Dankhert et al. (1976) found HBsAg in stained and unstained blood and marrow films and Kohn (1976) also drew attention to this hazard. Slides may be decontaminated with buffered formalin (p. 101).

Precautions against injection

Special precautions should be taken against needle-stick accidents. Needles should be removed from syringes before blood is discharged into specimen containers. Detaching needles is probably the commonest activity contributing to needle-stick injury (Collins and Kennedy, 1987) as well as a source of contaminated fingers. It is banned in many US hospitals. However, if necessary, needles can be removed safely, if needle guards or forceps are used. The obvious alternative is vacuum tube collection, when there is no need to transfer the blood (p. 147). Proper discard bins (see p. 85) are essential and should be where they are needed. They must not be overfilled.

Centrifugation; serum separation

Blood specimens should be centrifuged in sealed centrifuge buckets. Adaptors to hold large numbers of tubes and which fit into these buckets are sold by most centrifuge manufacturers (p. 88).

If serum is separated by pouring, the rim of the sample tube should be wiped with filter paper and soaked in hypochlorite or glutaraldehyde (p. 98).

Histopathology specimens

Small specimens, e.g. needle biopsies, will be fixed and decontaminated rapidly but larger pieces of tissue may require several days. If frozen section work is unavoidable precautions (see p. 250) should be taken and afterwards the instrument should be decontaminated (p. 183).

Spillage, decontamination and the disposal of waste

If blood or other infected material is spilled or splashed the procedures described on p. 181 should be followed.

Contaminated protective clothing should be autoclaved or bagged for hot-wash laundering. Gloves should be discarded into contaminated waste receptacles for autoclaving or incineration. If street clothing is contaminated (see p. 183) it should be sponged with hot detergent solution, possibly with glutaraldehyde depending on the nature of the material (not with hypochlorite, which bleaches) and laundered.

Waste from hepatitis/AIDS laboratories should receive the same treatment as that given in Chapter 7. Of particular note are the tissues used to wipe the sampling probes of automated equipment. Gloves should be worn and the waste placed in colour-coded bags for autoclaving or incineration.

Vaccination and post-exposure action

Vaccination against hepatitis B should by now be the norm. The recombinant vaccine is now available as a combined hepatitis A and B vaccine. Advice on hepatitis B vaccination is given by the British Medical Association (BMA, 1995) and McCloy (1997).

Percutaneous and mucocutaneous exposure should be reported immediately to the occupational health department. The affected part should be washed immediately with soap and water. Mucous membranes and conjunctivae should be irrigated thoroughly with water.

If the skin is accidentally punctured or skin lesions are contaminated immediate action is necessary. Bleeding should be encouraged under running water, a dressing applied and the accident reported. If the material involved is known to contain hepatitis virus or to be positive for HBsAg, hepatitis B immunoglobulin (HBIG) should be given at once. Otherwise, the material should be tested for HBsAg and the HBIG given only if it is positive.

TABLE 12.3 Summary of post-exposure prophylaxis against hepatitis B

Immune status of employee/HCW	Hepatitis B status of patient/source of exposure		
	Unknown*	Negative	S/E antigen positive
Unvaccinated	Vaccinate + or − HBIG	Vaccinate	Vaccinate + HBIG
Vaccinated responder:			
Anti-HBS < 10 mIU/ml	Booster	Booster	Booster + HBIG
Anti-HBS > 100/ml	No action	No action	No action
Non-responder to primary course (3 doses)	Booster doses +/− HBIG	No action or booster doses	HBIG + booster doses
Non-responder to primary course (6 doses)	HBIG	No action	HBIG

*Risk assessment will aid decision-making on requirement for HBIG (hepatitis B immune globulin),
+, with; −, without.
Reproduced from McCloy (1997) with permission of CAB International.

TABLE 12.4 Recommendations for chemoprophylaxis following occupational exposure to HIV-infected blood[1]

Type of exposure	Source materials	Prophylaxis	Recommended regimen[2]
Percutaneous	Blood[3]		
	Highest risk	Recommended	AZT + 3TC + IDV
	Increased risk	Recommended	AZT + 3TC ± IDV
	No increased risk	Offer	AZT + 3TC
	Fluid containing visible blood or other infectious fluid or tissue	Offer	AZT + 3TC
	Other body fluids	Not offer	
Mucous membrane	Blood	Offer	AZT + 3TC ± IDV
	Fluid containing visible blood or other infectious fluid or tissue	Offer	AZT + 3TC
	Other body fluids	Not offer	
Skin, increased risk[4]	Blood	Offer	AZT + 3TC ± IDV
	Fluid containing visible blood or other infectious fluid or tissue	Offer	AZT + 3TC
	Other body fluids	Not offer	

[1] Based on CDC (1996).
[2] AZR, zidovudine 100 mg 3 times daily; 3TC, lamivudine 150 mg 3 times daily; IDV, indivair 800 mg 3 times daily.
[3] Highest risk: deep injury with large volume of blood with high titre of HIV.
Increased risk: *either* exposure to large volume of blood or blood with high titre of HIV.
No increased risk: *neither* large volume of blood nor blood with high titre of HIV.
[4] For skin, risk is increased for exposures involving high titre of HIV, prolonged contact, contact over an extensive area or contact with broken skin.
Reproduced from Waldron (1997) with permission of CAB International.

Table 12.3 summarizes post-exposure prophylaxis against hepatitis B (McCloy, 1997) and Table 12.4 lists recommendations for chemoprophylaxis after occupational exposure to HIV-infected blood (Waldron, 1997).

Follow-up procedures should be commenced.

Chapter 13

Tuberculosis

Laboratory-acquired tuberculosis, both pulmonary and non-pulmonary, has been a matter of concern for many years (see Chapter 1). Many publications have presented measures to prevent, or at least minimize, infection (Fish and Spendlove, 1950; Long, 1951; Report, 1958; DH, 1970, 1978; Kubica and Dye, 1967; Collins, 1982; Collins and Lyne, 1976; Collins *et al.*, 1995, 1997; Richmond *et al.*, 1996) but as reported in Chapter 1 cases still occur.

The resurgence of tuberculosis after several years of declining incidence, perhaps not unconnected with the AIDS epidemic and the emergence of multi-drug-resistant strains of tubercle bacilli, has prompted the World Health Organization (WHO, 1996) to declare that the disease is now a global emergency. It follows that unless proper precautions are taken the numbers of cases of laboratory-acquired tuberculosis are likely to increase.

Even before microorganisms were classified into hazard groups, and *Mycobacterium tuberculosis* was placed in Group 3, recommendations were made that investigations involving tuberculous or potentially tuberculous material should be processed in a microbiological safety cabinet (e.g. Williams and Lidwell, 1957; Report, 1958). The (Howie) Code of Practice (DH, 1978) extended this to 'All sputum and other material that may contain tubercle bacilli even if examination for them is not requested' and required that the safety cabinet(s) should be in 'special accommodation' (not endorsed in later publications). This was probably prompted by the curious practice, noted at that time, that in some laboratories sputum specimens were sorted on the basis of the examination requested. If this was 'Tb' then the specimen was taken to the cabinet. If it was 'other organisms', even from the same patient, the sputum was examined on the open bench. Unfortunately, diagnoses and requests do not always match the bacteriology. The logistics of handling specimens other than sputum that might contain tubercle bacilli in a very large laboratory where many extrapulmonary samples yield tubercle bacilli has been questioned by Allen and Darrell (1981). This is not unreasonable. As such specimens rarely contain very large numbers of mycobacteria it might be considered a justifiable risk to culture them in a Level 2 laboratory and then remove positives to the Level 3 laboratory.

While homogenates and suspensions of tubercle bacilli should always be handled in an efficient safety cabinet, the requirement or recommendation that sputum should always be processed in one should also be reconsidered in developing countries where reliable safety cabinets, or the energy to use them, are not available. As pointed out in Chapter 5, an inefficient cabinet offers a greater hazard to the worker than open bench operations.

In laboratories and primary health-care facilities where bacteriological examination is limited to the preparation and examination of direct smears, the potential for aerosol generation from the sample is therefore limited, given reasonably good technique (see below) and adequate ventilation (open windows). On the other hand the laboratory worker may well be more exposed to infection from the community at large (at home, during travel to and from work and in public places) during the 16 or so hours of the day when not at work.

A risk assessment therefore may well indicate that the probability of acquiring pulmonary tuberculosis when preparing sputum smears is small. Even so technicians and assistants who prepare smears in these places should receive adequate instruction in handling the material.

Personal precautions

Protective clothing should be worn for all technical procedures. Gloves are not essential but are desirable for handling specimen containers (see below). Surgical masks are of little value unless they are of the close-fitting fibre type (p. 189).

The usual precautions against infection as described elsewhere in this book should be observed, especially those that minimise the dispersal of aerosols and hand-to-mouth exposure.

Sputum containers

As no really satisfactory container has been found (Chapter 6) it is more than likely that the outside of any container will be contaminated. Allen and Darrell (1983) isolated tubercle bacilli from the outsides of 16 of 279 containers (6.5%). The outsides of 41 others were contaminated with upper respiratory tract organisms. There is thus a strong case for great care in handling sputum containers, and even for disinfecting them on arrival in the laboratory; and also a case for wearing gloves.

Direct smear preparation

Rough handling of sputum, which is viscous, may result in the release of small amounts, but these, by their nature, are unlikely to become airborne unless the material is allowed to dry and is then disturbed. Films should not be prepared by squeezing sputum between two slides, drawing them apart, heating and repeating the process until the films are dry. This procedure might release large numbers of dried airborne particles. It is safer to spread small pieces of sputum gently with sticks or plastic loops. Sputum is difficult material to handle anyway, and the traditional wire loops are useless. Swab sticks and plastic loops are better. Glass tubes cut into 12–15 cm lengths are useful—one end is rounded to accept a rubber teat and the other end left sharp. When placed into sputum and rotated it will cut the material and some can be drawn up, using the rubber teat. The films should then be left to dry. They may then be fixed and stained. The organisms do not come off the slide into the air. The slides should be handled carefully, however, to avoid contaminating the fingers. Even fixed and stained slides may contain viable tubercle bacilli (Allen, 1981).

Homogenates and suspensions

Operations at this level, which generate aerosols, should be done only in better-equipped laboratories (usually Level 3), not at the primary health-care level. Efficient and well-maintained microbiological safety cabinets (MSCs) should therefore be in use.

The staff should be experienced workers, not new recruits, and they should have positive skin tests and adequate medical supervision (p. 191).

In the preparation of homogenates the sputum and reagent mixture should not be shaken vigorously. The Vortex mixer is safest, provided that the tubes or bottles are capped. The tubes or bottles should be opened in the safety cabinet. Special care is needed if trisodium phosphate is used as the reagent. A homogenate in this dries readily in the cap and around the rim during the long time necessary for digestion. This dried material may contain tubercle bacilli and it may be dispersed violently when the cap is removed.

Care is also needed when pasteur pipettes are used in neutralization procedures. It is very easy to stab a finger or to contaminate the pipette and then distribute bacilli on the cabinet floor to be picked up on the hands. Stabbing can be avoided if soft plastic pasteur pipettes are used. Pipetting may be avoided by using the single-dose neutralizing technique of Collins *et al.* (1995, 1997).

Homogenates should be centrifuged in tightly-capped bottles or tubes in sealed centrifuge buckets (p. 88) to avoid the wide dispersal of aerosols if a bottle breaks. The inoculation of culture media is best done with plastic pasteur pipettes.

Cultures in liquid media, especially those containing Tween 80, in which the organisms are dispersed rather than in clumps, are a particularly fruitful source of aerosols containing tubercle bacilli, particularly when the caps are removed. The current policy of providing specially-equipped laboratories to which myco-bacteria may be sent for identification and sensitivity testing removes many of the hazards of handling tubercle bacilli from clinical laboratories. Fewer and more experienced individuals are exposed to infection.

Accidental inoculation

Tuberculous lesions may result from the implantation of tubercle bacilli into tissues by accidental injection, e.g. during pasteur pipetting and animal inocula-tion and trauma, e.g. with scalpels during tissue trimming for section prepara-tion. References to incidents of this kind are given on p. 50 and by Grange *et al.* (1988).

Probably the most hazardous procedure under this heading was the inocula-tion of animals with tuberculous materials. Fortunately, improvements in cul-tural techniques have made animal tests largely unnecessary in clinical laboratories. If they must be done, for research purposes, the precautions described on p. 261 should be followed.

Tissue processing

Precautions must also be taken with tissues that are submitted for culture or histological examination for tubercle bacilli. Even formalin-fixed tissues may still contain viable tubercle bacilli (Kappel *et al.*, 1996). Spray-freezing material for sectioning in a cryostat is known to have dislodged infectious particles, which, when inhaled, have initiated positive Mantoux tests in operators (Vetter, 1997; see p. 252). In the cryostat itself infected ice and tissue particles may be dispersed and contaminate the inside of the machine.

The postmortem room

Tuberculosis may be acquired during autopsies by either the inhalation or the percutaneous route. This hazard is considered in Chapter 18.

Chapter 14

Prions: unconventional agents

Prions, also known as unconventional agents and slow viruses, are associated with some transmissible spongiform encephalopathies (TSEs), including, in humans, Creutzfeldt-Jakob disease (CJD), the Gerstmann-Straussler-Scheinker syndrome (GSS) and kuru. In animals they are associated with scrapie in sheep, bovine spongiform encephalopathy (BSE) in cattle and with other diseases of deer, elk and mink.

The new variant of the BSE agent (nvBSE) (Will *et al.*, 1996) has now been linked with a variant of CJD (nvCJD) (Bruce *et al.*, 1997; Hill *et al.*, 1997).

No confirmed cases of occupationally-transmitted TSEs have been reported but Miller (1988) has reported a possible transmission to a laboratory worker and the ACDP (1994) mentions two cases of CJD in ex-laboratory workers that are '... a matter for concern but association with work remains purely speculative.'

In view of the long period that may elapse between exposure and the onset of symptoms, and their irreversibility, the agents of CJD, GSS and kuru are placed in Hazard Group 3 in the EC Biological Agents Directive (EC, 1993). BSE and the new variant CJD (nvCJD) has now been placed in Group 3 (HSE, 1998). Exemption is permitted, however (see p. 56), and investigations on human TSEs may be done at Containment Level 2 with additional precautions (ACDP, 1994, 1995).

Potential sources of infection

Three degrees of infectivity in tissues and body fluids are indicated by ACDP (1994).

The highest titres have been found in tissues from the brain, spleen, spinal cord, dura mater, thymus, tonsil, eye, peripheral lymph nodes, placenta and membranes, and gut-associated lymphoid tissue.

Tissues that have occasionally been found to have moderate or low titres include major peripheral nerves, cerebrospinal fluid, adrenal gland, liver, lung and pancreas.

Materials thought unlikely to be infective in any species affected by TSEs include milk, semen, saliva, skin, urine, muscle, faeces, kidney and blood.

Precautions

Precautions additional to those specified for Level 2, or requiring emphasis, include the routine use of gloves, aprons and eye protection, avoiding sharps, avoiding the generation and dispersion of aerosols, e.g. when centrifuging (sealed buckets), and working, again as a routine, in microbiological safety cabinets.

Formalin-fixed tissues should be regarded as infectious even after prolonged exposure. Even formic acid fixation cannot be relied on to decontaminate tissues. Tissue processors should not be used because of problems of disinfection. Cryostats should not be used because the initial spray freezing may dislodge and disperse infectious particles from the surface of the tissue (p. 250).

Decontamination

Disinfection

Disinfectants known to be effective are formic acid, 95% freshly prepared sodium hypochlorite, 20 000 ppm available chlorine, and sodium hydroxide, 2 mol/l. Surfaces, instruments, etc. should be exposed to these for at least 1 hour (Bell, 1997). Other disinfectants (e.g. phenolics, aldehydes, β-propiolactone, alcohols) are not effective (Taylor (1991; Manuelidis, 1997).

Sterilization

The following autoclave cycles are said to be effective in a porous-load autoclave (ACDP, 1994):

- A single cycle at 134 ± 4°C for 18 min HTAT.
- Six separate successive cycles at 134 ± 4°C for 3 min HTAT.

Waste disposal

Waste, e.g. tissues and disposable materials should be incinerated, preferably after autoclaving as above.

Much has been written about TSEs in the past few years. The most useful reference that can be given here, however, are those of the Advisory Committee on Dangerous Pathogens (ACDP, 1994, 1997) and Bell (1997).

Chapter 15

Endoparasites

In the EU Directive the infective stages of members of four genera of protozoa and two species of helminths are in Hazard Group 3 (EC, 1990, 1993; ACDP, 1995). Some of them have caused laboratory-acquired infections (see Chapter 3). All other human endoparasites may be handled at Level 2. In the USA all these parasites may be handled at Level 2 (CDC/NIH, 1993). Apart from these, and the precautions outlined below for the individual parasites, an appendix to ACDP (1995) is useful. Herwaldt and Juranek (1995) give a number of case histories that illustrate the hazards.

Hazard Group 3 endoparasites

Leishmania spp.

Infections with *Leishmania donovani* and *braziliensis* may be acquired directly from the bites of sandflies (*Phlebotomus* spp.) or by percutaneous (needle-stick injuries) and mucocutaneous contact with cultured parasites. Gloves should be worn. Safety cabinets are unnecessary. Rooms need not be sealable for fumigation.

Naegleria fowleri

Naegleria fowleri which is responsible for meningoencephalitis, enters the human body through the olfactory neuroepithelium. Precautions must therefore include protection against the inhalation of droplets and aerosols. Face protection and work in safety cabinets are therefore necessary. No records of laboratory-acquired infections have been found.

Plasmodium falciparum

This, the agent of malignant tertian malaria, is the only plasmodium in Group 3. Infection may result directly from the bite of anophelene mosquitoes, and from percutaneous and mucocutaneous exposure to infected blood and cultures. Gloves should be worn. Safety cabinets are unnecessary. Rooms need not be sealable for fumigation.

Trypanosoma cruzi

This protozoan is the causative agent of Chagas' disease (South and Central America). Infective forms may be present in blood, cultures and in the faeces of vectors (triatomid bugs) and may enter the body by percutaneous or mucocutaneous exposure and possibly by aerosols. The organism does not survive outside the animal body or culture.

Detailed precautions for work with *T. cruzi* are given by Gutteridge *et al.* (1974) and Hudson *et al.* (1983) and these should be consulted by anyone who wishes to work with this parasite. In general it is recommended that staff should be screened for antibodies; there should be protocols for dealing with accidental exposure; protective clothing with close fitting sleeves, disposable if possible, should be provided, as well as good quality gloves (when working with vectors sleeves should be tucked into gloves), visors or face masks and goggles; shoes, not sandals should be worn; sealed buckets should be used for centrifugation. There should be Class I or Class II microbiological safety cabinets (parasites will not pass through HEPA filters). The guidelines include precautions for the maintenance and use of infected bugs.

Trypanosoma brucei rhodesiense

This is the agent of African trypanosomiasis (sleeping sickness) and is spread by the bite of the tsetse fly (*Glossina palpitans*). Laboratory workers may be infected by percutaneous and mucocutaneous contact with suspensions and cultures. Gloves should be worn but safety cabinets are unnecessary and rooms need not be sealable for fumigation.

Echinococcus granulosus

This species, along with *E. multilocularis* and *E. vogeli*, rarely causes human disease in the UK and no laboratory-acquired infections seem to have been have been reported anywhere.

Precautions are essential, however, in view of the serious consequences of infection. Infective eggs may be present in canine faeces. Protection of hands (gloves, washing) and avoidance of ingestion (hand-to-mouth route) are adequate. Safety cabinets are unnecessary. Rooms need not be sealable for fumigation.

Taenia solium

Taenia solium is the only tapeworm in Group 3. Infection is by ingestion of the eggs. Gloves should be worn. Safety cabinets are unnecessary. Rooms need not be sealable for fumigation.

Hazard Group 2 endoparasites

Toxoplasma gondii would seem to be the only Group 2 parasite of concern, although a few others have occasionally caused infections among laboratory workers.

Toxoplasma gondii

The infective stage is transmitted in the faeces and may also be in blood and exudates. The usual contact (gloves) and hand-to-mouth precautions are adequate. Safety cabinets are not necessary. Women of child-bearing age are advised not to work with this agent. Parker and Holliman (1992) consider that the risks associated with occupational exposure are overstated.

Other Hazard Group 2 parasites

The ACDP (1995) requires work with *Acanthamoeba* spp. which are spread by aerosols to be done in microbiological safety cabinets, and that gloves be worn for handling hookworms (*Ancylostoma* and *Necator* spp.) and *Schistosoma* spp.

Hands should be washed well with soap and water after handling faecal material. Most commercial chlorine and iodine disinfectants are effective against *E. histolytica* and *Giardia* but the oocysts of *Cryptosporidium* are resistant to all but those disinfectants that are safe to use on the skin (Herwaldt and Juranek, 1995).

Laboratory workers may show no obvious symptoms when infected with some parasites. The only evidence may be seroconversion.

Chapter 16

Cell lines

Cell lines (cultures) are biological agents within the definitions of the EC Biological Agents Directive (EC, 1990). They are used in diagnostic virology and in pharmaceutical production. They do not themselves pose a hazard to laboratory workers unless they contain latent pathogenic viruses or suffer extrinsic contamination by other pathogens. The cells then offer the same hazards as direct work with those agents.

Cell lines may be classified into three broad groups according to their provenance (Frommer *et al.*, 1993):

Cell line	*Source*
Primary	Grown directly from tissues and usually unable to be cultured beyond a limited number of generations.
Permanent (or continuous)	Will grow on indefinitely (> 70 generations) and are obtained from:

    (1) specific cell type isolated from cell of tumour origin;
    (2) mutants derived from primary lines;
    (3) virus modifications of primary lines;
    (4) recombinant DNA modifications of primary lines.

Hybridoma	Cell fusions of primary and permanent cell lines.

Hazards of cell lines

Cell lines may carry undesirable indigenous agents which can cause human disease, or be contaminated during propagation and use with adventitious agents or with contaminant in the culture media or additives.

Indigenous agents

Primary cell cultures may be contaminated with a wide variety of viruses: the agents of hepatitis A, B, C, D and E; human retroviruses including HIV; herpes viruses, e.g. Epstein-Barr and cytomegalovirus viruses; flaviviruses (e.g. yellow fever, Kyasanur Forest viruses; filoviruses (Marburg and Ebola viruses); simian haemorrhagic virus; rabies and polioviruses; herpes B virus (Diggelman, 1993) and lymphocytic choriomeningitis virus (Gregg, 1995). Viruses may also be released from cells derived from tumours and lymphoblastic cell lines transformed by the Epstein-Barr virus.

Hazards of this nature may be avoided by obtaining cell lines, and replacing them regularly, from properly regulated cell banks, e.g. the European Collection of Cell Cultures.

Exogenous contamination

Exogenous bacterial contamination is also a problem, arising from media and additives. Apart from pathogens and opportunists such as mycobacteria and brucellas, mycoplasmas are the most troublesome, both in laboratory and production lines, although the species so far isolated do not appear to be pathogenic to humans. McGarrity and Kotani (1985) reported that 12–15% of cell lines were contaminated with mycoplasmas.

Fetal or neonatal bovine serum may contain the agent of bovine spongiform encephalitis and in the UK the use of this material is strictly controlled.

Immortalization

Some cells are made 'immortal' and therefore continuous with the aid of viruses such as Epstein-Barr, Rous sarcoma, polyomas and SV40.

Precautions with cell lines

The World Health Organization (WHO, 1987) proposed a classification of cell lines on the basis of their likelihood of carrying viruses:
Low: cells derived from avian and invertebrate tissues;
Medium: mammalian non-haematogenous cells—fibroblasts and epithelial cells;
High: blood and bone marrow cells derived from humans or non-human primates, human pituitary cells, caprine and bovine cells, especially those of neural origin, and hybridoma cells when at least one fusion partner is of human or non-human primate origin.

A risk assessment will indicate the necessary containment level. In general, all manipulations involving mammalian cell lines should be carried out in Class II microbiological safety cabinets, under at least Level 2 conditions with appropriate personal precautions (see Chapter 3). If cells are deliberately inoculated then the containment level should be that appropriate for the hazard group of the agent.

The safe handling of cell lines in large-scale pharmaceutical work, including testing production lines for viruses, is outside the scope of this book and readers are referred to Beale (1992), Frommer *et al.* (1993), Minor (1993) and Onions (1994).

Chapter 17

Laboratory animals

This chapter is concerned only with those diseases and allergies to which laboratory workers may be exposed. Readers are referred elsewhere for the management of laboratory animals and animal houses. Any laboratory animal may be a symptomless carrier of a microorganism that is a pathogen of humans.

Two broad groups of vertebrate animals may be infected with diseases transmissible to laboratory workers:

- Those deliberately purchased or bred for research or as aids to diagnosis or identification of biological agents;
- Sick animals which require investigation.

Supply of laboratory animals

The first line of defence against infections acquired from laboratory animals is the selection of the supplier/breeder. In some countries, e.g. the UK, certain animals (mice, rats, hamsters, guinea pigs, rabbits, cats, dogs and non-human primates) must be obtained from or bred in an approved establishment (Home Office, 1986, 1990). It should be noted, however, that infection may be latent and some infected animals may be symptom free. Even then, serological screening is recommended (ACDP, 1995). It is not possible for suppliers to screen all animals for all infections, but this may be desirable in the larger laboratories, e.g. for hantaviruses and tick-borne encephalitis viruses, and in non-human primates for herpes simian B virus and the simian immunodeficiency virus (see Chapter 1).

Animals imported into Britain are usually subject to animal health legislation, and in some cases (e.g. simians) to quarantine. In the UK the *Importation of Dogs, Cats and Other Mammals Order 1974*, and the *Importation of Animals Order 1980* apply.

Animal house containment levels

As with laboratories (Chapter 3) the containment levels specify the kind of 'containment', i.e. accommodation and services, access, equipment and safety precautions for each hazard group of organisms that might be deliberately

258

TABLE 17.1 Summary of containment requirements for laboratory animal houses

Hazard group/Animal containment level	Precautions
1	As for Level 1 laboratories plus limited access, arthropod control, protective clothing and gloves
2	As for Level 1 laboratories and animal houses plus decontamination of waste and cages before washing, microbiological safety cabinets and personal protection devices
3	As for Level 2 laboratories and animal house plus controlled access
4	As for Level 3 laboratories and animal houses plus strictly limited acccess, waste decontamination before removal from facility, clothes changing rooms and shower

Adapted from CDC/NIH (1993), WHO (1993), ACDP (1995).

inoculated with microorganisms for research or diagnostic purposes. They are set out in full by the ACDP (1995, 1997b) for the UK and by the Centers for Disease Control and the National Institutes of Health (CDC/NIH, 1993) for the USA. They are summarized here in Table 17.1.

In applying these levels consideration must be given to the requirements of individual species, their behaviour (e.g. aggressiveness), their zoonoses and their endo- and ectoparasites.

Animals must, of course, be kept under humane conditions according to animal welfare legislation and recommendations (*Animals (Scientific Procedures) Act 1986*: ACDP, 1997) in the UK and the laboratory animals welfare regulations in the USA (NIH, 1985; National Research Council, 1985).

Zoonoses

There are several reports and discussions about infections acquired in animal houses, including those caused by dermatophytes (Mackenzie, 1961; Alteras, 1965), sporotrichosis (Norden, 1951; Meyer, 1957), tuberculosis (Lurie, 1930), rat-bite fever (Glenhill, 1967), lymphocytic choriomeningitis (Bowen *et al.* (1975), hantaviruses (Umenai *et al.* 1979; Tsai, 1987) and Graham (1988). The papers by Miller *et al.* (1987) and Fox and Lipman (1991) are useful sources of information about the potential infectious hazards of handling laboratory animals.

The diseases of laboratory, domestic and feral animals that are transmissible to humans (i.e. zoonoses) are listed in Table 17.2.

The agents may be acquired by laboratory workers (a) by exposure resulting from breaches in containment practices, and (b) from unknown agents, for which no containment protocols have been developed.

Sources and routes of infection

The sources of infection include blood, body fluids, faeces, urine, tissues and arthropod vectors. Exposure may be mucocutaneous (contact with skin or mucous membranes), percutaneous (sharps injuries, animal and insect bites and

TABLE 17.2 Zoonoses of laboratory animals and those encountered in veterinary diagnosis and research

Animals	Zoonoses
Mice, rats, voles	Salmonellosis, leptospirosis, pasteurellosis, rat-bite fevers, campylobacteriosis, listeriosis, lymphocytic choriomeningitis, hantavirus infections
Guinea pigs	Salmonellosis
Hamsters	Salmonellosis, campylobacteriosis, lymphocytic choriomeningitis, hantavirus infections
Rabbits	Salmonellosis, pasteurellosis
Ferrets	Salmonellosis, tuberculosis, pasteurellosis
Cats	Salmonellosis, pasteurellosis, cat scratch fever, tuberculosis, chlamydiosis, toxoplasmosis, toxocariasis, ringworms
Dogs	Salmonellosis, campylobacteriosis, pasteurellosis, leptospirosis, toxocariasis, hydatid disease
Sheep, goats	Anthrax, brucellosis, salmonellosis, *E. coli* O157 infection, erysipelas, Q fever, orf, ovine chlamydiosis, louping ill (ovine encephalitis), toxoplasmosis, cryptosporidiosis, hydatid disease, ringworms
Cattle	Salmonellosis, campylobacteriosis, leptospirosis, brucellosis, tuberculosis anthrax, *E. coli* O157 infection, Q fever, cryptosporidiosis, ringworms
Pigs	Salmonellosis, campylobacteriosis, brucellosis, *Streptococcus suis* infection, relapsing fever, ringworms
Horses	Glanders, vesicular stomatitis, ringworms
Non-human primates	Salmonellosis, shigellosis, tuberculosis campylobacteriosis, simian B virus infection, Marburg disease, other herpes virus infections, respiratory syncytial virus infection, helminthiasis
Armadillos	Relapsing fever
Birds	Salmonellosis, campylobacteriosis, *Mycobacterium avium* infection, avian chlamydiosis, Newcastle disease
Badgers	Tuberculosis (bovine)
Reptiles	Salmonellosis, mycobacteriosis
Fish	Listeriosis, mycobacteriosis

Adapted from Collins *et al.* (1997).

scratches), faecal-oral (after handling soiled animals, contaminated bedding, etc.), and by the inhalation of aerosols and contaminated dust.

Precautions against infection

Where the agent is known the appropriate containment level should be observed. Where it is not known the minimum should be Containment Level 2, unless the clinical history suggests infection with an agent in a higher group when a higher containment level should apply. Personal precautions are discussed in Chapter 8. These should be supplemented as the infectious agents are in living creatures, not in laboratory vessels. Protective clothing needs to be stronger than that used in laboratories and gloves should be more robust.

The dispersion of airborne organisms from the animals, their cages and their bedding should be minimized. Engineering design features, such as directional ventilation of caging and rooms is desirable but masks should be available. Although dust masks may be adequate in some circumstances (see under Allergies, below), masks that satisfy the British standard BS 6016 type 203 or BS EN type FFO2 or FFP3 or equivalent (BS, 1991; BS EN 1991; see also HSE, 1990b) should be used. It is advisable to cover the hair and to wear strong shoes.

The premises should be vermin proof and provided with insect screens and traps.

Consideration should be given to immunization of animal house staff (Chapter 8).

ANIMAL INOCULATION

Contamination of the operator and the environment may occur unless some precautions are taken, particularly with intradermal inoculations. Wedum (1953) and Hanel and Alg (1955) showed that the injection sites were contaminated as a result of leakage, but that a 30% reduction in the numbers of organisms could be obtained if the inoculation site was swabbed with disinfectant before and immediately after injection.

ACCIDENTS

The wide variety of accidents that may occur in animal houses is illustrated in Table 17.3, which shows the experience of the US National Animal Diseases Center (Miller *et al.*, 1987).

POSTMORTEM EXAMINATIONS

Autopsies on animals invariably generate aerosols. Those carried out on animals infected with Hazard Group 3 agents should be done in microbiological safety cabinets or isolators. There is a strong argument for applying this recommendation to agents in lower groups on the grounds of latent infections. The ACDP (1997) offers advice on the postmortem examination of animals infected with transmissible spongiform encephalopathy agents (see also Chapter 14).

TABLE 17.3 Agent/exposure/infection experience at the US National Animal Disease Center

Agent of exposure	Number of exposures	Number of infections resulting
Syringe accidents		
Autoinoculation	38	3
Spray	8	—
Animal autopsy		
Laceration with instruments	12	2
Splash/spray	6	—
Conjunctival exposure	4	2
Mouth pipetting	6	—
Animal contact	11	2
Glassware accidents		
Lacerations	2	—
Dropped culture	6	—
Equipment failure	2	—
Other	8	—
Unknown (?aerosols)	25	25
Total	128	128

From Miller *et al.* (1987).
Reproduced by permission of the American Industrial Hygiene Association.

DISPOSAL OF WASTE AND DEAD ANIMALS

All waste, and especially bedding, should be incinerated. Less bulky materials should first be autoclaved. Dead animals should be incinerated. The smaller animals should first be autoclaved.

Working with simians

The emergence of serious (Group 4) infections in monkeys and their transmission to humans (e.g. simian B, Marburg, and possibly Ebola viruses) has led to the adoption of special precautions for work with these animals. Probably the first and still valid set of such precautions was formulated by Hartley (1974); up-to-date guidance is now given by the (UK) Medical Research Council (MRC, 1990) and the Advisory Committee on Dangerous Pathogens (ACDP, 1997a).

Fortunately, only a few laboratories, worldwide, are engaged in work with these animals and the transport and laboratory use are well regulated in developed countries.

Allergy to laboratory animals

Allergy to laboratory animals (ALA) may manifest as urticaria and conjunctivitis resulting from skin contact, and rhinitis and/or asthma resulting from inhalation. The sensitizing agents are fur, feathers, dander, dried urine and dust in bedding containing any or all of these. The urine of rats, mice and guinea pigs contains allergenic proteins which are associated with asthma (Newman Taylor et al., 1977). Animal feeding stuffs may also contain allergenic spores.

In susceptible individuals the symptoms usually develop after exposure for 4–6 months.

Protection of staff

Individuals known to have allergies to any animals should not be employed in places where they are exposed.

The measures for protection again infection (see above) are usually effective in protecting against exposure to allergens, but special consideration should be given to protective clothing, including gloves, and the provision of masks. Industrial dust masks might be used for work with non-infected animals but it is best to supply workers who are at risk with those that conform with the standards indicated above or those of equivalent organizations. Masks should be worn during the changing and disposal of bedding as this is likely to release allergens, including spores of actinomycetes and fungi.

Monitoring

Legislation (e.g. in Europe) may require risk assessments and monitoring the animal environment. Simple particle counting is inadequate and such procedures as the radioallergosorbent test and enzyme-linked immunoassay (ELISA) with monoclonal antibodies should be used.

A booklet on allergy to laboratory animals is published by the Education Services Advisory Committee (HSE, 1990). The papers by Cockroft *et al.* (1981), Agrup *et al.* (1986) and Bryant *et al.* (1995) offer more detailed information. Useful information on allergy to laboratory animals is also given by Lipman and Newcomer (1989) and the HSE (1992).

Chapter 18

The postmortem room

A number of the infections mentioned in Chapter 1 were acquired by pathologists, technicians and lay assistants during autopsies. It may be argued that they were not 'laboratory acquired', but in the first four decades of this century pathology had not separated into several distinct disciplines and the staff moved freely between laboratory and mortuary. Today, autopsy work is restricted to histopathologists, forensic pathologists and their staff but still cannot be divorced from clinical laboratory activities.

Apart from the well-known story of Semmelweiss, the earliest report of an infection associated with postmortem examinations seems to be that of Wilks (1862) who described diseases of the skin—'verruca necrogenica'. Reports then followed about infections with blastomyces (e.g. Evans, 1903), tularaemia (Weilbacher, 1938), toxoplasmosis (Neu, 1967) and streptococci (reviewed by Hawkey *et al.*, 1980) and Wormald (1950) wrote of cases of salmonellosis, acquired by postmortem room staff after autopsies on patients known to be infected. More recently, Nolte *et al.* (1996) expressed concern about the possibility of the transmission of hantaviruses during autopsies.

Tuberculosis seems to be an occupational disease of pathologists and postmortem room staff. Alderson (1931) described an infection following a cut with a knife and 'inoculation tuberculosis' or 'prosector's finger' (see Stokes, 1925 and Minkowitz, 1969), resulting from cuts and pricks. Later, the incidence of pulmonary tuberculosis among doctors and medical students who were engaged in autopsy work caused some concern (see, e.g. Morris, 1946). That this is a continuing problem is evident from the papers of Sugita *et al.* (1989) and Templeton *et al.* (1995). Recently (Anon., 1995) there was a report about five people who were infected during autopsy.

Smith (1953), in an investigation in the UK covering 192 000 autopsies in which 9000 subjects had active tuberculosis, noted that only two pathologists and eight technicians acquired tuberculosis that may have been work related. Reid (1957), on the other hand, who compared the incidence of tuberculosis among mortuary workers with that in a control group reported that the observed:expected ratio was 9.1:1. Bogen *et al.* (1959) wrote of the transmission of tuberculosis post mortem.

Simpson (1965) was concerned about cases of tuberculosis first registered after death. Linel and Östberg (1966), Roberts (1971), Enarson *et al.* (1978), Katz *et al.* (1985) and Lundgren (1987) have all pointed to the hazards during autopsies of undiagnosed tuberculosis. Harrington and Shannon (1976) found

264

that the incidence of tuberculosis among those engaged in this kind of work was five times greater than in the general population. In a 2-year survey Grist and Emslie (1983) found that seven of 14 laboratory workers who had acquired tuberculosis had been involved in postmortem or mortuary work. Since then they have identified a further seven cases (Grist and Emslie, 1985, 1987, 1989, 1991).

Routes of infection

These are contact, either percutaneous or mucocutaneous, and inhalation of infected aerosols. Of these, the former is generally considered to be the most important in laboratory-acquired infections (Newsom *et al.*, 1983) but Hedwall (1940) found tubercle bacilli on towels, trays and mortuary tables. Bogen and Dunn (1941) exposed open petri dishes during postmortem examinations and recovered tubercle bacilli from them and Sloane (1942) exposed glass plate 20 cm above a tuberculous lung while it was sliced and also recovered tubercle bacilli. Tuberculosis in guinea pigs placed in cages near cadavers during autopsies was observed by Bogen (1959).

Mucocutaneous contact includes splashes into the eyes and onto the skin. Percutaneous contact is not confined to cuts and pricks with sharp instruments. The cut edges of bones and bone splinters can also penetrate the skin. Skin and mucous membranes, e.g. of the eyes, may receive blood splashes.

Aerosols are released during dissection of the cadaver, especially when saws and drills are use, and when organs are examined on side tables. Opening intestines is a fruitful source, as is the 'squelching' action when organs such as lungs are compressed for cutting.

Precautions against infection

Minimal protective clothing should include full length gowns, with arm protection, rubber or plastic aprons, suitable gloves (heavy duty or reinforced according to the nature of the work: see Chapter 8), rubber boots, visors or masks and goggles, and head covering (HSE, 1991b).

Covering severed rib ends with towels and using scissors, where possible, instead of knives are recommended by the National Research Council (1989). Bull *et al.* (1991) recommended that eye protection be worn during autopsies.

Altogether, these should afford reasonable protection against mucocutaneous and percutaneous contact in most cases.

Some protection against aerosol inhalation is offered by directional ventilation of the autopsy table (DH 1978) (i.e., the airflow should not be directed towards the operator's face). Air changes of the order of 10 per hour are recommended. Newsom *et al.* (1983) recommended, in addition, the provision of ventilated hoods for close dissection of organs. Class I and II microbiological safety cabinets may not be large enough and plastic isolators (Trexler and Gilmour, 1983) should be considered for potentially hazardous work.

High pressure sprays should not be used as they disperse aerosols and droplets.

Special precautions are recommended for opening the skull, e.g. in cases of

Creutzfeldt-Jakob disease (CJD). These include air-powered oscillating saws with remote exhaust ports and enclosing the head in a plastic bag into which the saw and hands are inserted through a hole (MacArthur *et al.*, 1986; ACDP, 1994; Bell, 1997))

Extra care is must be taken if it is considered necessary to conduct autopsies on patients known to have died of certain diseases (haemorrhagic fevers, hepatitis, AIDS, tuberculosis, spongiform encephalopathies, etc.), although in some cases a diagnosis is not made before death, e.g. with tuberculosis (Simpson, 1965), and autopsies conducted for forensic purposes. Working in plastic isolators may be indicated (Trexler and Gilmour, 1983; see p. 114). Detailed advice is given by the ACDP (1985, 1994, 1977a) and by MacArthur and Scheidermann (1987) and HSE (1991b).

Disinfection

Hypochlorite, 1000 ppm is suitable for 'clean' surfaces, but where there is blood a solution containing 10 000 should be used. Other disinfectants may not be suitable (see Chapters 7 and 14).

Waste disposal

Debris and disposable materials should be placed in colour-coded bags (p. 162) for autoclaving and incineration.

Chapter 19

Biotechnology: genetic modification

Biotechnology is concerned with the use of microorganisms and cells for the production of metabolic products for therapeutic and industrial purposes. It usually involves large scale processing.

This chapter is concerned only with the safe handling in the laboratory of microorganisms used in biotechnology and not with production or release into the environment. Nevertheless, the volumes used in biotechnology laboratory work are usually much greater than those clinical investigations and are usually of the order of 1–10 litres. The organisms are grown in closed containers known as fermenters.

There are two kinds of biotechnology: (1) that which uses naturally-occurring strains of microorganisms, and (2) that which uses genetically-modified microorganisms, prepared for similar reasons.

Naturally-occurring microorganisms

The microorganisms used in 'traditional' biotechnology are mostly strains in Hazard Group 1 and therefore generally regarded as harmless, although exposure to some of them may be associated with allergies (Duffus and Brown, 1985; Hambleton et al., 1992). The precautions required in handling these are no more than good microbiological practice and good occupational hygiene and safety procedures, with, of course reference to the COSHH regulations. A few microorganisms in higher groups are used, however, in the manufacture of vaccines and certain pharmaceuticals. Laboratory work with these requires, in addition, the same containment and precautions set out in Chapter 3 and detailed in later chapters.

Genetically-modified microorganisms (GMMs)

The Organization for Economic Cooperation and Development (OECD, 1986, 1992), the European Federation of Biotechnology (EFB; Frommer et al.,1989) and the World Health Organization (WHO, 1993) appear to agree that the potential risks associated with genetically-modified organisms are of the same order as those offered by naturally-occurring microorganisms—with reference, of course to the hazard groups of the hosts and inserts, and that biotechnology is a safe industry. Beringer (1997) points out that '... to date there have been no examples of workers being adversely affected by any genetically-modified organisms, although each year there are incidents of infections from known pathogens that are being handled by staff in hospital pathology laboratories.'

In some countries, however, genetic modification has become a political and ethical issue, and its regulation a growth industry. This is not the place to consider the the philosophy behind this development and only those issues that might affect laboratory-acquired infections and allergies are outlined, based on the EC (1990, 1994) Directives and the (UK) *Genetically Modified Organisms (Contained Use) Regulations* as amended by the *Genetically Modified Organisms (Contained Use)(Amended) Regulations 1996* and the views of the EFB.

Contained use is defined as any operation in which GMMs are '... cultured, stored, used, transported, destroyed or disposed of and for which physical barriers or a combination of physical barriers with chemical barriers or both, are used to limit their contact with the general population and the environment.'

A guide to the UK regulations is presented by the HSE (1996) and further guidance on good practice is given by the Advisory Committee on Genetic Modification (ACGM, 1997).

Classifications

The UK Regulations describe type A and type B operations:

Type A: The GMMs are used for teaching, research, development, non-industrial and non-commercial activities, requiring only good microbiological and good occupational safety and hygiene practices and where the agents can inactivated by standard laboratory procedures.

Type B: Operations other than type A. These are essential industrial, i.e., large scale, but laboratory work will be involved.

Other considerations for type B operations are:

(1) The vector and insert should not be self-transmissible and be poorly mobilizable.
(2) The vector and insert should be well characterized but only to a degree ... that they are unlikely to endow the GMM with a harmful phenotype.
(3) The GMM should not be capable of transferring resistance genes to other microorganisms if it could compromise disease treatment.
(4) The GMM should be as safe in the industrial setting as the parent organisms or have characteristics that limit survival and gene transfer.

The GMMs themselves are classified into two groups, I and II. Roman numerals are used to distinguish these groups from hazard groups, which use arabic numerals.

Group I

All three of the following criteria must be satisfied:

(1) The recipient/parental organism (the host) is unlikely to cause disease in humans, animals or plants (i.e. is essentially in Hazard Group I in the classification described in Chapter 3).

(2) The vector and insert do not endow the GMM with a phenotype likely to cause disease or any adverse effects of the environment.
(3) The (resulting) GMM is unlikely to cause disease in humans, animals or plants (i.e. is essentially in Hazard Group I in the classification described in Chapter 3).

(Our parentheses.)

Group II

This group includes any GMMs that do nor satisfy any of the above criteria.

Containment measures

Type A work with Group I GMMs, which offer no identifiable risk to human health, must satisfy the general requirements of the *Control of Substances Hazardous to Health Regulations 1994* (COSHH) but there is no need for health surveillance unless it is indicated for medical reasons.

Containment measures do apply to type B operations and GMMs. They are set out in the guide to the regulations (HSE, 1996) and ACGM (1997) as Containment Levels B2, B3 and B4. These are similar to but do not exactly equate with those designed for pathogens and described in Chapter 3.

Other requirements

The regulations require, in brief:

(1) risk assessments (see Chapter 11 of this book and below);
(2) a local genetic modification safety committee;
(3) advance notification to HSE of intention to use premises, and consent to do so;
(4) notification to HSE of individual genetic modification activities, and for some, consent;
(5) standards of occupational and environmental safety;
(6) notification of accidents and drawing up of emergency plans.

Risk assessments—'new' organisms

Biotechnology operations, may involve the use of microorganisms about which little is known, i.e. those never used before, newly isolated strains, mutants, and recombinants. The EFB Working Party on Safety in Biotechnology (Leleiveld *et al.*, 1995) therefore considered how the safety of such strains could be assessed. The following tests were considered.

Characterization

These include the normal taxonomic tests, with care to avoid guilt by association: an organism should not be regarded as a pathogen because other species in the same genus are harmful.

Pathogenicity

Tests include protein probes with monoclonal antibodies prepared against adhesins, toxins and other virulence factors.

Enzyme assay

Enzymes known to be associated with virulence include hyaluronidases, coagulases and siderophores.

Tests for fimbriae

These are known to be associated with the adhesion of bacteria to cells.

Serology

Tests with polyclonal and monclonal antibodies for antigens associated with pathogenicity.

Survival and growth in human serum

Some pathogens have this ability.

Gene probing

DNA-DNA hybridization, polymerase chain reactions and restriction-fragment-length techniques may be of assistance in the not too distant future.

Tissue culture tests

Much depends on the choice of cell line and dose applied. Even organisms known to be harmless may damage some cells.

Tests on animals

As pathogenicity to humans does not parallel that to animals this is an unreliable method unless strict parameters are imposed.

Allergens

Chemical assays in dust and the air may reveal the presence and amounts of these (mostly) water-soluble glycoproteins.

Toxic metabolites

Culture fluids may be tested for endotoxins by the *Limulus* or rabbit pyrogene methods.

A screening method, employing these tests was proposed by Lelieveld *et al.* (1995) and is shown in Table 19.1. This may enable an assessment to be made of the likelihood that the organism is of low, medium or high pathogenicity to

TABLE 19.1 Tentative screening scheme for new isolates

Screening step	Likelihood of pathogenicity to humans		
	Low	*Medium*	*High*
Source of isolate	Soil, water, air, cold blooded animals	Sewage, manure, warm blood animals	Human blood or tissue
Taxonomy (genus, species, strain, biochemical characteristic)[a]	No human pathogens known	Only one or few animal pathogens	Human or animal pathogens
Optimal growth temperature	< 30°C	31–35°C	36–40°C
Human serum required for growth	No	Doubtful	Yes
Haemolyses human red cells	No	No	Yes
Haemolyses animal red cells	No	Yes or doubtful	Yes
Toxins (endo-, afla, myco, ochra)	No	Doubtful	Yes
Adhesins, fimbriae	No	Doubtful	Yes
Enzymes associated with pathogenicity	No	Doubtful	Yes
Animal pathogenicity/toxicity[b]; high/ medium/low dose; route	Yes, with high dose	No, with high dose	Yes with high dose

[a] According to Bergey, etc.
[b] Appropriate animal.
Adapted from Lelieveld (1995) with permission of the Editors of *Applied Microbiology and Biotechnology.*

humans, and thus indicate appropriate containment levels (2, 3 or 4), although biological agents in Hazard Group 4 are not (at present) used in biotechnology.

Naked DNA and oncogenic viruses

Although there is no positive clinical evidence of transmission of either of these agents to laboratory workers (but see Malignant disease, p. 37) the potential for such transmission is recognised. Precautions and guidelines for working with them have been published (NIH, 1974a,b; 1979; HSE, 1997; see also Rayburn, 1990). In general, these are in accord with other precautions against laboratory-acquired infection.

References

Publications of the Department of Health, UK Health Departments and the Department of Health and Social Security are listed under DH. Those of the Health and Safety Commission and the Health and Safety Executive under HSE.

ACDP (1984). *Categorization of pathogens according to hazard and Categories of Containment.* Advisory Committee on Dangerous Pathogens. London: The Stationery Office.

ACDP (1985). Guidance for the use, testing and maintenance of laboratory and animal flexible film isolators. Advisory Committee on Dangerous Pathogens. London: Health and Safety Executive.

ACDP (1990). *Categorization of pathogens according to Hazard and categories of containment.* 2nd edn. Advisory Committee on Dangerous Pathogens. London: The Stationery Office.

ACDP (1994). *Precautions for work with the human and animal transmissible encephalopathies.* Advisory Committee on Dangerous Pathogens. London: The Stationery Office.

ACDP (1995a). *Categorisation of biological agents according to hazard and categories of containment.* 4th edn. Advisory Committee on Dangerous Pathogens. Sudbury, HSE Books.

ACDP (1995b). *Protection against blood-borne pathogens at work—HIV and hepatitis.* Advisory Committee on Dangerous Pathogens. Sudbury, HSE Books.

ACDP (1996). *Microbiological risk assessment: an interim report.* Advisory Committee on Dangerous Pathogens. London: The Stationery Office.

ACDP (1997a). *The management of simians in relation to infectious hazards to staff.* Advisory Committee on Dangerous Pathogens. Sudbury, HSE Books.

ACDP (1997b). *Working safely with research animals.* Advisory Committee on Dangerous Pathogens. Sudbury: HSE Books.

ACDP (1997c). *Infection risks to new and expectant mothers in the workplace.* Advisory Committee on Dangerous Pathogens. Sudbury: HSE Books.

ACDP (1997d). *Management and Control of viral haemorrhagic fevers.* Advisory Committee on Dangerous Pathogens. London: The Stationery Office.

ACGM (1993). *Guidelines for the risk assessment of operations involving the contained use of genetically-modified microorganisms.* ACGM/HSE/DE Note No. 7. Advisory Committee on Genetic Modification. London: The Stationery Office.

ACGM (1997). *Compendium of guidance on good practice for people working with genetically-modified organisms under containment conditions.* Advisory Committee on Genetic Modification. London: Health and Safety Executive.

ACHARD, C. (1929). Fievre typhoide contractee au laboratoire par la souillure des mains. *Bulletin of the Academy of Medicine Paris* **102**, 278–282.

AGRUP, G., BELIN, L., SJOSTED, L. *et al.* (1986). Allergy to laboratory animals in laboratory technicians and animal keepers. *British Journal of Industrial Medicine* **43**, 192–198.

AJMAL, M. (1969). A laboratory infection with *Erysipelothrix rhusiopathiae. Veterinary Record* **85**, 688.

AL-ASKA, A.K. & CHAGLA, A.H. (1989). Laboratory-associated Chagas disease. *Journal of Hospital Infection* **14**, 69–71.

ALBRECHT, J. (1967). Ungewohnlicher Verlauf einer Laboratoriumsinfektion durch *Salmonella typhi. Zentralblatt für Bakteriologie* Ab 1. Orig **204**, 299–301.

ALDERSON, H.E. (1931). Tuberculosis from direct inoculation with autopsy knife: report of a case. *Archives of Dermatology and Syphilology* **28**, 98–100.

ALEKSEEVA, A.A., LEBEDKA, W.V. & DUBNIAKOVA, W.M. (1959). Clinical aspects of Venezuelan equine encephalitis. *Zhurnal neuropatologii i Psikhiatrii* **59**, 313–320.

ALEXANDROFF, K. (1927). Case of laboratory infection with recurrent typhus (relapsing fever). *Vrachebnaya Gazeta* **31**, 765–767.

ALLBRITTEN, F.F., SHEELY R.F. & JEFFERS, W.A. (1940). *Haverhillia multiformans* septicaemia: in relation to Haverhill and rat-bite fevers. *Journal of the American Medical Association* **114**, 2360–2363.

ALLEN, B.W. (1977). A dual purpose gas burner for use in microbiological safety cabinets. *Medical Laboratory Sciences* **34**, 277–278.

ALLEN, B.W. (1981). Survival of tubercle bacilli in heat-fixed sputum smears. *Journal of Clinical Pathology* **34**, 719–722.

ALLEN, B.W. & DARRELL, J.H (1981). Extrapulmonary tuberculosis: a potential source of laboratory-acquired infection, *Journal of Clinical Pathology* **34**, 404–407.

ALLEN, B.W. & DARRELL, J.H. (1983). Contamination of specimen container surfaces during sputum collection *Journal of Clinical Pathology* **36**, 479–481.

ALLEN, R.K., PIERSON, D.L. & REDMAN, O.G. (1979). Cutaneous inoculation tuberculosis: prosector's wart occurring in a physician. *Cutis* **23**, 815–818.

ALTERAS, I. (1965). Human dermatophyte infections from laboratory animals. *Sabouraudia* **4**, 143–145.

AMOSS, H.L. (1931). Localization of brucella. *International Clinics* **4**, 93–98.

ANDERSEN, A.A. (1958). New sampler for the collection, sizing and enumeration of viable airborne particles. *Journal of Bacteriology* **76**, 471–484.

ANDERSON, S.G. (1946). A note of two laboratory infections with the virus of Newcastle diseases of fowls. *Medical Journal of Australia* **1**, 371.

ANDERSON, R.E., STEIN, L., MOSS, M. L. *et al.* (1952). Potential infection hazards of common bacteriological techniques. *Journal of Bacteriology* **64**, 473–481.

ANDREWES, C.H. (1940). Control of air-borne infection in air-raid shelters and elsewhere. *Lancet* **2**, 770–774.

ANGLIM, A.M., COLMER, J.E., LOVING, T.J. *et al.* (1995). An outbreak of needlestick injures in hospital employees due to needles piercing infectious waste containers. *Infection Control and Hospital Epidemiology* **16**, 470–476.

ANIDO, G. (1973). Australia antigen—transmission in laboratory. *New England Journal of Medicine* **288**, 160. *Animals (Scientific Procedure) Act 1986.* London: The Stationery Office.

ANON. (1944) A human case of pneumonic plague (laboratory infection). *Public Health Reports* **59**, 962.

ANON. (1945). Strain of *Brucella abortus* used for vaccination of calves: pathogenic for man. Annual Report, Albany, NY. Department of Health Division of Laboratories and Research.

ANON. (1969). *Annual Brucellosis Summary.* Atlanta: National Communicable Disease Center.

ANON. (1980). Tuberculosis infection associated with tissue processing. *California Medicine* **30**.

ANON (1981). Protective clothing in the laboratory. *Laboratory Equipment Digest* **19**, 67–69.

ANON. (1981). Tuberculosis infection associated with tissue processing. *Mortality and Morbidity Weekly Report* **30**, 73–74

ANON. (1989). Hepatitis B. *Hospital Hazardous Materials Management* **3**, 5.

ANON. (1994). Laboratory acquired invasive meningococcal disease. *Canadian Communicable Disease Reports* **20**, 12–13.

ANON. (1995). Tuberculosis. Five people infected during autopsy. *Hospital Infection Control* **22**, 85–86.

ANON. (1997). *British National Formulary.* Chapter 6, p. 310. London: British Medical Association and the Royal Pharmaceutical Society.

ANTOINE, H.M. MARX, R. & BARRE, A. (1965). Considerations cliniques et immunologiques a propos d'un cas de typhus murin (contamination de laboratoire). *Bulletin de la Medicin militaire francaise* **59**, 419–423.

ARLOING, S., COURMONT, P. & GATE J. (1910). Un cas de fievre de Malte; contagion de laboratoire. *Provence Medicale* **21**, 533.

ARONSON, P.R. (1962). Septicaemia from concomitant infection with *Trypanosoma cruzi* and *Neisseria perflava*; first case of laboratory-acquired Chagas' disease in the United States, *Annals of Internal Medicine* **57**, 994–1000.

AS (1994a). Australian Standard: *AS 2252.1. Part 1. Biolological Safety Cabinets (Class I) for personnel and environmental protection.* Sydney: Standards Association of Australia.

AS (1994b). Australian Standard: *AS 2252.1. Part 2. Biolological Safety Cabinets (Class II) for personnel and product protection.* Sydney: Standards Association of Australia.

AS (1994c). *Australian Standard: AS2647. Biolological Safety Cabinets—Installation and Use.* Sydney: Standards Association of Australia.

AS (1994d). Australian Standard: *AS 2252.2. Part 1. Laminar flow biolological Safety Cabinets (Class II) for personnel and product protection.* Sydney: Standards Association of Australia.

AS/NZ (1995). *Australian/New Zealand Standard AS/NZ 2243. Safety in Laboratories. Part 3. Microbiology.* Sydney: Standards Association of Australia.

ASHDOWN, L.R. (1992). Melioidosis and safety in the clinical laboratory. *Journal of Hospital Infection* 21, 301–306.

ASSOCIATION OF NATIONAL HEALTH SERVICE OCCUPATIONAL PHYSICIANS (1986). Health Assessment for Employment in the NHS, Physicians Guidance Note 9. Bath: Royal United Hospital.

BADGER, L.F., DYER, R.E. & RUMREICH, A. (1931). An infection of the Rocky Mountain spotted fever type. *Annals of Internal Medicine* 32, 982–987.

BAKER, A.S., PATON, B. & HAAF, J. (1989) Ocular infection; clinical laboratory considerations. *Clinical Laboratory Newsletter* 11, 97–101.

BALDWIN, A.H., McCALLUM, F. & DOULL, J. A. (1923). A case of pharyngeal diphtheria probably due to autoinfection from a diphtheritic lesion of the thumb. *Journal of the American Medical Association* 80, 1375.

BALL, M.J. & BOLTON, F.G. (1985). Effects on inactivation of HTLV-III on laboratory tests. *Lancet* ii, 99.

BALL, M.J & GRIFFITHS, D. (1985). Effects on chemical analysis of beta-propiolactone treatment of whole blood and plasma. *Lancet* i, 1160–1161.

BANERJEE, K., GUPTA, N.P. & GOVERDHAN, M.K. (1979). Viral infections in laboratory personnel. *Indian Journal of Medical Research* 69, 363–373.

BARBEITO, M.S., ALG, R.L. & WEDUM, A.G. (1961). Infectious bacterial aerosol from dropped petri dish cultures. *American Journal of Medical Technology* 27, 318–322.

BARBEITO, M.S. & BROOKEY, E.A. (1976). Microbiological hazards from the exhaust of a high vacuum sterilizer. *Applied and Environmental Microbiology* 32, 671–678.

BARBEITO, M.S. & GREMILLION, G.G. (1968). Microbiological evaluation of an industrial refuse incinerator. *Applied Microbiology* 16, 261–295.

BARBEITO, M.S. & TAYLOR, L.A. (1968). Containment of microbial aerosols in a microbiological safety cabinet. *Applied Microbiology* 16, 490–495.

BARCISZEWSKI, N. & DOMANSKI, E. (1951). A case of Weil's disease acquired in a laboratory. *Polski Lekarski* 6, 1550–1551.

BARDENWERPER, H.W. (1952). Human sickness caused by *Brucella abortus* strain 19. *Journal of the American Medical Association* 155, 970–971.

BARKIN, R.M., GUCKIAN, J.C. & GLOSSER, J.W. (1974). Infection by *Leptospira ballum*. A laboratory-associated case, *Southern Medical Journal* 67, 155–176.

BARKLEY, W.E. (1972). *Evaluation of controlled airflow systems for environmental safety in biomedical research.* PhD Thesis. University of Minnesota.

BARRY, M., RUSSI, M., ARMSTRONG, L. *et al.* (1995). Brief report: treatment of a laboratory-acquired Sabia virus infection. *New England Journal of Medicine* 333, 294–295.

BARWELL, C.F. (1955). Laboratory infection of man with virus of enzootic abortion of ewes. *Lancet* ii, 1369–1371.

BASSETT, D.J.C. (1971). Causes and prevention of sepsis due to Gram-negative bacteria: Common source outbreaks. *Proceedings of the Royal Society of Medicine* 64, 980–986.

BATCHELOR, B.I., BINDLE, R.J., GILKS, G.F. *et al.* (1992). Biochemical misidentification of *Brucella melitensis* and subsequent laboratory acquired infections. *Journal of Hospital Infection* 22, 159–162.

BAUM, G.L. & LERNER, P.I. (1970). Primary pulmonary blastomycosis: a laboratory acquired infection. *Annals of Internal Medicine* 73, 263–265.

BAUM, G.L. & SCHWARZ, J. (1959). North American blastomycosis. *American Journal of Medical Science* 238, 661–684.

BAUM, S.G., LEWIS, A.M., ROWE, W.P. *et al.* (1966). Epidemic non-meningitis lymphocytic-choriomeningitis virus infection. An outbreak in a population of laboratory personnel. *New England Journal of Medicine* 274, 934–936.

BAUMBERG, A. & FREEMAN, R. (1971). *Salmonella typhimurium* strain LT-2 is still pathogenic for man. *Journal of General Microbiology* 65, 99–100.

BAYER, R.A. (1982). Q fever as an occupational illness at the National Institutes of Health. *Public Health Reports* **97**, 58–60.

BEALE, A.J. (1992). Safe handling of mammalian cells on an industrial scale. In: *Safety in Industrial Microbiology and Biotechnology* (Eds C. H. Collins & A. J. Beale). pp. 153–160. Oxford: Butterworth-Heinemann.

BEAUMONT, L.R. (1987). The detection of blood on non-porous environmental surfaces, etc. *Infection Control* **8**, 424–426.

BECHTELSHEIMER, H., KORB, G. & GEDIEK, P. (1970). Die 'Marburgvirus' hepatitis. Untersuchungen bei Menschen und Meerschweinchen. *Virchows Archiv für pathologische Anatomie* **351**, 273–290.

BEEMAN, E.A. (1950). Q fever: an epidemiological note. *Public Health Reports.* Washington **65**, 88.

BELL, J. (1997) Managing risks from prions in the laboratory and post-mortem room. In: *Managing Biological and Chemical Risks* (Ed. D.R. Morgan) pp. 85–96. London: Medical Research Council and the Institute of Biology.

BELLER, K. (1949). Laboratoriumsinfektion mit dem Lansing-Virus. *Zentralblatt für Bakeriologie* Abt I Orig. **153**, 269–273.

BENDING, M.R. & MAURICE, P.D.L. (1980). Malaria: a laboratory risk. *Postgraduate Medical Journal* **56**, 344–345.

BENN, E.C. (1963). Smallpox in Bradford. *Proceedings of the Royal Society of Medicine* **56**, 343.

BERGOGNE-BEREZIN, E., CHRISTOL, D., ZECHOVSKY, N. *et al.* (1972). Pasteurelloses humaines par morsure; enquete epidemiologique en milieu de laboratoire, *Nouvelle Presse Medicale* **1**, 2953–2957.

BERINGER, J. (1997). Genetic manipulation; can genes really escape; does it matter? In: *Managing Biological and Chemical Risks* (Ed. D.A. Morgan) pp. 57–64. London: Medical Research Council and the Institute of Biology.

BERLANCA, J., JANNIN, P., HAMORY, N. *et al.* (1978). Laboratory-acquired endemic typhus—Maryland. *Morbidity and Mortality Weekly Report* **27**, 215–216.

BERNSTEIN, J.M. & CARLING, E.R. (1909). Observation on human glanders with a study of six cases and a discussion of the methods of diagnosis. *British Medical Journal* **1**, 315–325.

BERRY, G.P. & KITCHIN, S.F. (1931). Yellow fever accidentally acquired in the laboratory. A study of seven cases. *American Journal of Tropical Medicine* **11**, 365–434.

BERTOK, L., KEMENES, F. & SZARKA, G. (1960). A case of laboratory infection with *Leptospira canicula* adapted to rodents. *Orvosi hetilap* **101**, 1133–1134.

BEVERLEY, J.K.A., SKIPPER, E. & MARSHALL, S.C. (1955). Laboratory acquired toxoplasmosis. *British Medical Journal* **1**, 577.

BHATTI, A.R., DININNO, V.L., ASHTON, F.E. *et al.* (1982). A laboratory acquired infection with *Neisseria meningitidis. Journal of Infection* **4**, 241–252.

BIGGAR, R.J., SCHMIDT, T.J. & WOODALL, J.P. (1977). Lymphocytic choriomeningitis in laboratory personnel exposed to hamsters inadvertently infected with LCM virus. *Journal of the American Veterinary Medical Association* **171**, 829–832.

BIRNBAUM, D. & GROSCHE D.H.M. (1982) Transmission of infection via laboratory clothing. *Infection Control* **5**, 67–68.

BIRT, C. & LAMB, C. (1899). Mediterranean or Malta fever, *Lancet* **1**, 701–710.

BISCAY, V.M. & CARBONELLE, A.F. (1951). Estudios de brucellosis; autodescripcion de dos casos de infeccion de laboratorio. *Revista Medica Cubana* **62**, 151–161.

BLAGBURN, B.L. & CURRENT, W.L. (1983). Accidental infection of a laboratory worker with human cryptosporidium. *Journal of Infectious Disease* **148**, 772–773.

BLASER, M.J. & FELDMAN, R.A. (1980). Acquisition of typhoid fever from proficiency testing specimens. *New England Journal of Medicine* **303**, 1481–1483.

BLASER, M.J., HICKMAN, F.W., FARMER, J. *et al.* (1980). *Salmonella typhi*: the laboratory as a reservoir of infection. *Journal of Infectious Diseases* **142**, 934–938.

BLASER, M.J. & LOFGREN, J.P. (1981). Fatal salmonellosis originating in a clinical laboratory. *Journal of Clinical Microbiology* **13**, 855–858.

BLOOM, B. (1960). The hazard of orally pipetting tritium oxide. *Journal of Laboratory and Clinical Medicine* **55**, 164–167.

BLUMENBERG, W. (1937). Uber die Weilsche Krasnkheit als Laboratoriums und Stallinfektion. *Zentralblatt für Bakteriologie* Abt 1. Orig. **140**, 100–104.

BMA (1990). *A Code of Practice for the Disposal of Sharps.* London: British Medical Asociation.

BMA (1995). *A Code of Practice for Implementation of the UK Hepatitis B Immmunization Guidelines for the Protection of Patients and Staff.* London: British Medical Asociation.

BOGEN, E. (1959). Postmortem transmission of tuberculosis. *American Journal of Clinical Pathology* **31**, 343–344.

BOGEN, E & DUNN, W. (1941). Tubercle bacilli in air and dust. *American Review of Tuberculosis* **43**, 435–437.

BOHS (1993). *Laboratory Design Issues.* British Occupational Hygiene Society Technical Guide No 10. Leeds: H & H Scientifie Consultants.

BOISVERT, P.L. & FOUSEK, M.D. (1941). Human infection with *Pasteurella lepiseptica* following a rabbit bite. *Journal of the American Medical Association* **116**, 902–903.

BOND, W.W. (1984). Survival of hepatitis virus in the environment. *Journal of the American Medical Association* **251**, 397–398.

BOND, W.W., FAVERO, M.S. PETERSEN, N.J. *et al.* (1981). Survival of hepatitis B virus after drying and storage for one week. *Lancet* 1, 550–551.

BOND, W.W., PETERSEN, N.J. & FAVERO, M.S. (1977). Viral hepatitis B; aspects of environmental control. *Health Laboratory Science* **14**, 235- 252.

BOND, W.W., PETERSEN, N.J., FAVERO, M.S. *et al.* (1982). Transmission of type B viral hepatitis via eye inoculation of a chimpanzee. *Journal of Clinical Microbiology* **15**, 533–534.

BONE, J.M., TONKIN, R.W., DAVISON, A.M. *et al.* (1971). Outbreak of dialysis-associated hepatitis in Edinburgh 1969–1970. *Proceedings of the European Dialysis and Transplant Association* **8**, 189–197.

BOOTH, L. & ROWE, B. (1993). Possible occupational acquisition of *Escherichia coli* 0157 infection. *Lancet* **342**, 1298–1299.

BORGEN, L.O. (1953). Resistance of tubercle bacilli to isoniazid in vitro [Accidental self inoculation with tubercle bacilli]. *Journal of the Oslo City Hospitals* 3, 127–138.

BORGEN, L.O. & GAUSTAD, V. (1948). Infection with *Actinomyces muris rati (Streptobacillus moniliformis)* after bite of a laboratory rat. *Acta Medica Scandinavica* **130**, 189–198.

BORMANN, F.V. (1930). Eine Laboratoriumsinfektion mit Scharlach. *Zentralblatt fur Bakteriologie.* Abt 1. Orig. **117**, 460–463.

BORST, J.G.G., RUYS, A.C. & WOLF, J.W. (1948). Leptospirosis ballum in laboratory infection. *Nederlands Tijdschrift voor Geneeskunde* **92**, 2920–2922.

BORTSOV, V.N. (1976). Newcastle conjunctivitis (a case of laboratory infection). *Oftalmologie Zhurnal* **31**, 471–472.

BOURDILLON, R.B., LIDWELL, O.M. & THOMAS, J.C. (1941). A slit sampler for collecting and collecting air-borne bacteria. *Journal of Hygiene* **41**, 197–224.

BOUREE, P. & FOUQUET, E. (1978). Paludisme: contamination directe interhumain. *Nouvelle Presse* 7, 1965.

BOUVET, E. (1997) Phlebotomy. In: *Occupational Blood-borne Infections: Risks and Management.* (Eds C.H. Collins & D.A. Kennedy) pp. 101–112. Oxford: CAB International

BOWEN, G.S., CALISHER, C.H., WINKLER, W.G. *et al.* (1975). Laboratory studies of a lymphocytic choriomeningitis virus outbreak in man and laboratory animals. *American Journal of Epidemiology* **102**, 233–240.

BRAND, N. & KATHEIM, E.G. (1962). An outbreak of leptospirosis in Upper Galilee. *Israel Medical Journal* **21**, 61–65.

BREEN, R.E., LAMB, S.G. & OTAKI, A.T. (1958). Monkey bite encephalitis: report of a case with recovery. *British Medical Journal* 2, 22–23.

BRENNER, Z. (1987). Laboratory-acquired Chagas disease: comment. *Transactions of the Royal Society of Tropical Medicine and Hygiene* **81**, 527.

BRES, P. (1965). Infection humaine à virus Wesselbron par contamination au laboratoire. *Bulletin Societé Pathologie Exotique* **58**, 994–999.

BROOME, J.C & NORRIS, T.S. (1957). Failure of prophylactic penicillin to inhibit a human case of leptospirosis. *Lancet* 1, 721–722.

BROWN, T.M & NUNEMAKER, J.C. (1942). Rat bite fever: a review of the American cases and re-evaluation of etiology. *Bulletin of the Johns Hopkins Hospital* **70**, 201–237.

BRUCE, M.E., WILL, R.G., IRONSIDE, J.W. *et al.* (1996). Transmission to mice indicates that new variant CJD is caused by BSE agent. *Nature* **389**, 498–501.

BRUINS, S.C. & TIGHT, R.R. (1977). Laboratory-acquired gonococcal conjunctivitis. *Journal of the American Medical Association* **41**, 274–278.

BRUNER, D.W. (1946). A note of *Salmonella abortus-equi* infection in man. *Journal of Bacteriology* **52**, 147.

BRYAN, B.L., ESPANA, C.D., EMMONS, W.R. et al. (1975). Recovery from encephalomyelitis caused by Herpesvirus simiae. Archives of Internal Medicine 135, 368–70.

BRYANT, D.H., BOSCATA, L.M., MBOLOI, P.M. et al. (1995). Allergy to laboratory animals among animal handlers. Medical Journal of Australia 163, 415–418.

BS 3928 (1969). Method for the sodium flame test for air filters. London: British Standards Institution.

BS 5726 (1979). Specification for microbiological safety cabinets. London: British Standards Institution (superseded by BS 5726, 1992).

BS 4402 (1982). Specifications for safety requirements for laboratory centrifuges. London: British Standards Institution.

BS 6642 (1985). Specification for disposable plastics refuse sacks made of polyethylene. London: British Standards Institution.

BS 3316, Part 4. (1987). Code of practice for the design, specification, installation and commissioning of incineration plant for the destruction of hospital waste. London: British Standards Institution.

BS 5213 (1989). Specification for medical specimen containers for microbiology. London: British Standards Institution.

BS 7355 (1990). Specification for full face masks for respiratory protective devices and BS EN 143 1991 Specification for particle filters for use in respiratory protective equipment. London: British Standards Institution.

BS 4851 (1991). Specification for single-use labelled medical specimens. Containers for haematology and biochemistry. London: British Standards Institution.

BS 5726 (1992). Microbiological Safety Cabinets. Part 1. Specification for design, construction and performance prior to installation. Part 2. Recommendations for information to be exchanged between purchaser, vendor and installer, and recommendations for installation. Part 3. Specifications for performance after installation. Part 4. Recommendations for selection, use and maintenance. London: British Standards Institution.

BS 3970 (1996a). Sterilizing and disinfection equipment for medical products. Part 1. Specification for general requirements. Part 2 (1990). Specification for steam sterilizers for aqueous fluids in sealed rigid containers. Part 3 (1996). Specification for steam sterilisers for wrapped goods and porous loads. London: British Standards Institution.

BS 7320 (1996b). Specification for sharps containers. London: British Standards Institution.

BS 4005 (1996c). Specification for single-use sterile surgical gloves. London: British Standards Institution.

BS EN 143 (1991). Specification for particle filters for use in respiratory protective equipment. London: British Standards Institution.

BS EN 61010–1 (1993). Safety requirements for electrical equipment for measuring, control and laboratory use. General requiremnts. London: British Standards Institution.

BS prEN 1822–1 (1995a). High efficiency particulate air filters (HEPA and ULPA). Part 1. Requirements, testing and marking. Brussels: European Committee for Standardization.

BS EN 168 (1996). Personal eye protection. Specific requirements. London: British Standards Institution.

BS EN 829 (1997a). In vitro diagnostic systems. Transport packages for medical and biological specimens. Requirements, tests. London: British Standards Institution.

BS EN 867 (1997b). Non-Biological Systems for use in sterilisers. Part 1. General requirements. Part 2. Process indicators (Class A). Part 3. Specifications for Class B indicators for use in Bowie-Dick tests. London: British Standards Institution.

BS pr EN 12469 (1998). Biotechnology—performance criteria for safety cabinets. London: British Standards Institution.

BUCKLAND, R.E., DUDGEON, A., EDWARD, D.G. et al. (1945). Scrub typhus vaccine. Large scale production. Lancet 2, 734–737.

BUCHMEIER, M., ADAMS, E. & RAWLS, W.E. (1974). Serological evidence of infection by Pichinde virus among laboratory workers. Infection and Immunity 9, 821–823.

BULL, A.D., CHANNER, J., CROSS, R.D. et al. (1991). Should eye protection be worn when performing necropsies Journal of Clinical Pathology 44, 782.

BURKE-GAFFNEY, H.J.O. (1934). A human case of abortus fever due to laboratory infection. East African Medical Journal 12, 235–244.

BURMEISTER, R.W., TIGGERT, W.D. & OVERHOLT, E.L. (1962). Laboratory acquired pneumonic plague. Report of a case and review of previous cases. Annals of Internal Medicine 56, 789–800.

BURNE, J.C. (1970). Malaria by accidental inoculation, *Lancet* 4, 936.

BURNENS, A.P., ZBINDEN, R., KAEMPF, L. *et al.* (1993). A case of laboratory-acquired infection with *Escherichia coli* 0157:H7. *Zeitschrift für Bakteriologie* **279**, 512–517.

BURNET, E. (1925). Aperçu des acquisitions recentes sur la fievre mediterraneéne. *Bulletin de l'Institut Pasteur* **23**, 369–382.

BURNET, F.M. (1943). Human infection with the virus of Newcastle disease of fowls. *Medical Journal of Australia* **2**, 313–314.

BURNET, F.M. & FREEMAN, M. (1939). Note on a series of laboratory infections with the rickettsia of Q fever. *Medical Journal of Australia* **1**, 11–12.

BUSCHKE, A. (1913). Uber die Beziehung der Experimentell Erzeugten Tiersyphilis zur Menschlichen Lues. *Deutsche Medinische Wochenschrift* **39**, 1783–1785.

BUSH, J.D. (1943). Coccidioidomycosis. *Journal of the Medical Association of Alabama* **13**, 159–166.

BYRNE, E.B. (1966). Viral hepatitis. An occupational hazard of laboratory personnel. *Journal of the American Medical Association* **195**, 362–364.

CALIA, F.M., BARTELLONI, P.J. & McKINNEY, R.W. (1970). Rocky Mountain fever. *Journal of the American Medical Association* **211**, 2012–2014.

CALLENDER, M.E., WHITE, Y. & WILLIAMS, R. (1982). Hepatitis B infection in medical and health care personnel. *British Medical Journal* **284**, 324–326.

CALLISHER, C.H. & GOODPASTURE, H.C. (1975). Human infection with Bhanja virus. *American Journal of Tropical Medicine and Hygiene* **26** (6 part 1), 1040–1042.

CAMPBELL, E.P. & KETCHUM, W.H. (1940). Rocky Mountain spotted fever: an analysis of seven cases, including a laboratory infection. *New England Journal of Medicine* **233**, 540–543.

CANETTI, G., SAENZ, A., THIBIER, R. *et al.* (1951). Tuberculose de reinfection a bacilles streptomycine-resistants contracte au laboratoires. *Revue Tuberculose* **15**, 128–133.

CANNON, N.J., WALKER, S.P. & DISMUKES, W.A. (1972). Malaria acquired by accidental needle puncture. *Journal of the American Medical Association* **222**, 1425.

CARBONELLE B., CARBONELLE, P., FRUCHART, A. *et al.* (1975). Epidemiology and prevention of tuberculosis contamination in bacteriology laboratories. Result of a survey on 23 laboratories. *Revue Epidemiolique Med Sante Publique* 33, 417–428.

CARR, E.A. & KADULL, P.J. (1957). Persistence of *Bacterium tularense* in man in the absence of serious clinical illness. *Archives of Pathology* **64**, 382–384.

CARROLL, G.F., HALEY, L.D. & BROWN, J.M. (1977). Primary cutaneous coccidioidomycosis: a review of the literature and a report of a new case. *Archives of Dermatology* **113**, 933–936.

CARSTAIRS, K. & COATES, G. (1974). Potential laboratory hazard from vacuum tubes used for obtaining blood specimens, *Lancet* 2, 359–360.

CASALS, J., CURNEN, E.C. & THOMAS, L. (1943). Venezuelan equine encephalitis in man. *Journal of Experimental Medicine* **77**, 521–530.

CASEWELL, M.W., DESAI, N. & LEASE, E.J. (1986). The use of the Reuter centrifugal air sampler for the estimation of bacterial counts in different hospital locations. *Journal of Hospital Infection* **7**, 250–260.

CASEWELL, M.W., FERMIE, P.G. & SIMMONS, N.A. (1984). Bacterial air counts obtained with a centrifugal (RCS) sampler and a slit sampler—the influence of aerosols. *Journal of Hospital Infection* **5**, 76–82.

CDC (1974a). *Lab Safety at the Center for Disease Control.* Atlanta.

CDC (1974b). Rat bite fever—Texas and Virginia. *Morbidity and Mortality Weekly Report* **23**, 357–358.

CDC (1976c). *Classification of Etiological Agents on the Basis of Hazard.* 4th ed. Washington: Government Printing Office.

CDC (1977a). Fatal Rocky Mountain Spotted Fever—Georgia. *Morbidity and Mortality Weekly Report* **26**, 84.

CDC (1977b). Rabies in a laboratory worker—New York. *Morbidity and Mortality Weekly Report* **26**, 183–184.

CDC (1978). Laboratory-acquired endemic typhus. *Morbidity and Mortality Weekly Report* **27**, 215–216.

CDC (1979a). Laboratory-associated typhoid fever. *Morbidity and Mortality Weekly Report* **28**, 44.

CDC (1979b). Q fever at a university research centre—California. *Morbidity and Mortality Weekly Report* **28**, 333–334.

CDC (1980). Chagas' disease—Kalamazoo, Michigan. *Morbidity and Mortality Weekly Report* **29**, 147–148.

CDC (1981a). Classification of etiological agents on the basis of hazard. *Federal Register* **46**, 59379–59380.

CDC (1981b). Tuberculosis infection associated with tissue processing - California. *Morbidity and Mortality Weekly Report* **30**, 73–74.

CDC (1987a). Guidelines for the prevention of herpesvirus simiae (B virus) in monkey handlers. *Morbidity and Mortality Weekly Reports* **36**, 680–682, 687–689.

CDC (1987b). Recommendations for prevention of HIV transmission in health care settings. *Morbidity and Mortality Weekly Report* **36**, 1S-18S.

CDC (1988a). Agent summary statement for human immunodeficiency virus and report on laboratory-acquired infection with human immunodeficiency virus. *Morbidity and Mortality Weekly Report* **37** (SA), 1–22.

CDC (1988b). Update: universal precautions for prevention of transmission of human immunodeficiency virus, hepatitis B virus and other blood borne pathogens in health care settings. *Morbidity and Mortality Weekly Report* **37**, 377–383, 387–388.

CDC (1989). Guidelines for the prevention of transmission of human immunodeficiency virus and hepatitis B virus in health care and public safety workers. *Morbidity and Mortality Weekly Reports* **38** (Supp. 6), S3-S31.

CDC (1991). Laboratory-acquired meningococcemia—California and Massachsetts. *Morbidity and Mortality Weekly Report* **40**, 46–47, 53.

CDC (1992a). Seroconversion to simian immodeficiency virus in two laboratory workers. *Morbidity and Mortality Weekly Report* **39** (RR-1), 1–14.

CDC (1992b). Surveillance of occupationally-acquired HIV infection—United States 1981–1992. *Morbidity and Mortality Weekly Report* **41**, 823–825.

CDC (1994). Laboratory Management of Agents Associated with Hantavirus Pulmonary Syndrome: Interim Safety Guidelines. *Morbidity and Mortality Weekly Report* **43**, 1–7.

CDC/NIH (1993). *Biosafety in Microbiological and Biomedical Laboratories*. 3rd ed. (Eds J.Y. Richmond & R.W. McKinney). Washington: Government Printing Office.

CDSC (1991). Communicable Disease Surveillance Centre. *Brucella melitensis* laboratory-acquired infection. *PHLS Communicable Disease Reports* **1**, 37.

CEN prEN 819 (1995b). *In vitro diagnostic systems. Transport packages for medical and diagnostic specimens. Requirememts, tests.* Brussels: *European Committee for Standardization.*

CENTRAL HEALTH SERVICES COUNCIL (1968). *Report of the Joint Committee on the Care of the Health and Hospital Staff.* London: The Stationery Office.

CHACKO, C.W. (1966). Accidental human infection in the laboratory with the Nichols rabbit-adapted strain of *Treponema pallidum. Bulletin of the World Health Organization* 35, 809–810.

CHAPPLER, R.R., HOKE, A.W. & BORCHARDT, K.A. (1977). Primary inoculation with *Mycobacterium marinum. Archives of Dermatology* 113, 380.

CHARKES, N.D. (1959). Haemagglutination test in tularemia; results in 56 vaccinated persons with laboratory acquired infection. *Journal of Immunology* **83**, 213–220.

CHATIGNY, M.A. (1961). Protection against infection in the microbiological laboratory devices and procedures. In: *Advances in Microbiology.* (Ed. W.W. Umbreit). London: Academic Press.

CHATIGNY, M. A. & CLINGER, D. I. (1969). Contamination control in aerobiology. In: An Introduction to Experimental Aerobiology (Eds R. L. Dimmick & A. B. Akers). New York: Wiley.

CHATIGNY, M.A., DUNN, S., ISHIMARU, K. *et al.* (1979). Evaluation of a Class III biological safety cabinet for enclosure of an ultracentrifuge. *Applied & Environmental Microbiology* **38**, 934–939.

CHATIGNY, M.A., SARSHAD, A.A, & PIKE, G.R. (1970). Design and evaluation of a system for thermal decontamination of process air. *Biotechnology and Bioenginering* **12**, 483–500.

CHATTOPADHYAY, B. & THOMAS, E. (1978). Bacterial contamination of laboratory forms. *Journal of Clinical Pathology* 10, 1004–1005.

CHEN, S.K., VESLEY, D., BROSSEAUU, L.M. *et al.* (1994). Evaluation of single-use masks and respirators for the protection of health care workers against mycobacterial aerosols. *American Journal of Infection Control* **22**, 65–74.

CHENEY, J.E. & COLLINS, C.H (1995). Formaldehyde disinfection in laboratories: limitations and hazards. *British Journal of Biomedical Science* **52**, 195–201.

CHICK, E.W., BAUMAN, D.S., LAPP, N.L. *et al.* (1972). A combined field and laboratory epidemic of histoplasmosis. Isolation from bat faeces in West Virginia. *American Review of Respiratory Disease* **105**, 968–971.

CHIEN, J.T.T. & WIGGINS, M.L. (1954). Self-inoculation with *Mycobacterium tuberculosis* and *Pseudomonas aeruginosa* by a diabetic woman. *American Review of Tuberculosis* **69**, 818–823.

CHIN, J. (1998). Throat infection with toxigenic *Corynebacterium diphtheriae*. *Communicable Disease Reports* **8**, 7.

CHUNG, H.L. (1931). An early case of kala-azar, possibly oral infection in the laboratory. *National Medical Journal of China* **17**, 617–621.

CLARK, R.P. (1997) Standards for safety cabinets. *Nature* **390**, 550.

CLARK, R.P. & GOFF, M.R. (1981). The potassium iodide method for determining protection factors in open fronted microbiological safety cabinets. *Journal of Applied Bacteriology* **51**, 439–460.

CLARK, S., LACH, V. & LIDWELL, O.M. (1981). The performance of the Biotest RCS centrifugal air sampler. *Journal of Hospital Infection* **2**, 181–186.

CLARK, R.P. & MULLEN, B.J. (1978). Airflows in and around linear downflow 'safety' cabinets. *Journal of Applied Bacteriology* **45**, 131–135.

CLARK, R.P., OSBORNE, R.W.E., PRESSEY, D.C. *et al.* (1990). Open fronted safety cabinets in ventilated laboratories. *Journal of Applied Bacteriologu* **69**, 338–358.

CLEARKIN, P.A. (1928). A case of rat bite fever contracted in the laboratory. *Kenyan East African Medical Journal* **5**, 196–200.

COATES, D. & DEATH, J.E. (1978). Sporicidal activity of mixtures of alcohol and hypochlorite. *Journal of Clinical Pathology* **31**, 148–152.

COCKCROFT, A., McCARTHY, P., EDWARDS, J. *et al.* (1981). Allergy in laboratory animal workers. *Lancet* i, 827–830.

COHEN, B.J., COURUCE, A.M., SCHWARZ, T.F. *et al.* (1988). Laboratory infection with parvovirus B19. *Journal of Clinical Pathology* **41** 1027–1028.

COLE, J.S., STOLL, R.W. & BULGER, R.J. (1969). Rat bite fever. Report of three cases. *Annals of Internal Medicine* **71**, 979–981.

COLLINS, C.H. (1959). The effect of mechanical shaking on the concentration of sputum for the cultivation of the tubercle bacillus. *Journal of Medical Laboratory Technology* **9**, 217–219.

COLLINS, C.H. (1964). *Microbiological Methods*. pp.79,119,229. London: Butterworths.

COLLINS, C.H. (1972). Flaming wire loops. *Institute of Medical Laboratory Sciences Gazette* **16**, 243.

COLLINS, C.H. (1974). Laboratory-acquired infections. In: *The Prevention of Laboratory-acquired Infection*. PHLS Monograph No. 6. London: The Stationery Office.

COLLINS, C.H. (1976). The bacteriologist's loop: a biohazard. *Institute of Medical Laboratory Sciences Gazette* **20**, 55–56.

COLLINS, C.H. (1980a). The hazards of mouth pipetting. *Institute of Medical Laboratory Sciences Gazette* **24**, 301–302.

COLLINS, C.H. (1980b). Instruction in laboratory safety. *Medical Laboratory World* **4**, 14–19.

COLLINS, C.H. (1982). Laboratory-acquired tuberculosis. *Tubercle* **63**, 151–155.

COLLINS, C.H. (1993). *Laboratory-acquired Infections*. 3rd ed. Oxford: Butterworth-Heienemann.

COLLINS, C.H. (1994). Opinion: Infected laboratory waste. *Letters in Applied Microbiology* **19**, 61–62.

COLLINS, C.H. (1997). Bacterial and other agents of blood-borne infections. In: *Occupational Blood-borne Infections*. (Eds C.H. Collins & D.A. Kennedy). pp. 17–26. Oxford: CAB International.

COLLINS, C.H., AW, T.C. & GRANGE, J.M. (1997) *Microbial Diseases of Occupations, Sports and Recreations*. Oxford: Butterworth-Heinemann.

COLLINS, C.H. & BEALE, A.J. (1992). *Safety in Industrial Microbiology and Biotechnology*. Oxford: Butterworth-Heinemann

COLLINS, C.H., GRANGE, J.M. & YATES, M.D. (1997) *Tuberculosis Bacteriology*. 2nd edn. Oxford: Butterworth-Heinemann.

COLLINS, C.H. & GUNTHORPE, W.J. (1981). Centrifuges in safety cabinets. *Institute of Medical Laboratory Sciences Gazette* **25**, 230–231.1

COLLINS, C.H & JOHNS, W.E. (1998) Home-made microbiological safety cabinets in the microbiological laboratory: a hazard warning. *Biomedical Scientist* **42**, 296–297.

COLLINS, C.H. & KENNEDY, D.A. (1987). A review: Microbiological hazards of occupational needlestick and 'sharps' injuries. *Journal of Applied Bacteriology* **62**, 385–402.

COLLINS, C.H. & KENNEDY, D.A. (1993). *The Treatment and Disposal of Clinical Waste*. Leeds: Science Reviews.

COLLINS, C.H. & KENNEDY, D.A. (Eds) (1997). *Occupational Blood-borne Infections*. Oxford: CAB International.

COLLINS, C.H. & LYNE, P.M. (1976). *Microbiological Methods*. 4th ed. p. 316. London: Butterworths.

COLLINS, C.H., LYNE, P.M. & GRANGE, J.M. (1995) *Collins and Lyne's Microbiological Methods*. 7th ed. pp. 35,36,110,263,413. Oxford: Butterworth-Heinemann.

COLLINS, C.H. & YATES, M.N. (1982). The use of a flexible film isolator in a diagnostic laboratory. *Laboratory Practice* September 1982, pp. 15–17

COMMISSION ON ACUTE RESPIRATORY DISEASES (Fort Bragg, N. Carolina) (1946). A laboratory outbreak of Q fever caused by the Balkan grippe strain of *Rickettsia burnetii*. *American Journal of Hygiene* **44**, 123–157.

COMMITTEE OF PUBLIC ACCOUNTS. 17th Report Session, 1981–1982. London: The Stationery Office.

CONOMY, J.P., LEIBOVITZ, A., McCOMBS, W. *et al.* (1977). Airborne rabies encephalitis. *Neurology* **27**, 67–69.

Control of Substances Hazardous to Health Regulations 1994. London: The Stationery Offfice.

COOK, E.B.M. (1961). Safety in the Public Health Laboratory. *Public Health Reports* **76**, 51.

COOK, I.J.Y. (1972). The collection of specimens and choice of containers with special reference to leakage and aerosol tests. *The Medical Technologist* 2, No. 12 (December).

COOPER, H.R. (1948). Tularemia; report of a case. *US Navy Medical Bulletin* **48**, 102–103.

COOPER, W.C., GREEN, I.J. & FRESH, J.W. (1964). Laboratory infection with louping ill virus. A case study, US Naval Medical Research Unit No. 2. Research Report MR005.091201.

COWAN, S.T. (1951). In: *Freezing and Drying*. Symposium of Institute of Biology. No. 1. London.

CRANE, J.T. & RICHMOND, J.Y. (1993). Design of biomedical laboratory facilities. In: *Laboratory Safety. Principles and Practice.* 2nd ed. (Eds D.O. Fleming, J.H. Richardson, J.I. Tulis & D. Vesley). Washington: American Society for Microbiology.

CRAVITZ, L. & MILLER, W. R. (1950). Immunologic studies with *Malleomyces mallei* and *Malleomyces pseudomallei. Journal of Infectious Disease* **86**, 46–51.

CRONER (1997). Respiratory protection. In: *Croner's Handbook of Occupational Hygiene.* (Eds B. Harvey & G. Crockford). Sections 8.11.2, 8.11.3). Kingston: Croner Publications.

CROOK, B. (1995). Inertial samplers: biological perspectives. In: *Bioaersosols Handbook.* (Eds C.S. Cox & C.A. Wathes). London: Lewis.

CROSHAW, B. (1981). Disinfectant testing, with particular reference to the Rideal-Walker and Kelsey-Sykes tests. *In: Disinfectants, Their Use and Evaluation of Effectiveness* (Eds C.H. Collins, M.C. Allwood, S.F. Bloomfield & A. Fox). pp. 1–16. London: Academic Press.

CROSS, J.H., HSU-KUO, M.Y. & LIEN, J.C. (1973). Accidental human infection with *Plasmodium cynomolgi bastianelli. South East Asian Journal of Tropical Medicine & Public Health* 4, 481–483.

CULLLIFORD. B.J. (1981). *The Examination and Typing of blood Stains.* pp. 247–284. Washington: US Government Printing Office.

CURET, L.B. & FAUST, J.C. (1972). Transmission of a fever from experimental sheep to laboratory personnel. *American Journal of Obstetrics & Gynecology* **114**, 566–568.

DADSWELL, J.V. (1983). Laboratory acquired shigellosis. *British Medical Journal* **286**, 58.

DAILY TELEGRAPH (1982a). Hospital defects waste 830m. 31 May, 1981.

DAILY TELEGRAPH (1982b). Hospital design faults will cost millions. 21 September 1982.

DALRYMPLE-CHAMPNEYS, W. (1960). *Brucella Infections and Undulant Fever in Man.* London: Oxford University Press, pp. 40–41.

DANDEWATE, C.N., WORK, T.H., WEBB, J.K.G. *et al.* (1969). Isolation of Ganjam virus from a human case of febrile illness. A report of a laboratory infection and serological survey of human sera from three different states of India. *Indian Journal of Medical Research* **57**, 975–980.

DANKHERT, J., UITENMUIS, J., POSTMA, A. *et al.* (1976). HBsAg hazard in blood and marrow smears. *Lancet* 1, 1083–1084.

DARLOW, H.M. (1959). Sputtering in bunsen flames. *Lancet* 1, 651.

DARLOW, H.M. (1969). *Safety in the Microbiology Laboratory.* In: Methods in Microbiology I. (Eds J.R. Norris & D.W. Ribbons). pp. 164–204. London: Academic Press.

DARLOW, H.M. (1972). Safety in the Microbiology Laboratory: An Introduction. In: *Safety in Microbiology* (Eds D.A. Shapton & R.G. Board). pp. 1–19. London: Academic Press.

DAVIDSON, W.L. & HUMMELER, K. (1961). B virus infection in man. *Annals of the New York Academy of Sciences* **85**, 970–979.

DAVISON, G., NEUBAUER, C. & HURST, E.W. (1948). Meningo-encephalitis in man due to louping ill virus. *Lancet* 2, 453–457.

DE (1993) Department of the Environment. *Waste Management Paper No. 25: Clinical Waste.* London: The Stationery Office.

DEATH, J.E., HALLIN, B.E. & HARPER, E.J. (1982). Decontamination of automated laboratory equipment. *Journal of Clinical Pathology* **35**, 580–581.

DENTON, J.F., DI SALVO, A.F. & HIRSCH, M.L. (1967). Laboratory-acquired North American blastomycosis. *Journal of the American Medical Association* **199**, 935–936.

DESMYTTER, J., LE DUC, J.W., JOHNSON, K.M. *et al.* (1983). Laboratory rat associated outbreak of haemorrhagic fever with renal syndrome due to Hantaan-like virus in Belgium. *Lancet* 2, 1445–1448.

DH (1970). *Precautions Against Tuberculosis Infection in the Diagnostic Laboratory.* HM 70/60. London: Department of Health.

DH (1972). *Safety in Pathology Laboratories.* London: Department of Health.

DH (1974). Hazard from a Laminar Flow Cabinet, Health Equipment Information SO, 7/74 (January 1974).

DH (1975). *Report of the Working Party on the Laboratory Use of Dangerous Pathogens.* Cdmnd. 6054. London, The Stationery Office.

DH (1976). Dangerous Pathogens Advisory Group. *Control of Laboratory Use of Pathogens Very Dangerous to Humans.* London: Department of Health.

DH (1978). *Code of Practice for the Prevention of Infection in Clinical Laboratories and Post-mortem Rooms.* Department of Health. London: The Stationery Office.

DH (1979). Health Service Development. *Code of Practice for the Prevention of Infection in Clinical Laboratories and Post-mortem Rooms.* Training of safety officers (infection). RSCO RETO 79/16. London: Department of Health.

DH (1980a). *Report of the Investigation into the Causes of the 1978 Birmingham Smallpox Occurrence* (Chmn R. A. Shooter). London: The Stationery Office (House of Commons Paper 79880. No 668).

DH (1980b) Bulletin 1 of the Interim Advisory Committee: Code of Practice for the Prevention of Infection in Clinical Laboratories. London: Department of Health.

DH (1985). Possible infection risk to laboratory staff from human blood-based coagulation-deficient plasma. Safety Information Bulletin No. 23. SIB (85)30. London: Department of Health.

DH (1990). *Guidance for Health Care Workers: Protection against Infection with HIV and Hepatitis Viruses.* London: The Stationery Office.

DH (1991). *Hospital Building Note No. 15.* (Revised), London: Department of Health.

DH (1992a) Glutaraldehyde disinfectants: use and management. Advisory Bulletin SAB(92)17. London: Department of Health.

DH (1992b) *Immunization against Infectious Diseases.* London: The Stationery Office.

DH (1993a). Preparation of heavy suspensions of *Neisseria meningitidis* on the open bench. H C (Hazard) (93)1. Department of Health.

DH (1993b). *Protecting Health Care Workers and Patients from Hepatitis B.* London: Department of Health.

DICKIE, H.A. & MURPHY, M.E. (1955). Laboratory infection with *Histoplasma capsulatum. American Review of Tuberculosis* **72**, 690–692.

DICKSON, E.C. (1937). 'Valley fever' of the San Joaquin Valley and fungus coccidioides. *Californian and Western Medicine* **47**, 151–155.

DICKSON, E.C. & GIFFORD, M.A. (1938). Coccididioides infection. *Archives of Internal Medicine* **62**, 853–871.

DIENE, B.B. WALLACE, R., ASHTON, F.E. *et al.* (1976). Gonococcal conjunctivitis: accidental infection. *Canadian Medical Association Journal* **115**, 609–612.

DIETER, L.V. (1926). A case of tularaemia in a laboratory worker. *Public Health Reports* **41**, 1355–1357.

DIETZMAN, D.E., FUCCILLO, D.A., WEST, F.J. *et al.* (1973). Conjunctivitis associated with Coxsackie B1 virus in a laboratory worker. *American Journal of Ophthalmology* **75**, 1045–1046.

DIGGELMANN, H. (1994) Hazard potential from viruses and oncogenes. In: *Biosafety of Mammalian Cells.* Proceedings of the Basel Forum on Biosafety, October 1993. pp. 15–18. Basel: Agency for Biosafety Research.

DISCOMBE, G. (1985). Laboratory design. *Bulletin of the Royal College of Pathologists* No. 51, pp. 7–8.

DIVO, A. & LUGO, A. (1952). Un caso de parotitis human por virus de Newcastle (infeción de laboratorio). *Bol Inst Inv Vet Caracas* **4**, 644–649.

DOLAN, M.M., KLIGMAN, A.M., KOBYLINSKI, P.G. *et al.* (1958). Ringworm epizootics in laboratory mice and rats: experimental and accidental transmission of infection. *Journal of Investigative Dermatology* **30**, 23–25.

DONOVAN, J.W. (1974). The first case of laboratory acquired hepatitis? *Transactions of the Royal Society for Tropical Medicine and Hygiene* **68**, 259.

DOUVIN, C., SIMON, D., ZINELABINE, H. *et al.* (1990). An outbreak of hepatitis B in an endocrinology unit traced to a capillary blood sampling device. *New England Journal of Medicine* **322**, 57–60.

DOWSETT, E.G. & HEGGIE, J.F. (1972). A protective pathology laboratory coat. *Lancet* 1, 1271.

DOYLE, L. GALLAGHER, K., HEATH, B.S. *et al.* (1989). An outbreak of infectious conjunctivitis spread by microscopes. *Journal of Occupational Medicine* **31**, 758–762.

DRAESE, K.D. (1939). Uber Laboratoriumsinfektion mit Typhusbazillen und anderen Bakterien. *Archiv für Hygiene und Bakteriologie* 121, 232–291.

DRITZ, S., BLACK, A., HINE, C. *et al.* (1979). Q fever at a university research center—California. *Morbidity and Mortality Weekly Report* **28**, 333–334.

DROUHET, E., SEGRETAIN, G. & MARIAT, F. (1974). Coccidioidomycosis infection of a laboratory worker. *Bulletin de la Societe Mycolique de France* **3**, 163–165.

DUFFUS, J.H. & BROWN, C.M (1985). Health aspects of biotechnology. *Annals of Ocupational Health* **29**, 1–12.

DURAY, P.H., FLANNERY, B. & BROWN, S. (1981). Tuberculous infection from preparation of frozen sections. *New England Journal of Medicine* **305**, 167.

DURIN, E. (1984). HFRS after a wild rodent bite in the Haute Savoie and risk of exposure to Hantaan-like virus in a Paris laboratory. *Lancet* 1, 676–677.

DYER, R.E. (1938). A filter passing infectious agent isolated from ticks. IV. Human infection. *Public Health Reports* **53**, 2277–2282.

DYKEWICZ, C.A., DATO, V.M. & FISHER-HOCH, S.P. (1992). Lymphocytic choriomeningitis outbreak associated with nude mice in a research institute. *Journal of the American Medical Association* **267**, 1349–1353.

EBRING, F. (1969). Artifizielle Superinfektionen mit Tuberkllbakterien unter INA-Behandlung. *Praxis der Pneumologie* **23**, 256–260.

EC (1990). Commission of the European Communities. *Council Directive on the Protection of Workers related to Exposure to Biological Agents at Work.* 90679/EEC. Brussels: European Commission.

EC (1990/94) Council Directive 90/219/EEC on the Contained Use of Genetically Modified Micro-organisms, as amended by Council Directive 94/51/EEC. Brussels: European Commission.

EC (1993). Commission of the European Communities. *Council Directive on the Classification of Biological Agents.* (93/88/EEC). Brussels: European Commission.

EDLICH, R. (1995). Emergency first aid guide. In: *Laboratory Safety. Principles and Practice* (Appendix). (Eds D.O. Fleming, J.H. Richardson, J.I. Tulis & D. Vesley). 2nd edn. pp. 375–379. Washington: American Society for Microbiology.

ELLINGSON, H.V., KADULL, P.J., BOOKWALTER, H.L. *et al.* (1946). Cutaneous anthrax. Report of twenty five cases. *Journal of the American Medical Association* **131**, 1105–1108.

EMERIBE, A.O. (1988). Gambiense trypanosomiasis acquired from a needle scratch. *Lancet* i, 470.

EMOND, R.T.D. (1978). Isolation, monitoring and treatment of a case of Ebola virus infection. In: *Ebola Virus Haemorrhagic Fever.* (Ed. R. Pattyn). pp. 27–32. Amsterdam: Elsevier/North Holland Biomedical Press.

EMOND, R.T., EVANS, B., BOWEN, E.T. *et al.* (1977). A case of Ebola virus infection. *British Medical Journal* 2, 541–544.

ENARSON, D.A. GRZYBOWSKI,S. & DORKEN, E. (1978) Failure of diagnosis as a factor in tuberculosis mortality. *Canadian Medical Association Journal* **118**, 1520.

ENGBAEK, H.C., VERGMANN, B. & BUNCH-CHRISTENSEN, K. (1977). Pulmonary tubercu-losis due to BCG in a technician employed in a BCG laboratory. *Bulletin of the World Health Organization* **55**, 517–520.

Environmental Protection Act 1990. London: The Stationery Office.

ESKEY, C.R. & HAAS, V.H. (1962). Plague in the Western part of the United States. *Public Health Bulletin* No. 254. Washington: US Public Health Service.

EVANS, A.C. (1947). Brucellosis in the United States. *American Journal of Public Health* **37**, 139–151.

EVANS, C.G.T. & HARRIS-SMITH, R. (1970). The POMEC: an apparatus for growing dense cultures of pathogenic microorganisms. In: *Automation, Mechanization and Data-handling in*

Microbiology. (Ed. A Baillie & R.J. Gilbert). London: Academic Press

EVANS, C.G.T., HARRIS-SMITH, R. & STRATTON, J.E.D. (1972). The use of safety cabinets in the prevention of laboratory acquired infection. In: *Safety in Microbiology* (Eds D. A. Shapton & R. G. Board). pp. 21–35. London: Academic Press.

EVANS, M.R. HENDERSON, D.K. & BENNETT, J.E (1990). Potential for laboratory exposure to biohazardous agents found in blood *American Journal of Public Health* **80**, 423–427.

EVANS, N. (1903). A clinical report of a case of blastomycosis of the skin from accidental inoculation. *Journal of the American Medical Association* **40**, 1772–1775.

EVANS, T.G. & PEARSON, R.D. (1988). Clinical and immunological responses following accidental inoculation of *Leishmania donovani. Transactions of the Royal Society of Tropical Medicine and Hygiene* **828**, 854–856.

EVERALL, P.H. & MORRIS, C.A. (1976). Failure to sterilize in plastic bags. *Journal of Clinical Pathology* **29**, 1132.

EYLES, D.E., COATNEY, G.R. & GETZ, M.E. (1960). Vivax-type malaria parasite of macaques transmissible to man. *Science* **131**, 1812–1813.

EYRE, J.W.H. (1913). *Bacteriological Technique.* Philadelphia: Saunders.

FALLON, R. (1986). Identifying 'high risk' laboratory specimens. *Journal of Clinical Pathology* **37**, 811.

FARMER, T.W. & JANEWAY, C.P. (1942). Infections with the virus of lymphocytic choriomeningitis. *Medicine* **21**, 1–63.

FARRELL, E. (1939). Weil's disease: a compensable infection in New York State. *New York State Journal of Medicine* **39**, 1969–1971.

FAVA, A. (1909). Un cas de sporotrichose conjunctivale et palpebrale primitives. *Annales d'oculistique, Paris* **141**, 338–343.

FELDMAN, H.A. (1968). Toxoplasmosis. *New England Journal of Medicine* **279**, 1370–1375.

FELLOWS, O.N., DIMOPOULLOS, G.T. & CALLIS, J.J. (1957). Isolation of vesicular stomatis virus from an infected laboratory worker. *American Journal of Veterinary Research* **16**, 623–626.

FELTZ, E.T. & McALLISTER, R. (1964). Effect of a major disaster on virology research laboratory. *Journal of the American Medical Association* **189**, 143–144.

FIELD, P.R., MOYLE, C.G. & PARNELL, P.M. (1972). The accidental infection of a laboratory worker with *Toxoplasma gondii. Medical Journal of Australia* **2**, 197–198.

FIELITZ, H. (1910). Ueber einer Laboratoriumsinfektion mit dem sporotrichum de Bearmanni. *Zentralblatt für Bakteriologie* etc. Abt. 1. Orig. 55, 361–370.

FIERER, J., BAZELEY, P. & BRAUDE, A.I. (1973). Herpes B virus encephalomyelitis presenting as an ophthalmic zoster. *Annals of Internal Medicine* **79**, 225–228.

FIESE, M.J. (1958). *Coccidiodomycosis.* pp. 77–91. Springfield, IL: Thomas.

FINDLAY, G. M. (1932). Rift Valley fever or enzootic hepatitis. *Transactions of the Royal Society for Tropical Medicine* **25**, 229–265

FINDLAY, G.M., DUNLOP, J.C. & BROWN, H.C. (1931). Observations on epidemic catarrhal jaundice. *Transactions of the Royal Society for Tropical Medicine* **25**, 7–28.

First Aid at Work Regulations 1981. London: The Stationery Office.

FISCHER, J.B. & KANE, J. (1973). *Coccidioides immitis*: a hospital hazard. *Canadian Journal of Public Health* **64**, 276–278.

FISH, C.H. & SPENDLOVE, G.A. (1950). Safety measures in a tuberculosis laboratory. *Public Health Reports* **65**, 466–467.

FITCH, K.M., ALVAREZ, L.P., MEDINA, R.A. *et al.* (1995). Occupational transmission on HIV in health-care workers. *European Journal of Public Health* **5**, 175–186.

FITZGERALD, J.J., JOHNSON, R.C. & SMITH, M. (1976). Accidental laboratory infection with *Treponema pallidum*, Nichols strain. *Journal of the American Venereal Disease Association* **3**, 76–78.

FLEWETT, T.H. (1980). Safety in the virology laboratory. In: *Recent Advances in Clinical Virology*, 2 (Ed. A. P. Waterson). pp. 169–187. Edinburgh: Churchill Livingstone.

FLOWERS, A.I. & HALL, C.F. (1962). Erysipelas infection in turkeys and laboratory workers. *Southwest Veterinarian* **16**, 39- 41.

FONSECA, V., HINSON. J., PAPPAS, A. *et al.* (1997). An erbium:YAG laser to obtain capillary blood without a needle for point-of-care laboratory testing. *Archives of Pathology and Laboratory Medicine* **121**, 685–686.

FOORD, N. & LIDWELL, O.M. (1975). Airborne infection in a fully air-conditioned hospital. *Journal of Hygiene* **75**, 15–56.

FORTNER, J. (1936). Der Stand der Psittakoseforschung und bekampfung. *Berliner Tieraierztliche*

Wochenschrift **52**, 405–409.

FORTNER, J. & PFAFFENBERG, R. (1934). Uber das gehaufte Wiederauftreiten der Psittakose. I. *Zeitschrift für Hygiene und Infektionskrankheiten* **116**, 397–416.

FORTNER, J. & PFAFFENBERG, R. (1935). Uber das gehaufte Wiederauftreiten der Psittakose. II. Mittelilung. *Zeitschrift für Hygiene und Infektionskrankheiten* **117**, 286–287

FOTHERGILL, L.D., DINGLE, J.H., FARBER, S. *et al*. (1938). Human encephalitis caused by the virus of the eastern variety of equine encephalitis. *New England Journal of Medicine* **219**, 411.

FOTHERGILL, L.D., DINGLE, J.H., FARBER, S. *et al*. (1939). Western equine encephalomyelitis in a laboratory worker. *Journal of the American Medical Association* **113**, 206–207.

FOURNIER, J. (1960). Une zoonose qui gagne du terrain: la melioidose. *Medecin d'Egypte* **9**, 23–54.

FOX, J.G. & LIPMAN, N.S. (1991). Infections transmitted by large and small animals. *Infectious Diseases Clinics of North America* **5**, 131–163.

FRAME, J.D., BALDWIN, J.M., GOCKE, D. J. *et al*. (1970). Lassa fever, a new virus disease of man from West Africa. *American Journal of Tropical Medicine & Hygiene* **19**, 670–676.

FRANCIS, E. (1922). Tularemia Francis 1921. A new disease of man. *Hygiene Laboratory Bulletin* No. 13O. Washington: Government Printing Office.

FRANCIS, E. (1925). Tularemia. *Journal of the American Medical Association* **84**, 1243–1250.

FRANCIS, E. (1936). Immunity in tularemia. *Public Health Reports* **51**, 397–398.

FRANCIS, E. (1937). Sources of infection and seasonal incidence of tularemia in man. *Public Health Reports* **52**, 103–113.

FRANCIS, T. & MAGILL, R.P. (1935). Rift Valley Fever. A report of three cases of laboratory infections. *Journal of Experimental Medicine* **62**, 433–448.

FRAZER, S.C. (1972). Safety in hospital laboratory design. *Laboratory Practice* **21**, 85–90, 96.

FREEDMAN, D.O., MACLEAN, J.D. & VILORIA, J.B. (1987). A case of laboratory-acquired *Leishman donovani* infection: evidence for primary dissemination. *Transactions of the Royal Society for Tropical Medicine and Hygiene* **81**, 118–119.

FREYMAN, M.W. & BANG, F.B. (1948). Human conjunctivitis due to Newcastle virus in the USA. *Bulletin of the Johns Hopkins Hospital* **84**, 409–413.

FRICKE, W. (1919). *Schutzmassnahmen bei bakteriologischem und serologischem Arbeiten.* Jena: Gustav Fischer.

FRIEDMAN, U. (1928). Das scharlachproblem. *Klinische Wochenschrift* **7**, 2321–2325.

FROMMER, W. and a Working Party of the European Federation of Biotechnology (1989). Safe biotechnology. 3. Safety precautions for handling microorganisms of different risk classes. *Applied Microbiology and Biotechnology* **30**, 541–552.

FROMMER, W. and a Working Party of the European Federation of Biotechnology (1993). Recommendations for safe work with animal and human cell culture concerning potential human pathogens. *Applied Microbiology and Biotechnology* **43**, 389–393.

FURCOLOW, M.L. (1961). Airborne histoplasmosis. *Bacteriological Reviews* **25**, 301–309.

FURCOLOW, M.L. (1965). Environmental aspects of histoplasmosis. *Archives of Environmental Health* **10**, 4–10.

FURCOLOW, M.L., GUNTHEROTH, W.G. & WILLIS, M.J. (1952). The frequency of laboratory infections with *Histoplasma capsulatum*. *Journal of Laboratory & Clinical Medicine* **40**, 182–187.

GAENSSLEN, R.E. (1983) *Sourcebook in Forensic Serology, Immunology and Biochemistry.* Washington: National Institute of Justice.

GAHYLLE, D. (1924). Le lapin attenue-t-il la virulence pour l'homme, due treponeme pale? *Comptes rendus de la Societe de Biologie* **91**, 911–914.

GAIGER, S.H. (1913). Glanders in man. *Journal of Comparative Pathology and Therapeutics* **26**, 223–236.

GALE, G.L. (1957). Accidental infection with tubercle bacilli in laboratory technicians. *Canadian Medical Association Journal* **76**, 646–648.

GANDSMAN, E.J., AALESTAD, H.G., OUIMEL, T.C. *et al*. (1997). Sabia virus incident at Yale University. *American Industrial Hygiene Association Journal* **58**, 51–53.

GARDNER, J.F. & PEEL, M.M. (1991). *Introduction to Sterilization and Disinfection.* 2nd ed. London: Churchill Livingstone.

GARNER, J.F. & MASTERSON, R.G. (1990). Specimen transport audit. *Journal of Clinical Pathology* **43**, 712–713.

GARNHAM, P.C.C., MOLINARI, V. & SHUTE, P.G. (1962). Differential diagnosis of bastianelli and vivax malaria *Bulletin of the World Health Organization* **27**, 199–202.

GAUGHWIN, M.D., COWANS, E., AI, R. *et al.* (1991). Bloody needles; the volume of blood transferred in situations of needle stick injuries and shared use of syringes for injection of intravenous drugs. *AIDS* **5**, 1025–1027.

GEAR, J.H.S. & BECKER, L.H. (1938). A case of typhus fever contracted in the laboratory from a virus isolated from rats. *South African Medical Journal* **12**, 57–60.

Genetic Modification (Contained Use) Regulations 1992 as amended 1996. London: The Stationery Office.

GEORGIOU, P.R. & YOUNG, E.J. (1991). Prolonged incubation in brucellosis. *Lancet* **337**, 1543.

GERBERDING, J.L., HOPEWELL, P.C. & KAMINGSKY, L.S. (1985). Transmission of hepatitis B without transmission of AIDS by needlestick. *New England Journal of Medicine* **312**, 56.

GERSHON, R.M. & ZIRKIN, B.G. (1993). Behavioral factors in safety training. In: *Laboratory Safety Practices and Principles.* (Eds D.O. Fleming, J.H. Richardson, J.I. Tulis & D. Vesley). 2nd edn. pp. 269–278. Washington: American Society for Microbiology.

GERVIN, J.L. & WILLIS, D.D. (1973). Absolute containment of preoperative ultracentrifuge in hepatitis research. In: *Proceedings of the National Cancer Institute Symposium on Centrifuge Biohazards.* Cancer Research Safety Monograph Series, Volume 1. Frederick, MD: Littel Bionetics.

GHOSH, H.K. (1982). Laboratory-acquired shigellosis. *British Medical Journal* **285**, 695–696.

GIBSON, J. (1955). Safety in a tuberculosis laboratory, Medical Technicians Bulletin Supplement. *US Armed Forces Medical Journal* **4**, 181.

GILBERT, R. & COLEMAN, M.B. (1928). Recent cases of undulant fever in New York State. *Journal of Infectious Disease* **43**, 273–279.

GILCHRIST, M.J.R. (1995) Biosafety precautions for airborne pathogens. In: *Laboratory Safety. Principles and Practice.* (Eds D.O. Fleming, J.H. Richardson, J.I. Tulis & D. Vesley). 2nd edn. pp. 67–76. Washington: American Society for Microbiology.

GILKES, C.F., LAMBERT, H.P., BROUGHTON, E.S. *et al.* (1988). Failure of penicillin prophylaxis in laboratory-acquired leptospirosis. *Postgraduate Medical Journal* **64**, 236–238.

GILLESPIE, E.H. & GIBBONS, S.A. (1975). Autoclaves and their dangers and safety in laboratories. *Journal of Hygiene* **75**, 475–487.

GILMAN, H.L. (1944). Undulant fever caused by *Brucella abortus* strain 19. *Cornell Veterinian* **34**, 193–194.

GLASER, J.B. & GORDON, A. (1985). Inoculation of cryptococcus without transmission of acquired immune deficiency syndrome. *New England Journal of Medicine* **313**, 266.

GLENHILL, A.W. (1967). Rat bite fever in laboratory personnel. *Laboratory Animals* **1**, 73–76.

GOEBEL, S. (1916). Beitrage zur Frage der Sogenannter Weilschen Krankheit. *Medizinische Klinic* **12**, 381–383.

GOLD, H. & FITZPATRICK, F. (1942). Typhus fever in a previously vaccinated laboratory worker. *Journal of the American Medical Association* **119**, 1415–1416.

GOLD, H. & HAMPIL, B.L. (1942). Equine encephalomyelitis in a laboratory technician with recovery. *Annals of Internal Medicine* **16**, 556–559.

GOLDMAN, J.M., TREXLER, P.C., SPIERS, A.S.D. *et al.* (1976). The use of plastic isolators to prevent infection in neutropenic patients. *Postgraduate Medical Journal* **S2**, 558–562.

GOLEY, A.F., ALEXANDER, A.D., THIEL, J.F. *et al.* (1960). A case of human infection with *Leptospira mini. Public Health Reports* **75**, 922–924.

GOPAL RAO, G., SAUNDERS, B.W. & MASTERTON, R.C. (1996) Laboratory-acqquired verotoxin-producing *Escherichia coli* infection. *Journal of Hospital Infection* **33**, 228–229.

GOPAUL, D.L., BROWN, S. & JASKOT, E. (1986). Accidental infection by *Brucella abortus. Canadian Journal of Medical Technology* **48**, 36–38.

GRACE, J.T. & MIRAND, E. A. (1963). Human susceptibility to a simian tumour virus. *Annals of the New York Academy of Science* l08, 1123–1129.

GRAETZ, F. & DELBANCO, E. (1914). Beitrage sum Studium der Histo-Pathologie for experimentellen Kaninchensyphilis, *Medizinische Klinik* **10**, 420.

GRAHAM, C.J. YAMAUCHI, T. & ROUNTREE, P. (1988). Q fever in animal laboratory workers: an outbreak and its investigation. *American Journal of Infection Control* **17**, 345–348.

GRAMMONT-CUPILLARD, M., BERTHET-BADETTI, L. *et al.* (1996). Brucellosis from sniffing cultures. *Lancet* **348**, 1733–1734.

GRANGE, J.M., NOBLE, W.C., YATES, M.D. *et al.* (1988) Inoculation mycobacterioses. *Clinical and Experimental Dermatology* **13**, 211–220.

GREEN, H.L. & LANE, W.R. (1964). *Particulate Dusts, Smokes and Mists.* London: Butterworths.

GREEN, H.N. (1941). Laboratory infection with *Brucella abortus. British Medical Journal* 1, 478–479.

GREEN, R.N. & TUFFNELL, P.C. (1974). Laboratory-acquired melioidosis. *American Journal of Medicine* **44**, 599–605.

GREEN, T.W. (1950). Aureomycin therapy of human psittacosis. *Journal of the American Medical Association* **144**, 237–238

GREEN, T.W. (1951). Reinfection brucellosis: a report of two cases. *Archives of Internal Medicine* **35**, 717–721.

GREEN, T.W. & EIGELSBACH, H.T. (1950). Immunity in tularemia: report of two cases of proved reinfection. *Archives of Internal Medicine* **85**, 777–782.

GREENBAUM, S.S. (1937). Chancre of lip in a laboratory technician. *Urologic and Cutaneous Review* **41**, 488–489.

GREGG, M.B. (1975). Recent outbreaks of lymphocytic choriomeningitis in the United States of America. *Bulletin of the World Health Organization* **52**, 549–553.

GRIST, N.R. (1975). Hepatitis in clinical laboratories; a three-year survey. *Journal of Clinical Pathology* **28**, 255–259.

GRIST, N. R. (1976). Hepatitis in clinical laboratories, 1973–1974. *Journal of Clinical Pathology* **29**, 480–483.

GRIST, N.R. (1978). Hepatitis in clinical laboratories, 1975- 1976. *Journal of Clinical Pathology* **31**, 415–417.

GRIST, N. R. (1980). Hepatitis in clinical laboratories, 1977–1978. *Journal of Clinical Pathology* **33**, 471–473.

GRIST, N.R. (1981a). Hepatitis and other infections in clinical laboratory staff 1979. *Journal of Clinical Pathology* **34**, 655–658.

GRIST, N. R. (1981b). Hepatitis infection in clinical laboratory staff. *Medical laboratory Sciences* **38**, 103–109.

GRIST, N.R. (1983). Infections in British clinical laboratories 1980–81. *Journal of Clinical Pathology* **36**, 121- 126.

GRIST, N.R. & EMSLIE, J.A.N. (1985). Infections in British clinical laboratories 1982–83. *Journal of Clinical Pathology* **38**, 721–725.

GRIST, N.R. & EMSLIE, J.A.N. (1987). Infections in British clinical laboratories, 1984–85. *Journal of Clinical Pathology* **40**, 826–829.

GRIST, N.R. & EMSLIE, J.A.N. (1989). Infections in British clinical laboratories, 1986–87. *Journal of Clinical Pathology* **42**, 677–681.

GRIST, N.R. & EMSLIE, J.A.N. (1991). Infections in British clinical laboratories, 1988–89. *Journal of Clinical Pathology* **44**, 667–669.

GROSS, H.T.(1940). Erysipeloid. A report of thirteen cases among veterinary students at Kansas State College. *Journal of the Kansas Medical Society* **41**, 329–332.

GROSS, L. (1971). Transmission of cancer in man. *Cancer* **23**, 785–788.

GRUBER, G. B. (1949). Zur Frage der Tuberkulose bei Mitgliedern pathologischer Institute. *Zentrablatt für Allgemeine Pathologie* **85**, 129–134.

GRUNER, E., BERNASCONI, E., GALEAZZI, R.L. *et al.* (1994). Brucellosis: an occupational hazard for medical personnel. Report of five cases. *Infection* **22**, 33–36.

GRUNKE, W. (1933). Infektion als Berufskrankheit. *Zeitschrift für arztliche Fortbildung* **30**, 453–457.

GUGEL, E.A. & SANDERS, M.E. (1986). Needlestick transmission of human colonic adenocarcinoma. *New England Journal of Medicine* **316**, 1487.

GUNTHORPE, W.J. (1987). First aid in the laboratory. In: *Safety in Clinical and Biomedical Laboratories* (Ed. C.H. Collins). pp. 133–150. London: Chapman & Hall.

GUSTAFSON, D.A. & MOSES, H.E. (1951). Isolation of Newcastle disease virus from the eye of a human being. *Journal of the American Veterinary Medical Association* **118**,1–2.

GUTTERIDGE, W.E., COVER, B. & COOKE, A.J.D. (1974). Safety precautions for working with *Trypanosoma cruzi. Transactions of the Royal Society of Tropical Medicine and Hygiene* **68**,161.

GUY, W.H. & JACOB, F.M. (1927). Granuloma coccidioides. *Archives of Dermatology and Syphilology* **16**, 308–311.

HABOBOU-SALA, P. (1932). Piqure operatoire a streptococque hemolytique jungules par la vaccinotherapie. *Tunisie Medicale* **26**,78–79.

HACKNEY, R. W., RUTALA, W. A., THOMANN, C. A. *et al.* (1985). Report of a laboratory-acquired *Neisseria gonorrhoeae* infection. XXVIIIth Biological Safety Conference, Salk Institute for Biological Studies, La Jolla, California.

HADLER, S.C, DOTTO, I.L., MAYNARD, J.E. *et al.* (1985). Occupational risk of hepatitis B infection in hospital workers. *Infection Control* **6**, 24–31.

HAEDICKE, T. A. (1947). Typhoid fever in vaccinated laboratory workers. *Journal of Infectious Disease* **80**, 113–116.

HALEY, C. REFF, V.J. & MURPHY, K.F. (1989). Report of a possible laboratory-acquired HIV infection. Abstr. 5th International Conference on AIDS, Montreal. (Cited by Fitch, 1995.)

HALL, C.V. (1975). A biological safety centrifuge. *Health Laboratory Science* **12**, 104–106.

HALL, C.J., RICHMOND, S.J., CAUL, E.O *et al.* (1982). Laboratory acquired outbreak of Q fever acquired from sheep, *Lancet* 1, 1001–1006.

HAMADEH, G.N., TURNER, B.W., TRIBLE, W. *et al* (1992). Laboratory outbreak of Q fever. *Family Practitioner* **35**, 683–685.

HAMBLETON, P., BENNETT, A.M. & LEAVER, G. (1992). Biosafety monitoring devices for biotechnology processes. *Trends in Biotechnology* (TIBTECH) **10**, 192–199.

HAMBURGER, M. & KNOWLES, H. C. (1953). *Streptobacillus moniliformis* infection complicated by acute bacterial endocarditis. Report of a case in a physician following bite of a laboratory rat. *Archives of Internal Medicine* **92**, 216–220.

HAMEL, E. (1931). Etat actuel de la question de la psittacose et de la lutte contre cette maladie. *Bulletin de l'office international d'hygiene publique* **23**, 1047–1058.

HAMMERSCHMIDT, J. (1924). Accidental infection with diphtheria. *Munchen medizinische Wochenschrift* **71**, 1755.

HANDSFIELD, H.H., CUMMINGS, M.J. & SWENSON, P.D. (1987). Prevalence of antibody to human immunodeficiency virus and hepatitis B surface antigen in blood samples submitted to a hospital laboratory. *Journal of the American Medical Association* **258**, 3395–3397.

HANEL, E. & ALG, R.L. (1955). Biological hazards of common laboratory procedures. II. The hypodermic syringe and needle. *American Journal of Medical Technology* **21**, 343–346.

HANEL, E. & KRUSE, R.H. (1967). Laboratory-acquired mycoses. Fort Detrick: Miscellaneous Publications No. 28. Ad-665376.

HANSON, R.P. & BRANDLEY, C.A. (1957). Epizootiology of vesicular stomatitis. *American Journal of Public Health* **47**, 205–2009.

HANSON, W.L., DEVLIN, R.F. & ROBERTSON, E.L. (1974). Immunoglobulin levels in a laboratory-acquired case of human Chagas diseases. *Journal of Parasitology* 60, 532–533.

HANSON, R.P., RASMUSSEN, A.F., BRANDLEY, C.A. *et al.* (1950). Human infection with the virus of vesicular stomatitis. *Journal of Laboratory and Clinical Medicine* 36,751–758.

HANSON, R.P., SULKIN, S.E., BUESCHER, E.L. *et al.* (1967). Arbovirus infection of laboratory workers. *Science* **158**, 1283–1286.

HARDING, L. & LIBERMAN, D.F. (1995). Epidemiology of laboratory-associated infections. In: *Laboratory Safety. Principles and Practice.* (Eds D.O. Fleming, J.H. Richardson, J.I. Tulis & D. Vesley). 2nd edn. pp. 7–18. Washington: American Society for Microbiology.

HARDY, A.V., HUDSON, M.G. & JORDAN, C.G. (1927). The skin as a portal of entry in *Brucella melitensis* infections. *Journal of Infectious Disease* **45**, 271–281.

HARPER, G.J. (1981). Contamination of the environment by special purpose centrifuges used in clinical laboratories. *Journal of Clinical Pathology* **34**, 1114–1123.

HARPER, G.J. (1983). Assessment of environmental contamination arising from use of equipment for carrying out the ELISA technique. *Journal of Clinical Pathology* **36**, 110–113.

HARPER, G.J. (1984a). Evaluation of sealed containers for use in centrifuges by a dynamic microbiological test. *Journal of Clinical Pathology* **37**, 1134–1139.

HARPER, G.J. (1984b). An assessment of environmental contamination arising from the use of some automated equipment in microbiology. *Journal of Clinical Pathology* **37**, 802–804.

HARRELL, A. & CURTIS, A. C. (1959). North American blastomycosis. *American Journal of Medicine* **27**, 750–766.

HARRINGTON, J.S., AW, T.C. & GARDNER, K. (1998). *Occupational Health: a Pocket Consultant.* 4th ed. Oxford: Blackwell.

HARRINGTON, J.M. & SHANNON, H.S. (1976). Incidence of tuberculosis, hepatitis, brucellosis and shigellosis in British medical laboratory workers. *British Medical Journal* 1, 759–762.

HARRINGTON, J.M. & OATES, D. (1984). Mortality study of British pathologists, 1974–1984. *British Journal of Industrial Medicine* **41**, 188–191.

HARRINGTON, J.M. & SHANNON, H.S. (1977). Survey of safety and health care in British medical laboratories. *British Medical Journal* 1, 626–628.

HARSTAD, J. B., DECKER, H. M., BUCHANAN *et al.* (1967). Air filtration of submicron virus aerosols. *American Journal of Public Health* **57**, 2186–2193.

HARTLEY, E.C. (1966). 'B' virus in monkey and man *British Veterinary Journal* **122**, 46–50.

HARTLEY, E.C. (1968). Human disease hazards from the laboratory monkey. *Veterinary Annual*, pp. 27–31.

HARTLEY, E.C. (1974). Primate Disease Hazards and their Prevention. In: *The Prevention of Laboratory Acquired Infection*. (Eds C.H.Collins, E.G. Hartley, & R. Pilsworth) pp. 51–55. London: The Stationery Office.

HARTUNG, F. & SALFELDER, K. (1962). Histoplasmosis with fatal outcome as an occupational disease in a mycologist. *Internationales Archiv für Gewerbepathologie* 19, 270–289.

HARVEY, R.W.S., PRICE, T.H. & JOYNSON, D.H.M. (1976). Observations on environmental contamination in a microbiological laboratory. *Journal of Hygiene* 76, 91–95.

HATCH, T.F. (1961). The distribution and deposition of inhaled particles in the respiratory tract. *Bacteriological Reviews* 25, 237–240.

HAWKEY, P.M., PEDKAR, S.J. & SOUTHALL, P.J. (1980). *Streptococcus pyogenes*: a forgotten hazard in the mortuary, *British Medical Journal* 281, 1085.

HAYES, G.S. & HARTMAN, T.C. (1943). Lymphocytic choriomeningitis: Report of a laboratory infection. *Bulletin of the Johns Hopkins Hospital* 73, 275–286.

HAYES, E.R., KIDD, R.E. & COWAN, D.W. (1950). Rat bite fever due to *Streptobacillus moniliformis*. *Journal Lancet (Minneapolis)* 70, 394–395.

HAYMAKER, W., SATHER, G.E. & HAMMON, W.M. (1955). Accidental Russian Spring Summer viral encephalitis; cases occurring in two laboratory workers. *Archives of Neurology and Psychiatry* 73, 609–630.

Health and Safety at Work etc. Act, 1974. London: The Stationery Office.

Health and Safety (First Aid) Regulations 1981. London: The Stationery Office.

HEALTH CANADA (1996). *Laboratory Safety Guidelines*, 2nd ed. Ottawa: Laboratory Centre for Disease Control.

HECKERT, R.A., BEST, M., JORDAN, L.T. *et al.* (1997). Efficacy of vaporised hydrogen peroxide against exotic animal viruses. *Applied and Environmental Microbiology* 63, 3916-3918.

HEDWALL, E. (1940). The incidence of tuberculosis among students at Lund University. *American Review of Tuberculosis* 41, 770–780.

HELLMAN, A. (1969). *Biohazard Control and Containment in Oncogenic Virus Research*. Atlanta: US Department of Health, Education and Welfare.

HELWIG, F.C. (1940). Western equine encephalitis following accidental inoculations with chick embryo virus. *Journal of the American Medical Association* 115, 291–292.

HENCKE, C.B. (1973). Containment recommendation and prototype equipment for ultracentrifuges in cancer research. In: *Proceedings of the National Cancer Institute Symposium on Centrifuge Hazards*. Cancer Research Safety Monograph Series Volume 1. Frederick, MD: Litton Bionetics.

HENNESSEN, W. (1968). A haemorrhagic disease transmitted from monkeys to man. *National Cancer Monographs* 29, 161–71.

HEPTONSTALL, J., PORTER, K. & GILL, N.O. (1995). Occupational transmission of HIV. Summary of Published Reports. PHLS AIDS Centre (CDSC), London.

HERBERT, W.J., PARRATT, D., VAN MEIRVENNE, N. *et al.* (1980). An accidental laboratory infection with trypanosomes of defined stock. *Journal of Infection* 2, 113–124.

HERMENTIN, K., HASSL, A., PICHER, O. *et al.* (1989). Comparison of different serotests for specific *Toxoplasma* IgM antibodies (ISAGA, SPIHA, IFAT) and detection of circulating antigen in two cases of toxoplasma infection. *Zentralblatt für Bakteriologie, Mikrobiolgie und Hygien Abt 1. orig.* 270, 534–541.

HERNANDEZ-MORALES, F. (1946). Brucellosis: a review of clinical manifestations and with presentations of twelve cases occurring in Puerto Rico. *Puerto Rico Journal of Public Health* 22, 3–24.

HERR, A. & BRUMPT, L. (1939). Un cas aigu de maladie de Chagas contracte accidellement on contact de triatomes mexicain. *Bulletin de la Societe de Pathologie exotique* 32, 566–571.

HERWALDT, B.L & JURANEK, D.F.D. (1997). Protozoa and helminths. *In: Laboratory Safety. Principles and Practice*. (Eds D.O. Fleming, J.H. Richardson, J.I. Tulis & D. Vesley). 2nd edn. pp. 77–92. Washington: American Society for Microbiology.

HILL, A. (1971). Accidental infection of man with *Mycoplasma caviae*. *British Medical Journal* 2, 711–712.

HILL, A.F., DESBRUSLOIS, M., JOINER, S. *et al.* (1996). The same prion strain causes nv CJD and BSE. *Nature* 389, 448–450.

HILLEMAN, M.R. & TAYLOR, R.O. (1958). A safe high speed blender for processing infectious materials. *Journal of Laboratory and Clinical Medicine* 51, 977–980.

HILLIS, W.D. (1961). Viral hepatitis associated with sub-human primates. *Transfusion* 3, 445–454.

HINMAN, A.R., KRADER, D.W., DOUGLAS, R.G. *et al.* (1975). An outbreak of lymphocytic choriomeningitis virus infections in medical centre personnel. *American Journal of Epidemiology* **101**, 103–110.

HIRSCHBRUCK, M. & THIEM, H. (1918). Aud der Bakteriologischen Anstalt fur Loth ringen in metz. Uber Rhurbazillen vom Typus Schmitz. *Deutsche Medizinische Wochenschrift* **44**, 1353–1354.

HOERL, D. (1988). Typhoid fever acquired in a medical teaching laboratory. *Laboratory Medicine* **19**, 166–168.

HOFFLIN, J.M., SADLER, R.H., ARAUJ, F.G. *et al.* (1987). Laboratory-acquired Chagas disease. *Transactions of the Royal Society of Tropical Medicine and Hygiene* **81**, 437–440.

HOFFMAN, P.N. & KENNEDY, D.A. (1997). Treatment and decontamination of blood spills. In: *Occupational Blood-borne Infections: Risks and Management.* (Eds C.H. Collins & D.A. Kennedy). pp. 249–256. Oxford: CAB International.

HOFFMAN, P.N., LARKIN, D. & SAMUEL, D. (1989). Needlestick and needleshare—the difference. *Journal of Infectious Disease* **160**, 545–546.

HOGAN, M.J. & ZIMMERMAN, L.E. (1962). Conjunctiva. *Ophthalmic Pathology.* 2nd edn. Philadelphia: Saunders.

HOLLSTROM, V. E. & HARD, S. (1953). A fatality from BCG vaccination. *Acta Dermatologica Venereologica* **33**, 159–160.

HOLM, K. (1924). Ueber eine Falle von Infection mit Malaria tropica an der Leiche. *Klinische Wochenschrift* **3**, 1633–1634.

HOLMES, G.P., HILLIARD, J.K., KLONTZ, K.C. *et al.* (1990). B virus (*Herpesvirus simiae*) infection in humans; epidemiological investigation of a cluster. *Annals of Internal Medicine* **11**, 833–839.

HOLMES, M.B., JOHNSON, D.L., FIUMARA, N.J. *et al.* (1980). Acquisition of typhoid fever from proficiency testing specimens. *New England Journal of Medicine* **303**, 519–521.

HOLTON, J. & PRINCE, M. (1986). Blood contamination during venepucture and laboratory manipulation of specimen tubes. *Journal of Hospital Infection* **8**, 178–183.

HOME OFFICE (1989) *Code of Practice for the Housing and Care of Animals used in Scientific Procedures.* London: The Stationery Office.

HOME OFFICE (1990) *Guidance on the Operation of the Animals (Scientific Procedures) Act 1986.* London: HMSO.

HORNIBROOK, J. W. & NELSON, K. R. (1940). An institutional outbreak of pneumonitis. *Public Health Reports* **55**, 1936–1944.

HOTCHIN, J., SIKORA, R., KINCH, W. *et al.* (1974). Lymphocytic choriomeningitis in a hamster colony causes infection in hospital personnel. *Science* **185**, 1173–1174.

HOWE, C. & MILLER, W.R. (1947). Human glanders. Report of six cases. *Annals of Internal Medicine* **26**, 93–115.

HOWE C., MILLER, E.S., KELLY, E.H. *et al.* (1947). Acute brucellosis among laboratory workers. *New England Journal of Medicine* **236**, 741–747.

HOWIE, J.W. & COLLINS, C.H. (1980). The Howie Code for preventing infection in clinical laboratories. Comment on some general criticisms and specific complaints. *British Medical Journal* **2**, 1071–1074.

HSE (1981). Formaldehyde. HSE Toxicity Review. London: Health and Safety Executive.

HSE (1982). Pre-employment Health Screening. Guidance Note MS2O, Health and Safety Executive. London: The Stationery Office.

HSE (1986). *A Guide to the Reporting of Injuries, Diseases and Dangerous Occurrences Regulations 1985.* Sudbury: HSE.

HSE (1990a). *First Aid at Work Regulations 1981.* Revised Code of Practice. Sudbury: HSE Books.

HSE (1990b). Education Services Advisory Committee. *What you should know about allergy to laboratory animals.* Sudbury: HSE Books.

HSE (1991a). Health Services Advisory Committee. *Safe Working and the Prevention of Infection in Clinical Laboratories.* London: The Stationery Office.

HSE (1991b). Health Services Advisory Committee. *Safe Working and the Prevention of Infection in the Mortuary and Post-mortem Room.* London: The Stationery Office.

HSE (1992a). Health Services Advisory Committee. *Safe Disposal of Clinical Waste.* Sudbury: HSE Books.

HSE (1992b). Education Services Advisory Committee. *Health and safety in animal facilities.* London: The Stationery Office.

HSE (1992). *Formaldehyde. HSE Toxicity Review.* Sudbury: HSE Books.

HSE 1993). *A Step by Step Guide to COSHH Assessments.* Sudbury: HSE Books.

HSE (1994). *Preventing Asthma at Work.* Sudbury: HSE Books.

HSE (1995). *General COSHH Approved Code of Practice. Carcinogens ACOP and Biological Agents ACOP.* L5. Sudbury: HSE Books.

HSE (1996). *A Guide to the Genetically Modified Organisms (Contained Use) Regulation 1992,* as amended in 1996. Sudbury: HSE Books.

HSE (1997a). Working Safely at Containment Level 3 - Videotape. Sudbury: HSE.

HSE (1997b) *General COSHH ACOP, carcinogens ACOP and Biological agents ACOP.* Sudbury: HSE Books.

HSE (1998a). *Control of Substances Hazardous to Health Regulations 1994. Approved List of Biological Agents.* 3rd ed. (Categorization, 1988.)

HSE (1998). *Glutaraldehyde and you. General Guidance for the Health Care Sector.* Sudbury: HSE Books.

HSU (1943). A case of accidentally infected bubonic plague. *Chinese Medical Journal* **62a**, 112–113.

HUANG, C.H., HUANG, C.Y., CHU,L. W. *et al.* (1948). Pneumonic plague. A report of recovery in a proved case. *American Journal of Tropical Medicine* **28**, 361–371.

HUDDLESON, I.F. (1926). Is *Bacterium abortus* pathogenic for human beings? *Journal of the American Medical Association* 86, 943–944.

HUDDLESON, I.F. & MUNGER, M. (1940). A study of an epidemic of brucellosis due to *Brucella melitensis. American Journal of Public Health* 30, 944–945.

HUDSON, L., GROVER, F., GUTTERIDGE, W.E. *et al.* (1983). Suggested guidelines for work with live *Trypanosoma cruzi. Transactions of the Royal Society of Tropical Medicine and Hygiene* **77**, 416–419.

HUEBNER, R.J. (1947). Report of an outbreak of a fever at the National Institute of Health. *American Journal of Public Health* 37, 431–440.

HULL, R.N. (1973). Biohazards associated with simian viruses. In: *Biohazards in Biological Research* (Eds A. Hellman, M.N. Oxman & R. Pollack). Cold Spring Harbor Laboratory Press.

HUMMELER, K., DAVIDSON, W.L., HENLE, W. *et al.* (1959). Encephalomyelitis due to infection with herpes virus simiae (herpes B-virus). A report of two fatal laboratory acquired cases. *New England Journal of Medicine* **261**, 64–68.

HUMPHREYS, F.A. & GUEST, W.A. (1932). Undulant fever contracted in the laboratory. *Canadian Medical Association Journal* **27**, 616–619.

HUNT, D.L. (1997). Epidemiology of blood-borne infections. In: *Occupational Blood-borne Infections: Risks and Management.* (Eds C.H. Collins & D.A. Kennedy). pp. 267–286. Oxford: CAB International.

HUNT, D.L. (1997) Review of the OSHA Regulations on blood-borne infections. In: *Occupational; Blood-borne Infections.* (Eds C H. Collins & D.A. Kennedy). pp. 267–286. Oxford: CAB International.

HUNTER, D. (1936). *Saints and Martyrs. Lancet* 2, 1131–1134.

HUNTER, M.C., KEENEY, A.H. & SIGEL, M.M. (1951). Laboratory aspects of an infection with Newcastle disease virus in man, *Journal of Infectious Disease* **88**, 272–277.

IAMLT (1992). *A Curriculum for a Course in Health and Safety for Medical Laboratory Workers.* Stockholm: International Association of Medical Laboratory Technologists.

IATA (1994). *Dangerous Goods Regulations.* Montreal: International Air Transport Association.

IEC (1990) *Safety requirements for electrical equipment for measuring, control and laboratory use.* Geneva: International Electrotechnical Commission. (see also BS EN 061010–1 (1993).

IFCC (1990). Guidelines for selection of safe laboratory centrifuges and their safe use. International Federation of Clinical Chemistry. *Journal of Automated Chemistry* 13, 221–229.

IMLS GAZETTE (1980). Mouth pipetting. Correspondence 24, 406, 512, 560.

Importation of Dogs, Cats and other Mammals Order 1974. London: The Stationery Office.

Importation of Animals Order 1980. London: The Stationery Office.

ISAACSON, M., PROZESKY, O.W., JOHNSON, K.M. *et al.* (1978). *Ebola Virus Haemorrhagic Fever.* p.245. Amsterdam: Elsevier/North Holland Biomedical Press.

ISHIZAKI, H., IKEDA, M. & KURATA, Y. (1979). Lymphocutaneous sporotrichosis caused by accidental inoculation. *Journal of Dermatology* 6, 321–323.

ISO (1994) Draft International Standard ISO/DIS/ 6710.3 for Single Use Containers for Venous Blood Specimen Collection. Geneva: International Standards Office.

ISSA (1999). *Control of Risks in Work with Biological Agents. Part 2. In the Laboratory.* Heidelberg:

International Social Security Association—Section for the Prevention of Occupational Risks in the Chemical Industry.

IWANOWA, D.A. (1928). Ein Fall von Laboratoriumsinfektion mit Ruckfallifieber durch die Conjunctiva. *Klinische Wochenschrift* **7**, 1742–1743.

JACOBSON, J.T., ORLOB, R.B. & CLAYTON, J.L. (1985). Infection acquired in laboratories in Utah. *Journal of Clinical Microbiology* **21**, 486–489.

JAGGER, J. & BENTLEY, M. (1997). Clinical laboratories: percutaneous exposure. In: *Occupational Blood-borne Infections: Risks and Management*. (Eds C.H. Collins & D.A. Kennedy). pp. 75–86. Oxford: CAB International.

JAMA (1936). Obituary: Bacteriologist dies of meningitis. (Anna Pabst. Death attributed to meningitis contracted while conducting experiments in the laboratories of the National Institutes of Health). *Journal of the American Medical Association* **106**, 129.

JAMA (1950). Tuberculosis in laboratory workers. *Journal of the American Medical Association* **143**, 478.

JAWETZ, E.T., HANNA, L., SONNE, M. *et al.* (1959). Laboratory infection with adenovirus type 8. *American Journal of Hygiene* **69**, 13.

JEANSELME, E. & CHEVALIER, P. (1910). Chancres sporotrichosiques des doigts produits par la morsure d'un rat inocule de sporotrichose. *Bulletin Memoriale de Medicale Hopital (Paris)* **30**, 176–178.

JEANSELME, E. & CHEVALIER, P. (1911). Transmission de la sporotrichose a l'homme par les morsures d'un rat blanc inocule avec une nouvelle variety de Sporotrichum. Lymphangite gommeuse ascendante. *Bulletin Memoriale de Medicale Hopital (Paris)* **31**, 287–301.

JEANSELME, E., HUET, L. & HOROWITZ, E. (1928). Quatre ca de gommes et ulcerations sporotrichosiques accidentelles, survenues a la suite d'intradermo-reactions. *Bulletin de la Societe françoise de dermatologie et de syphilogie* **35**, 416–422.

JELINKOVA-SKALOVA, E. (1974). Laboratory infection with the virus of Omsk haemorrhagic fever with neurological and psychiatric symptomatology. *Ceskoslovenska Epidemiologie, Microbiologie, Immunologie* **23**, 590–593.

JENNIS, F. & MAZO, A. (1971). A human case of bacteraemia due to *Vibrio fetus*. *Pathology* **3**, 263–265.

JENNISON, M.W. (1942) *Aerobiology*. American Association for the Advancement of Science. Publ No. 17. p.106.

JENSEN, J.B., CAPPS, T.C. & CAVLIN, J.M. (1981). Clinical drug-resistant falciparum malaria acquired from cultured parasites. *American Journal of Tropical Medicine and Hygiene* **30**, 523–524.

JERVIS, G.A. & HIGGINS, G.H. (1973). Russian spring-summer encephalitis; clinicopathologic report of a case in a human. *Journal of Neuropathology and Experimental Neurology* **12**, 1–10.

JOFFE, B. & DIAMOND, M.T. (1966). Brucellosis due to self-inoculation. *Annals of Internal Medicine* **65**, 564.

JOHNSON, H.N. (1944) Isolation of *Bacterium tularense* from the sputum of an atypical case of tularaemia. *Journal of Laboratory and Clinical Medicine* **29**, 903–905.

JOHNSON, J.E. & KADULL, P.J. (1966). Laboratory-acquired Q fever. *American Journal of Medicine* **41**, 391–403.

JOHNSON, J.E. & KADULL, P.J. (1967). Rocky Mountain Spotted Fever in the laboratory. *New England Journal of Medicine* **277**, 842–847.

JOHNSON, J.E., PERRY, J.E., FEKETY, F.R. *et al.* (1964). Laboratory acquired coccidioidiomycosis: a report of 210 cases. *Annals of Internal Medicine* **60**, 941–956.

JOHNSON, K.M., VOGEL, J.E.P. & PERALTA, P.H. (1966). Clinical and serological response to laboratory-acquired human infection by Indiana type vesicular stomatitis virus. *American Journal of Tropical Medicine and Hygiene* **15**, 244–246.

JOIRIS, E. (1950). Infection de laboratoire a *Brucella abortus*. *Acta Clinica Belgica* **5**, 277–278.

JONES, B.P.C. (1996) Fumigation and management of containment level 3 facilities. *PHLS Microbiology Digest* **12**, 169–171.

JONES, O.R., PLATT, W.D. & AMILL, L.A. (1949). Miliary tuberculosis caused by intravenous self-infection of tubercle bacilli. *American Review of Tuberculosis* **60**, 514–519.

JONES, L., RISTOW, S., YILMA, T. *et al.* (1986). Accidental human vaccination with vaccine virus expressing nucleoprotein gene. *Nature* **319**, 543.

JONES, P., HAMILTON, P.J., OXLEY, A. *et al.* (1985). Anti-HTLV positive laboratory reagents *Lancet* i, 1458–1459.

JUSTINES, G.A. & SHOPE, R.G. (1969). Wesselbron virus infection in a laboratory worker with virus recovery from a throat washing. *Health Laboratory Science* **6**, 46–49.

KAO, H.S, ASHFORD, D.A., McNEIL, M.M. *et al.* (1997). Descriptive profile of tuberculin skin testing programs and laboratory-acquired tuberculosis infections in public health laboratories. *Journal of Clinical Microbiology* 45, 1361–1364.

KADULL, P.J., REAMES, H.R., CORIELL, L.L. *et al.* (1950). Studies on tularemia. *Journal of Immunology* 65, 425–435.

KAFFKA, A. & RIETH, H. (1958). Laboratoriumstiere els Uhrsache eine einer Berufsdermatomykose und Massnahmen zur Verhutung Wider Pilzinfektion. *Zentralblatt fur Bakteriologie etc.* Abt. I Orig. 171, 319–321.

KAMELAM, A. & THAMBIA, A. S. (1979). *Trichophyton simiae* infection due to laboratory accident. *Dermatologica* 159, 180- 181.

KAPPEL, T.J., REINARTZ, J.J., SCMIDT, J.L. *et al.* (1996). Viability of *Mycobacterium tuberculosis* in formalin-fixed autopsy tissue. *Human Pathology* 327, 14361–1364.

KAPPELER, R., BARUNDUN, S., LUTHI, H. *et al.* (1961). On a laboratory *Leptospira ballum* infection. *Schweizer Medinische Wochenscrift* 91, 811–812.

KARIMOV, S.K. (1975). Case of a laboratory infection with the Crimean haemorrhagic fever virus. *Zhurnal Mikrobiologie, Epidemiologie und Immunobiologie* 5, 136–137.

KARTMAN, L., QUAN, S.F. & LECHLEITNER, R.R. (1962). Die-off of a Gunnison's prairie dog colony in central Colorado. II. Retrospective determination of plague inspection in flea vectors, rodents and man. *Zoonosis Research* 1, 201–224.

KATHE, J. & MOCHAMAN, H. (1962). Die Albinoratte als Infektionsquelle für Erkrankungen an Morbus Weil. *Monatschafte für Veterinämedizin* 17, 17–31.

KATZ, I., ROSENTHAL, T. & MICHAELI, D. (1985). Undiagnosed tuberculosis in hospital patients. *Chest* 87, 70.

KELSEY, J.C. & MAURER, I. (1966). An in-use test for hospital disinfectants. *Monthly Bulletin of the Ministry of Health and Public Health Laboratory Service* 25, 180–184.

KENNEDY, D.A. (1987). Water fog as a medium for visualization of airflows. *Annals of Occupational Hygiene* 31, 255–259

KENNEDY, D.A. (1988a). *Studies in Laboratory Acquired Infection with Particular Reference to Equipment.* PhD Thesis, University of London.

KENNEDY, D.A. (1988b). Equipment-related hazards. In: *Safety in Clinical and Biomedical Laboratories.* (Ed. C.H. Collins). pp. 11–46. London: Chapman & Hall.

KENNEDY, D.A. (1997). Detection of surface and air-borne blood contamination. In: *Occupational Blood-borne Infections: Risks and Management.* (Eds C.H. Collins & D.A. Kennedy). pp. 89–100. Oxford: CAB International.

KENNEDY, D.A. & COLLINS C.H. (1998). Clinical laboratories: mucocutaneous exposure. In: *Occupational Blood-borne Infections: Risks and Management.* (Eds C.H. Collins & D.A. Kennedy). pp. 173–190. Oxford: CAB International.

KENNEDY, D.A., STEVENS, J.F. & HORN, A.N. (1988). Clinical laboratory environmental contamination: use of a fluorescent-bacterial tracer. *Journal of Clinical Pathology* 41, 1229–1332.

KENNY, M.T. & SABLE, F.L. (1968). Particle size distribution of *Serratia marcescens* aerosols created during common laboratory procedures and simulated laboratory accidents. *Applied Microbiology* 16, 1146–1156.

KEW, M.C. (1973) Possible transmission of serum (Australia antigen positive) hepatitis via the conjunctiva. *Infection and Immunity* 7, 823–824.

KHABBAZ, R.F., HENEINE, W., GEORGE, J.R. *et al.* (1994). Brief report: infection of a laboratory worker with simian immunodeficiency virus. *New England Journal of Medicine* 330, 172–177.

KIBBLER, C.C. (1997). Universal precautions and the advent of standard precautions. In: *Occupational Blood-borne Infections: Risks and Management.* (Eds C.H. Collins & D.A. Kennedy). pp. 287–298. Oxford: CAB International.

KIKUTH, W. & BOCK, W. (1949). 23 Falle von Laboratoriumsinfektionen mit Q-Fieber. *Medizinische Klinik* 44, 1056–1060.

KILEY, M.P. (1992). Clinical laboratory safety, biohazard surveillance and infection control. In: *Clinical Laboratory Medicine.* (Eds R.C. Tilton, A. Balows, D.C. Hohnadel & R.F. Reiss). St Louis: Mosby.

KISSKALT, K. (1915). Laboratoriumsinfektionen mit Typhusbazillen. *Zeitschrift für Hygiene und Infektionskrankheiten* 50, 145–162.

KISSKALT, K. (1929). Laboratoriumsinfektionen mit Typhusbazillen und anderen Bakterien. *Archiv für Hygiene und Bakteriologie* 101,137–160.

KISSLING, R.E., MURPHY, F.A. & HENDERSON, B.E. (1970). Marburg virus. *Annals of the New York Academy of Science* 174, 932–945.

KITCHEN, S.F. (1934). Laboratory infections with the virus of Rift Valley. *American Journal of Tropical Medicine* **14**,547–564.

KLAPES, N.N. (1990). New applications of chemical germicides: hydrogen peroxide. *ASM International Symposium on Chemical Germicides,* Atlanta, GA: Washington: American Society of Microbiologists.

KLAPES, N.A. & VESELY, D. (1990). Vapor-phase hydrogen peroxide as a surface decontaminant and sterilant. *Applied and Environmental Microbiology* **56**, 32–40.

KLEINSCHMIDT, A. & CHRIST, P. (1959). *Leptospira ballum* als Ursache einer Laboratoriumsinfektion. *Zeitschrift für Immunitätsforschung* **117**,107–113.

KLUTSCH, K., HUMMER, N., BRAUN, H. *et al.* (1965). Zur Klinik der Coccidiomykose. *Deutsche Medizinische Wochenschrift* 90, 1498–1501.

KNOBLOCH, J. & DEMAR, M. (1997), Accidental *Leishmania mexicana* infection in an immunosuppressed laboratory technician. *Tropical Medicine and International Health* **2**, 1152–1155.

KOBAYASKI, R. (1931). Studies on *Bacillus dysenteriae. Kruse Kitasato Archives of Experimental Medicine* **8**, 99–173.

KOCH, O. (1951). Zur tuberkulosen Berufserkrankung des Artes, besonders der Pathologen. *Tuberkulosearzt* **5**, 498–502.

KOCH, R. (1886). In: *Selected Essays on Microparasites in Disease* (Ed. G. L. Laycock). London.

KOHN, N.J. (1976) Blood smears and hepatitis. *Lancet* 2, 226.

KOPROWSKI, H. & COX, H.R. (1947). Human laboratory infection with Venezuelan equine encephalomyelitis virus. Report of four cases. *New England Journal of Medicine* **236**, 647-654.

KORTHOF, G. (1937). Tamme ratten also bron voor besmetting met Weil Leptospirae. *Nederlands tijdschrift voor geneeskunde* **81**, 4571–4574.

KOSINA, F. & KOLOUCH, Z. (1975). Q fever laboratory infection. *Casopis lekaro ceskych* **114**,134–136.

KRASSNITSKY, O., PESENDORFER, F. & WEWALKA, F. (1974). Hepatitis und Laboratorium. *Das medizinische Laboratorium (Stuttgart)* **27**, 77–81.

KRUG, E.S. & GLEN, H.R. (1953). Case report of anthrax acquired in a college research laboratory. *Journal Lancet (Minneapolis)* **73**, 506–508.

KRUSE, R.H. (1962). Potential aerogenic laboratory hazards of *Coccidioides immitis. American Journal of Clinical Pathology* **37**, 150–158.

KRUSE, R.H., PUCKET, W.H. & RICHARDSON, J.H. (1991). Biological safety cabinetry. *Clinical Microbiology Reviews* **4**N, 207–241.

KUBICA, G.P. & DYE, W.E. (1967). *Laboratory Methods for Clinical and Public Health Mycobacteriology.* US Publication No 1547. Washington DC: US Department of Health Education and Welfare.

KUCHARSKI, J.K., SZUSZKO, B. & MARDARWICZ, C. (1960). A case of laboratory tetanus. *Polski tygodnik lekarski* **15**, 263–265.

KUEHNE, R.W., SAWYER, W.D. & GOCHENOUR, W.S. (1962). Infection with aerosolized attenuated Venezuelan equine encephalomyelitis virus. *American Journal of Hygiene* **75**, 347–350.

KUH, C. & WARD, W.E. (1950). Occupational virus hepatitis, an apparent hazard for medical personnel. *Journal of the American Medical Association* **143**, 631–635.

KULAGIN, S.M., FEDOROVA, N.I. & KETILADZE E.S. (1962). Laboratory outbreak of haemorrhagic fever with renal syndrome. *Zhurnal Mikrobiologie, Epidemiologie i Immunologie* **33**,121–126.

KUNZ, L.J. & EWING, W.H. (1965). Laboratory infection with a lactose-fermenting strain of *Salmonella typhi. Journal of Bacteriology* **89**, 1629.

KURL, D.N. (1981). Laboratory-acquired human infection with Group A type 5O streptococci. *Lancet* 2, 752.

LACEY, J. & DUTKIEWICZ, J. (1994). Bioaerosols and occupational lung diseases. *Journal of Aerosol Science* **25**, 1371–1404.

LACEY, J., PEPYS, J. & CROSS, T. (1972). Actinomycete and fungus spores in air as respiratory allergens. In: *Safety in Microbiology* (Eds D.A. Shapton & R.G. Board). pp. 151–184. London: Academic Press.

LACH, V.H. (1985). Performance of the surface air system air samplers. *Journal of Hospital Infection* **6**, 102–107.

LACH, V.H., HARPER, G.J. & WRIGHT, A.E. (1983). An assessment of some hazards associated with the collection of venous blood. *Journal of Hospital Infection* **4**, 57–63.

LACH, V.H. & WRIGHT, A.E. (1981). The testing of HEPA filters fitted to microbiological safety cabinets. *Journal of Hospital Infection* **2**,385–388.

LAKE, G.C. & FRANCIS, E. (1922). Tularemia Francis 1921. Six cases of tularemia occurring in laboratory workers. *Public Health Reports* **37**,392–413.

LANCET (1949). Leptospirosis in Denmark. 1, 742–743.

LANCET (1962). Death of a Porton scientist. 2, 463.

LANCET (1967). Disease transmitted from monkeys to man. 2, 1129–1130.

LANCET (1971). Marburg disease. 2, 31.

LANDAY, M.E. & SCHWARZ, J. (1971). Primary cutaneous blastomycosis. *Archives of Dermatology* **104**, 408–411.

LANGMUIR, A.D. (1961). Epidemiology of airborne infection. *Bacteriological Reviews* **25**, 173–181.

LANPHEAR, B.P. (1994). Trends and patterns in the transmission of blood-borne pathogens to health care workers. *Epidemiological Reviews* **16**, 10–14.

LARSEN, K. & LEBEL, H. (1943). A small laboratory epidemic of typhus fever in Copenhagen. *Acta medica Scandinavica* **115**, 524–536.

LARSH, H.W. & SCHWARZ, J. (1977). Accidental inoculation blastomycosis. *Cutis* **19**, 334–335.

LAUER, J.L., VAN DRUNEN, N.A., WASHBURN, J.W. *et al.* (1979). Transmission of hepatitis B virus in clinical laboratory areas. *Journal of Infectious Disease* **140**, 513–536.

LEDINGHAM, J.C.G. & FRAZER, F.R. (1924). Tularemia in man from laboratory infections. *Quarterly Journal of Medicine* **17**,365–383.

LEE, H.W. & JOHNSON, K.M. (1982). Laboratory-acquired infections with Hantaan virus, the etiologic agent of Korean haemorrhagic fever. *Journal of Infectious Disease* **146**, 645–651.

LEES, R. (Ed.) (1993). *Design, Construction and Refurbishment of Laboratories.* Vol 2. Chichester: Ellis Horwood.

LEIFER, E., GOCKE, D.J. & BOURNE, H. (1970). Lassa fever. A new virus disease of man from West Africa. II. Report of a laboratory acquired infection. *American Journal of Tropical Medicine and Hygiene* **19**, 677–679.

LELIEVELD, H.L.M. and the Working Party on Safety in Biotechnology of the European Federation of Biotechnology (1995). Safe biotechnology. Part 6. Safety assessment, in respect of human health, of microorganisms used in biotechnology. *Applied Microbiology and Biotechnology* **43**, 389–393.

LEMIERRE, A. & AMEUILLE, P. (1938). (Self inoculation with tubercle bacilli), cited by Pike, 1979.

LENNETTE, E.H., MEIKLEJoHN, G. & THELEN, H.M. (1948). Treatment of Q fever in man. *Annals of the New York Academy of Science* **51**, 331–342.

LENNETTE, E.H. & KOPROWSKI, H. (1943). Human infection with Venezuelan equine encephalomyelitis virus. A report of eight cases of infection acquired in the laboratory. *Journal of the American Medical Association* **123**, 1088–1095.

LENNOX, V.A. & ACKERMAN, V.P. (1986). Aerosols from the catalase test. *Pathology* **18**, 481.

LEPINE, P. & SAUTTER, V. (1938). Contamination de laboratoire avec le virus de la choriomeningite lymphocytaire. *Annals de l'Institute Pasteur* **61**, 519–526.

LEVADITI, C. & MARIE, A. (1919). Etude sur le treponeme de la paralysie generale. *Annals de l'Institut de Paris* **33**, 741–776.

LEVY, B.S., HARRIS, J.C., SMITH, J.L. *et al.* (1977). Hepatitis B in ward and clinical laboratory employees of a general hospital. *American Journal of Epidemiology* **106**, 330–335.

LEWIN, W., BECKER, B.J.P. & HORWITZ, B. (1948). Two cases of pneumonic plague. *South African Medical Journal* **22**, 699–703.

LEWIS, A.M., ROWE, W.P., TURNER, H.C. *et al.* (1965). Lymphocytic choriomeningitis virus in hamster tumour. Spread to hamsters and humans. *Science* **150**, 363–364.

LEWIS, S. M. & WARDLE, J.M. (1978). An analysis of blood specimen container leakage. *Journal of Clinical Pathology* **31**, 888–892.

LIBERMAN, D.F. & GORDON, J.G. (Eds) (1989). *Biohazards Management Handbook.* New York: Dekker.

LICHT, W. (1972). The movement of aerosol particles. *Journal of the Society of Cosmetic Chemists* **23**, 657–678.

LIDWELL. O.M. (1970). Mikroorganismer: levende stof i luflen. In: *Termisk og atmosfaerisk indeklima* (Ed. N. Jomassen). Copehagen: Plyteknisk Forlag.

LIEBOWITZ, S., GREENWALD, L., COHEN, I. *et al.* (1949). Serum hepatitis in a blood bank worker. *Journal of the Arnerican Medical Association* **140**, 1331.

LINELL, F. & ÖSTBERG, G. (1966) Tuberculosis in an autopsy material. *Scandinavian Journal of Respiratory Diseases* **47**, 200–208.

LIND, A. (1957). Ventilated cabinets in a tuberculosis laboratory. *Bulletin of the World Health Organization* **16**,448- 453.

LINK, V.B. (1951). Plague. *American Journal of Tropical Medicine* **3**, 452–457.

LINK, V.B. (1955). *A History of Plague in the United States*. Public Health Monographs No. 26. Washington. US Public Health Service.

LIPMAN, N.S. & NEWCOMER, C.E. (1989). Hazard control in the animal house. In: *Biohazards Management Handbook*. (Eds D.F. Liberman & J.C. Gordon). pp. 107–150. New York: Dekker.

LIPPELT, H. (1951). Spezielle Fragen zur Rickettsier. *Zentralblatt für Bakteriologie* Ab. 1 Orig. **159**, 29.

LIPPINCOTT, L.S. (1925). A case of of bacillary dysentery contracted in the laboratory. *Journal of the American Medical Association* **85**, 901.

LISELLA, F.S. & THOMASTON, S.W. (1995). Chemical safety in the microbiology laboratory. In: *Laboratory Safety. Principles and Practice*. 2nd ed. (Eds D.O. Fleming, J.H. Richardson, J.I. Tulis & D. Vesley). pp. 247–256. Washington: American Society for Microbiology.

LISIEUX, T., COIMBRA, T.L., NASSAR, E.S. *et al.* (1994). New arena virus in Brazil. *Lancet* **343**, 391–392.

LLOYD, G. & JONES, N. (1986). Infections of laboratory workers with Hantaan virus acquired from immunocytomas propagated in laboratory rats. *Journal of Infection* **12**, 117-125.

LO GRIPPO, G.A. & HAYASHI, H. (1973). Incidence of hepatitis or Australia antigenaemia among laboratory workers. *Health Laboratory Science* **10**, 157–162.

LOFFLER, W. & MOOSER, H. (1942). Zum Ubertragungsmodus des Fleckfebers beobachtungen anlasslich einer Laboratoriurns-gruppeninfektion. *Schweizer Medizinsche Wochenschrift* **72**,755–761.

LONG, E.R. (1951). The hazard of acquiring tuberculosis in the laboratory. *American Journal of Public Health* **41**, 782–787.

LOONEY, J.M. & STEIN, T. (1950). Coccidioidomycosis; the hazard involved in diagnostic procedures, with report of a case. *New England Journal of Medicine* **242**, 77–82.

LOT, F. & ABITEBOUL, D. (1993). Infections professionales par le VIH en France. Le point au 31 Decembre 1993. *Bulletin Epidemiologique Hebdomadaire* **25**, 111–113.

LOVE, F.M. & JUNGHERR, E. (1962). Occupational infection with virus B of monkeys. *Journal of the American Medical Association* **179**, 804–806.

LOWE, C.G. & FAIRLY, N.H. (1931). Observations on laboratory or hospital infection with yellow fever in the United Kingdom. *British Medical Journal* 1, 125.

LUBARSCH, O. (1931). *Ein bewegtes Gelehrtenleben*. p. 68. Berlin: Julius Springer.

LUDLAM, G. B. & BEATTLE, C. P. (1963). Pulmonary toxoplasmosis. *Lancet* 2, 344–349.

LUNDGREN, R., NORMAN, E & ÅSBERG, I. (1987). Tuberculosis infection transmitted at autopsy. *Tubercle* **68**, 147–150.

LURIE, M. B. (1930). Air-borne contagion of tuberculosis in an animal room. *Journal of Experimental Medicine* **51**, 743–751.

LUZZI, G.A., BRINDLE, R., SOCKET, P.N. *et al.* (1993). Brucellosis: imported and laboratory-acquired cases, and an overview of treatment trials. *Transactions of the Royal Society for Tropical Medicine and Hygiene* **87**, 138–141.

MacARTHUR, S. & SCHNEIDERMAN, H. (1986). Autopsy removal of brain in AIDS: a new technique. *Human Pathology* **15**, 172–177.

MacARTHUR, S. & SCHNEIDERMAN, H. (1987). Infection control and autopsy of persons with the immunodeficiency virus. *Human Pathology* **15**, 172–177.

McCARTHY, L.J. (1978). Gonorrhoea of the eye in an adult. *Lancet* 1, 51.

McCLOY, E. (1997). Immunization and post-exposure prophylaxis. In: *Occupational Blood-borne Infections: Risks and Management*. (Eds C.H. Collins & D.A. Kennedy). pp. 233–248. Oxford: CAB International.

McCOLLUM, R.W. (1962). Armed Forces Epidemiological Board: Reappraisal of viral hepatitis in chimpanzees. *Military Medicine* **127**, 994–996.

McCOY, G.W. (1930). Accidental psittacosis infection among personnel of the hygienic laboratory. *Journal of Infectious Disease* **55**, 156–167.

McCOY, G.W. (1934). Psittacosis among the personnel of the hygienic laboratory. *Journal of Infectious Disease* **55**, 156–167.

McCOY, G.W. & CHAPMAN, C.W. (1912). Studies of plague, a plague-like disease and tuberculosis among rodents in California, *Public Health Bulletin* No. 53.

McCULLOCH, N.B. (1963). Medical care following accidental infection of *Brucella abortus* strain-l9 in man. *Journal of the American Medical Association* **143**, 617–618.

McCULLOCH, T., WEIR, J.C. & CLAYTON, F.H. (1907). In: *Report of the Mediterranean Fever Commission* Part VII, p. 253.

McDADE, J.J., SABEL, F.L., AKERS, R.L. *et al.* (1968). Microbiological studies on the performance of a laminar airflow biological cabinet. *Applied Microbiology* **16**, 1086–1092.

McGARRITY, G.J. & KOTANI, H. (1985). Cell culture mycoplasmas. In: *The Mycoplasmas*. (Eds S. Razin & M.F. Barile). New York: Academic Press.

MACKENZIE, D.W.R. (1961). *Trichophyton mentagrophytes* in mice; infections of humans and incidence among laboratory animals, *Sabouraudia* **1**, 178–182.

MACKENZIE, D. (1992). Clean white coats spread mutant microbes. *New Scientist* **133**, 11.

McKINNEY, R.W., WASSERMANN, B., CARPENTER, M. *et al.* (1985). Possible laboratory-acquired *Bordetella pertussis* infections. XXVIIIth Biological Safety Conference, Salk Institute for Biological Studies, La Jolla, California.

MAGNUSSON, J.H. (1951). Clinical aspects of toxoplasmosis. *Nordisk Medicin* **45**, 344–349.

MAGRUDER, G.B., GORDON, F.B., QUAN, A.L. *et al.* H.R. (1963). Accidental human trachoma with rapid diagnosis by cell culture technique. *Archives of Ophthalmology* **69**, 300–303.

MALLORY, D. (1913). Cited in *The Bacteriology of Diphtheria* (Eds G. H. Nuttall & G. S. Grahman Smith). p.120. Cambridge: Cambridge University Press.

Management of Health and Safety at Work Regulations 1992. London: The Stationery Office.

MANTKELOW, B.W. & RUSSELL, R.R. (1960). Human ringworm associated with *Trichophyton mentagrophytes* in guinea pigs, *New Zealand Medical Journal* **59**, 488.

MANULELIDIS, L. (1997). Decontamination of Creutzfeldt-Jakob disease and other transmissable agents. *Journal of Neurovirology* **3**, 62–65.

MARCHOUX, E. (1934). Un cas d'inoculation accidentelle du bacille de Hansen en pays nonlepreux, *International Journal of Leprosy* **2**, 1–6.

MARIMATHU, T. (1980). Type B viral hepatitis in medical laboratory technologists. *South African Journal of Medical Laboratory Technology* **26**, 29–31.

MARTIN, L. & PETTIT, A. (1916). Trois cas de spirochetose icterohemorragique en France, *Bulletin Academie Medicale Paris* **76**, 247–253.

MARTIN-MAZUELOS, E., NOGALES, M.C., FLOREZ, C. *et al.* (1994) Outbreak of *Brucella melitensis* amomng microbiology laboratory workers. *Journal of Clinical Microbiology* **31**, 2035–2036 .

MARTINI, G.A, & SCHMIDT, H.A. (1968). Spermatogenic transmission of Marburg virus. *Klinische Wochenschrift* **46**, 398–400.

MATTHEWS, J.A. (1985). *An evaluation of test methods for microbiological safety cabinets.* Thesis. London: Council for National Academic Awards.

MATYSIAK-BUDNIK, T., BRIET, F., HEGMAN, M. *et al.* (1995). Laboratory-acquired *Helicobacter pylori* infection. *Lancet* **346**, 489–490.

MAURER, I.M. (1972). The management of laboratory discard jars. In: *Safety in Microbiology* (Eds D. A. Shapton & R. G. Board). pp. 53–60. London: Academic Press.

MAY, K.R. & HARPER, G.J. (1957). The efficiency of various liquid impinger samplers in bacterial aerosols, *British Journal of Industrial Medicine* **14**, 287–297.

MDA (1996). *Latex Sensitisation in the Health Care Setting (Use of Latex Gloves).* MDA DB 9601. London: Medical Devices Agency.

MDA (1997). *Evaluation Report. Thirteen Lancing Devices. Part 1. Laboratory Study.* MDA/9/22. London: Medical Devices Agency.

MDA (1998a). *Evaluation Report. Thirteen Lancing Devices.* MDA/98/05. London: Medical Devices Agency.

MDA (1998b) Steriliser test safety. Safety Notice SN 9810. London: Medical Devices Agency.

MEERS, P.D., CALDER, M.W., MAZHAR, M.M. *et al.* (1973). Intravenous infusion of contaminated dextrose solution. *Lancet* **2**, 1184–1192.

MEIKLEJOHN, G. & LENNETTE, E. H. (1950). Q fever in California. *American Journal of Hygiene* **52**, 54.

MELNICK, J.L., CURNEN, E.C. & SABIN, A.B. (1948). Accidental laboratory infection with human dengue virus, *Proceedings of the Society for Experimental Biology and Medicine* **68**, 198–200.

MERGER, C. (1957). Hazards associated with the handling of pathogenic bacteria. *Canadian Journal of Medical Technology* **18**, 122–125.

MERRILL, J.T. (1981). Evaluation of selected aerosol control measures on flow sorters. *Cytometry* **1**, 342–345.

MESELSON, M., GUILLEMIN, J., HUGH-JONES, M. *et al.* (1994). The Sverdlovsk anthrax outbreak of 1979. *Science* **266**, 1202–1208.

METCHNIKOFF, E. & ROUX, E. (1905). Etudes experimentales sur la syphilis. *Annales de Institute Pasteur Paris* **19**, 673–698.

METCHNIKOFF, E. & ROUX, E. (1906). Etudes experimentales sur la syphilis. *Annales de Institute Pasteur Paris* **20**, 785–800.

MEYER, G. (1957). Uber zwei Laboratoriumsinfektion mit *Trichophyton mentagrophytes*: Ausgehend von spontan Erkrankten Meerschweinchen. *Mykosen* **1**, 70–73

MEYER, K.F. (1915). The relation of animal to human sporotrichosis. *Journal of the American Medical Association* **65**, 579–585.

MEYER, K.F. (1943). Observations on the pathogenesis of undulant fever. In: *Essays in Biology American Medical Association* **65**, 579–585.

MEYER, K.F. (1950). Modern theory of plague. *Journal of the American Medical Association* **144**, 982–985.

MEYER, K.F. & EDDIE, B. (1941). Laboratory infections due to brucella. *Journal of Infectious Diseases* **68**, 24–32.

MEYER, K.F. & GEIGER, J.C. (1935). The increasing importancre of brucellosis as an occupational hazard. *Journal of the American Veterinary Medical Association* **86**, 280–286.

MIKHAIL, J.S. & TATTERSALL, W.H. (1954). Self-inflicted tuberculosis following BCG vaccination. *Tubercle* **35**, 220–221.

MIKOL, E.V., HORTON, R., LINCOLN, N.S. *et al.* (1952). Incidence of pulmonary tuberculosis among employees at a tuberculosis hospital. *American Review of Tuberculosis* **66**, 16.

MILLER, D.C. (1988). Creutzfeldt-Jacob disease in histopathology technicians. *New England Journal of Medicine*, **318**, 853–854.

MILLER, C.D., SONGER, J.R. & SULLIVAN, J.F. (1987). A twenty-five year review of laboratory-acquired human infections at the National Animal Diseases Center. *American Industrial Hygiene Association Journal* **48**, 271–275.

MILZER, A. & LEVINSON, S.O. (1942). Laboratory infection with the virus of lymphocytic choriomeningitis. *Journal of the American Medical Association* **120**, 27–30.

MIMS, C.A. (1982). *The Pathogenesis of Infectious Disease.* 2nd edn. London Academic Press.

MINKOWITZ, S., BRANDT, L.J., RAPP, Y. *et al.* (1969). 'Prosector's wart' (cutaneous tuberculosis) in a medical student. *American Journal of Clinical Pathology* **5l**, 260–263.

MINOR, P.D. (1994). Ensuring safety and consistency in cell culture production processes: viral screening and inactivation. *Trends in Biotechnology (Tibtech)* **12**, 257–261.

MOCHAMANN, H. & SCHMUTZLER, R. (1956). Erfolgreiche Prophylaxe durch Antibiotika bei einer Laboratoriumsinfektion mit virulenter Weil-Leptospiren. *Zentralblatt fur Bakteriologie* Ab. 1. Orig. **165**, 148–155.

MOLTKE, O. & POULSEN, K.A. (1929b). Zwei Falle Vermutlicher Laboratoriumsinfektionen mit scarlatina. *Zeitschrift für Immunitalsforschung* **64**, 157–166.

MONTES, J., RODRIGUEZ, M.A., MARTIN, T. *et al.* (1986). Laboratory acquired meningitis caused by *Brucella abortus* strain 19. *Journal of Infectious Disease* **154**, 915–916.

MOORE, B. (1971). Handling infectious material in the laboratory, *Annals of Clinical Biochemistry* **8**, 136–142.

MORGAN, C. (1987). Import of animal viruses oppposed after accident at laboratory. *Nature* **328**, 8.

MORRIS, C.A. & EVERALL, P.H. (1972). Safe disposal of air discharged from centrifuges. *Journal of Clinical Pathology* **25**, 742–744.

MORRIS, E.J. (1960). A survey of safety precautions in the microbiological laboratory. *Journal of Medical Laboratory Technology* **17**, 70–81.

MORRIS, R.T. (1913). A case of systemic blastomycosis. *Journal of the American Medical Association* **61**, 2043–4044.

MORRIS, S.J. (1946). Tuberculosis as an occupational hazard during medical training. *American Review of Tuberculosis* **54**, 140–158.

MORSE, J.L., RUSS, S.B., NEEDY, C.F. *et al.* (1962). Studies of viruses of the tick-borne encephalitis group. *Journal of Immunology* **88**, 240–242.

MOSES, A.M. (1997). Dealing with hazardous chemicals. In: *Managing Biological and Chemical Risks* (Ed. D.R. Morgan.) pp. 45–50. London: Medical Research Council and the Institute of Biology.

MOSS, W.L. & CASTENADA, M. (1928). Malta fever: a laboratory infection in the human. *Transactions of the Association of American Physicians* **42**, 272–284.

MOST, H. (1973). *Plasmodium cynomolgi* malaria: accidental human infection. *American Journal of Tropical Medicine & Hygiene* **22**, 151–158.

MRC (1990). *The management of simians in relation to infectious hazards to staff.* London: Medical Research Council.

MRC (1996). *Risk Assessment of Work with Chemical, Biological and Ionising Radiation Hazards.* MRC Health and Safety Policy Note A3. London: Medical Research Council.

MULLER, H.E. (1988a). Risikofaktoren und Risikoabschätzungen in Tuberkuloselaboratien. Ergebnisse einer Unfrage. *Laboratoriumsmedizin* **12**, 284–289.

MULLER, H.E. (1988b). Laboratory-acquired mycobacterial disease. *Lancet* ii, 331.

MUNTER, E.J. (1945). Pneumonic plague. Report of a case with recovery. *Journal of the American Medical Association* **128**, 281–283.

MURPHY, L.C. & EASTERFAY, D.B.C. (1961). Rift Valley fever; a zoonosis. *Proceedings of the United Livestock Sanitary Association* **65**, 397–412.

MURRAY, J.F. & HOWARD, D.H. (1964). Laboratory-acquired histoplasmosis. *American Review of Respiratory Disease* **89**, 631–640.

MUSTAFFA-BABJEE A., LATIF ABRAHIM, A. & TEH, S. K. (1976). a case of human infection with Newcastle disease. *South East Asian Journal of Tropical Medicne and Public Health* **7**, 622–623.

MYERS, J.A. (1941). Tuberculosis in students. *American Review of Tuberculosis* **44**, 479-486.

MYERS, J.A., DIEHL, H.S., BOYNTON, R.E. *et al.* (1941). Tuberculosis among students and graduates in medicine. *Annals of Internal Medicine* **14**, 1575–1594.

NABARRO, J.D.N. (1948). Primary pulmonary coccidioidomycosis; a case of a laboratory infection in England. *Lancet* 1, 982–984.

NAGLER, E.P. & KLOTZ, M. (1958). A fatal B virus infection in a person subject to recurrent herpes labialis. *Canadian Medical Association Journal* **79**, 743–745.

NAKHLA, L.S. & CUMMINGS, R.F. (1981). A comparative evaluation of a new centrifugal air sampler (RCS) with a slit sampler (SAS) in a hospital environment. *Journal of Hospital Infection* **2**, 261–266.

NAMIKAWA, H. (1929). Uber zwei falle von accidenteller Recurrensinfection im Laboratorium, und Veründerung der Virulenz durch Menschen-Passage. *Taiwan Igakkai Zasshi* **297**, 65.

NAPOLI, V.M. & MCGOWAN, J.E. (1987). How much blood is in a needlestick? *Journal of Infectious Disease* **155**, 828.

NASZ, I., DAN, P. & KULCSA, R. G. (1963). Accidental laboratory infections with adenovirus, type 8. *Acta microbiologica Academiae scientiarum hungarica* **10**, 53–57.

NATIONAL RESEARCH COUNCIL (1985). *Guide for the Care and Use of Laboratory Animals.* NIH publication 83–23. Washington: Government Printing Office.

NATIONAL RESEARCH COUNCIL (1989). *Biosafety in the Laboratory. Prudent Practices for the Handling and Disposal of Infectious Materials.* Washington: National Academy Press.

NAUCK, E. G. & WEYER, F. (1949). Laboratoriumsinfektionen bei Q-fieber. *Deutsche Medizinische Wochenschrift* **74**, 198–204.

NEU, H.C. (1967). Toxoplasmosis transmitted at autopsy, *Journal of the American Medical Association* **202**, 844–845.

NEUFELD, F. & LEVINTHAL, W. (1932). Schutz gegen Laboratoriumsinfektion bei Psittakosearbeiten, *Zentralblatt fur Bakteriologie* Abt. I Orig. **125**, 254–256.

NEWITT, A.W., KOPPA, T.M. & GUDAKUNST, D.W. (1939). Water-borne outbreak of *Brucella melitensis* infection, *American Journal of Public Health* **29**, 738–743.

NEWMAN TAYLOR, A., LONGBOTTOM, J.L. & PEPYS, J. (1977). Respiratory allergy to urine proteins of rats and mice. *Lancet* ii, 847–849.

NEWMAN TAYLOR, A. (1997). Occupational asthma and byssinosis. In: *Occupational Lung Disorders* (Ed. W.R.Parkes) pp.710–754. Oxford: Butterworth-Heinemann.

NEWSOM, S.W.B. (1979a). Performance of exhaust-protective (Class I) biological safety cabinets. *Journal of Clinical Pathology* **32**, 576–583.

NEWSOM, S.W.B. (1979b). Class II (laminar flow) biological safety cabinets. *Journal of Clinical Pathology* **32**, 505–513

NEWSOM, S.W.B., ROWLANDS, C., MATTHEWS, J. *et al.* (1983). Aerosols in the mortuary. *Journal of Clinical Pathology* **36**, 127–132.

NEWSOM, S.W.B. & WALSINGHAM, B.M. (1974). Sterilization of the biological safety cabinet. *Journal of Clinical Pathology* **27**, 921–924.

NEWSOM, S.W.B. (1976). *Laboratory Infections. Their control by containment.* MD Thesis. London: University of London.

NICHOLAS, J. (1893). Sur un cas de tetanos chez l'homme par inoculation accidentelle des produits solubles du bacille de Nicolaier. *Compte Rendus de l'Acadmie des Sciences Paris* **9**, 844–846.

NICOLLE, C. (1906). Une observation de fievre Mediterannee par contamination de laboratoire. *Archives de l'Institut Pasteur de Tunisie* **1**, 155–158.

NICOLLE, C. (1935). A propos de six cas de typhus murin contractes au cours de recherche. *Archives de l'Institut Pasteur de Tunisie* **24**, 99–113.

NIGG, C. (1962). Subclinical infection in melioidosis. *Bacteriological Proceedings* **62**, 91.

NIH (1974) *NIH Biosafety Guide.* Public Health Service, National Institutes of Health. Washington: Government Printing Office.

NIH (1978). National Institutes of Health. *Laboratory Safety Monograph. Supplement to the NIH Guidelines for Recombinant DNA Research.* Bethesda, MD: US Department of Health Education and Welfare, National Institutes of Health.

NIH (1979) *Laboratory Safety Monograph, National Institutes of Health.* Washington: Government Printing Office.

NIH (1985). *Guide for the Use and Care of Laboratory Animals.* US Department of Health and Human Welfare. Washington: Government Printing Office.

NIKODEMUSZ, I. (1975). Laboratory infections. *Orvosi Hetilap* **116**, 2243–2245.

NILZEN, A. & PALDROCK, H. (1953). A laboratory infection caused by *Histoplasma capsulatum. Acta Dermatologia Venereologica* **33**, 329–341.

NOLTE, K.B., FOUCAR, K. & RICHMOND, J.Y. (1996). Hantavirus biosafety issues in the autopsy room and laboratory. Concerns and recommendations. *Human Pathology* **27**, 1253–1254.

NORAZAH, A., MAZLAH, A., CHEONG, Y.M. *et al.* (1995). Laboratory-acquired murine typhus; a case report. *Medical Journal of Malaysia* **50**, 177–179.

NORDEN, A. (1951). Sporotrichosis: clincal and laboratory features and a serological study in experimental animals and humans. *Acta pathologia microbiologia Scandinavica* Suppl. **89**, 3–119.

NSF 49 (1983). *Class II Laminar Flow Biohazard Cabinetry.* Ann Arbor: National Sanitation Foundation.

O'BRIEN, P.J. (1962). A naturally acquired and a laboratory acquired case of brucellosis. *Medical Journal of Australia* **2**, 377–378.

OATES, K. DEVERILL, C.E.A., PHELPS, M. *et al.* (1983). Development of a laboratory autoclave system. *Journal of Hospital Infection* **4**, 181–190.

OATES, J.D. & HODGKIN, U.G. (1981). Laboratory-acquired campylobacter enteritis. *Southern Medicine* **74**, 83.

OBENOUR, R.A. (1969). Case report. North American blastomycosis. *Journal of the Tennessee Medical Association* **62**, 324–327.

OECD (1992). *Recombinant DNA Safety Considerations.* Paris: Organization for Economic Co-operation and Development.

OGATA, N. (1931) Aetiologie der Tsutsugamushikrankheit: *Rickettsia tsutugamushi. Zentralblatt für Bakteriologie.* Abt. 1 Orig. **122**, 245–253.

OKAMOTO, R. & MASAYAMA, S. (1937). Uber einen Fall von Ubergangsform des in Laboratorium Infizierten Fleckfiebers. *Transactions of the Society of Pathology (Japan)* **27**, 602–605.

OKUNYO, Y. (1982). Serological studies on a case of laboratory-acquired dengue infection. *Biken Journal* **25**, 163–170.

O'LEARY, P.A. & HARRISON, M.W. (1941). Inoculation tuberculosis. *Archives of Dermatology* **44**, 371.

OLCERST, R.B. (1987). Microscopes and ocular infections. *American Industrial Hygiene Association Journal* **48**, 425–431.

OLIPHANT, J.W., GORDON, D.A., MEIS, A. *et al.* (1949). Q fever in laundry workers, presumably transmitted from contaminated elothing. *American Journal of Hygiene* **45**, 76–82.

OLIPHANT, J.W. & PARKER, R.R. (1948). Q fever: three cases of laboratory infection. *Public Health Reports, Washington* **63**, 1364–1370.

OLITSKY, P.K. & CASALS, J. (1952). Viral encephalitides. In: *Viral and Rickettsial Infections of Man* (Ed. T.M. Rivers). 2nd edn. pp. 214–266. Philadelphia: Lippincott.

OLITSKY, P.K. & MORGAN, I.M. (1939). Protective antibodies against equine encephalomyelitis virus in the serum of laboratory workers. *Proceedings of the Society for Experimental Biology and Medicine* **41**, 212–215.

OLLE-GOIG, J.E. & CANELAR-SOLER, J. (1987). An outbreak of *Brucella melitensis* infection by airborne transmission among laboratory workers. *American Journal of Public Health* **77**, 335–338.

OLSON, C.L., GAINES, S. & HOOK, E.W. (1961). Laboratory-acquired typhoid fever; infection with a laboratory strain of *Salmonella typhosa* isolated 41 years earlier. *Bulletin of the Johns Hopkins Hospital* **109**, 125–133.

ONIONS, D. (1994) The safety evaluation of cell lines used in biotechnology: screening for adventitious agents. In: *Biosafety of Mammalian Cells*. Proceedings of the Basel Forum on Biosafety, October 1993. pp. 27–36. Basel: Agency for Biosafety Research.

ONSTAD, G.C. (1971). Primary pulmonary blastomycosis. *Annals of Internal Medicine* **74**, 146.

OPENSHAW, P.J.M., ALWAN, W.H., CHERRIE, A.M. *et al.* (1991). Accidental infection of laboratory worker with recombinant vaccinia virus. *Lancet* **338**, 459.

ORTELL, S. (1975). Listeria during pregnancy and excretion of listerias by laboratory workers. *Zentralblatt für Bakteriologie* 1 (A 231), 491.

OSHA (1991). US Occupational Safety and Health Administration. Occcupational exposure to blood-borne pathogens, final rule. *Federal Register* **56**, 64175–64182.

OSTER, C.N., BURKE, D.S., KENYON, R. *et al.* (1977). Laboratory-acquired Rocky Mountain spotted fever. The hazard of aerosol transmission. *New England Journal of Medicine* **297**, 859–863.

OVERHOLT, E.L., TIGERTT, W.D., KADULL, P.J. *et al.* (1961). An analysis of forty-two cases of laboratory-acquired tularemia. *American Journal of Medicine* **3O**, 785–806.

OVERHOLT, E. L. & HORNICK, R.B. (1964). Primary cutaneous coccidioidomycosis. *Archives of Internal Medicine* **114**, 149–153.

OYA, A. (1975). Biohazards in the field of microbiology. *Bibliothek Hematologie* No. 40. pp. 771–773. Basel: Karger.

PAINE, T.F. (1946). Infection in man following inhalation of *Serratia marcescens, Journal of Infectious Disease* **79**, 226.

PALCA J. (1987). Lab worker infected with AIDS virus. *Nature* 329, 92.

PALMER, P.E. & McFADDEN, S.W. (1968). Blastomycosis; a report of an unusual case. *New England Journal of Medicine* **279**, 975–983.

PALMER, D., PERRY, K.R., MORTIMER, P.P. *et al.* (1991). Fifteen HBsAg screening assays, MDA evaluation. Report No MDA/95/92. London: Medical Devices Agency.

PALMER, J.D. & RICKETT, J.W.S. (1992). The mechanisms and risks of surgical glove perforation. *Journal of Hospital Infection* **22**. 279–286.

PANETH, L. (1915). The prevention of laboratory infections. *Medizinische Klinik* **11**, 1398–1399.

PAPP, K. (1957). The eye as a portal of infection. *Bulletin of Hygiene*, **24**, 969–971.

PARKER, R.R. (1938). Rocky Mountain spotted fever. *Journal of the American Medical Association* **110**, 1185–1188.

PARKER, S.L. & HOLLIMAN, R.E. (1992). Toxoplasmosis and laboratory workers: a case control assessment of risk, *Medical Laboratory Sciences* **49**, 103–106.

PARKER, R.R. & SPENCER, R.R. (1926). Six additional cases of laboratory infection of tularemia in man, *Public Health Reports* **41**, 1341–1354.

PARKES, W.R. (1994). Morphology of the respiratory tract. In: *Occupational Lung Disorders* 3rd ed. pp. 1–17. (Ed. R.W. Parkes) Oxford: Butterworth-Heinemann.

PARKES, W.R. (1994). Aerosols, their deposition and clearance. In: *Occupational Lung Disorders* 3rd ed. pp. 35–49. (Ed. R.W. Parkes) Oxford: Butterworth-Heinemann.

PARRY, S.H., ABRAHMAM, S.N., FEAVERS, M. *et al.* (1981). Urinary tract infection due to laboratory-acquired *Escherichia coli*: relation to virulence. *British Medical Journal* **282**, 949–950.

PATTERSON, W.C., MOTT, L.O. & JENNEY, E.W. (1958). A study of vesicular stomatitis in man. *Journal of the American Veterinary Medical Association* **133**, 57–62.

PATTISON, C.P., BOYER, K.M., MAYNARD, J.E. *et al.* (1974). Epidemic hepatitis in a clinical laboratory - possible association with computer card handling. *Journal of the American Medical Association* **230**, 854–857.

PAUL, M., HIMMESLSTEIN, J., WEISTEIN, S. *et al.* (1989). Ocular infection and the industrial use of microscopes. *Journal of Occupational Medicine* **31** 763–766.

PEERBOOMS, P.G.H, VAN DOORNUM, G.J.J., VAN DEUTEKOM, H. *et al.* (1995). Laboratory-acquired tuberculosis. *Lancet* **345**, 1311–1312.

PENNER, J.L., HENNESSY, J.N., MILLS, S.D. *et al.* (1983). Application of serotyping and chromosomal restriction endonuclease digent analysis in investigating a laboratory-acquired case of *Campylobacter jejuni* enteritis. *Journal of Clinical Microbiology* **18**, 1429–1429.

PERCH, B. (1947). On a laboratory infection with *Salmonella senegal, Acta pathologia microbiologia Scandinavica* **24**, 399–400.

Personal Protective Equipment at Work Regulations 1992. London: The Stationery Office.

PETHER, J.V.S., THURLOW, J., PALFREYMAN, T.G. *et al.* (1993). Acute hantavirus infection presenting as hypersensitivity vacuolitis with arthropathology. *Journal of Infection* **26**, 75–77.

PETITHORY, J. & LEBEAU, G. (1977). Contamination probable de laboratoire par *Plasmodium falciparum*. *Bulletin de la Societe de Pathologie exotique* **70**, 371–375.

PHILLIPS G. & OLD, D.C. 1997). Laboratory-acquired VTEC infection. *Journal of Hospital Infection* **35**, 72

PHILLIPS, G.B. (1961). *Microbiological Safety in US and Foreign Laboratories*. Technical Report No. 35. US Army Chemical Corps, Biological Laboratories, Fort Detrick, Frederick, Maryland.

PHILLIPS, G.B. (1969). Control of microbiological hazards in the laboratory. *American Industrial Hygiene Association Journal* **30**, 170–176.

PHILLIPS, G.B. & BAILEY, S.P. (1966). Hazards of mouth pipetting. *American Journal of Medical Technology* **32**, 127–129.

PHILLIPS, G.B., NOVAK, F.E. & ALG, R.L. (1955). A portable, inexpensive plastic safety hood. *Applied Microbiology* **3**, 216

PHILLIPS, G. B. & REITMAN, M. (1956). Biological hazards of common laboratory procedures. IV The inoculating loop. *American Journal of Medical Technology* **22**, 16–17.

PHILLIPS, I., MEERS, P.D. & D'ARCY, P.F. (1976). *Microbiological Hazards of Infusion Therapy*. Lancaster: MTP Press.

PHLS (1978). Autoclaving practice in microbiological laboratories. Report of a survey. Public Health Laboratory Service. *Journal of Clinical Pathology* **31**, 418–422.

PHLS (1981). Specifications for laboratory autoclaves. The Public Health Laboratory Service Subcommittee on Laboratory Autoclaves. *Journal of Hospital Infection* **2**, 377–384.

PIERCE, E.C., PIERCE, J.D. & HULL R.N. (1958). B virus. Its current significance: Description and diagnosis of a fatal human infection. *American Journal of Hygiene* **68**, 242–250.

PIKE, R.M. (1976). Laboratory-associated infections. Summary and analysis of 3921 cases. *Health Laboratory Science* **13**, 105- 114.

PIKE, R.M. (1978). Past and present hazards or working with infectious hazards. *Archives of Pathology and Laboratory Medicine* **102**, 333–336.

PIKE, R.M. (1979). Laboratory-associated infections: incidence, fatalities, causes and prevention. *Annual Review of Microbiology* **33**, 41–66.

PIKE, R.M. & SULKIN, S.E. (1952). Occupational hazards in microbiology. *Science Monthly* **75**, 222–228.

PIKE, R.M., SULKIN, S.E. & SCHULZE, M.L. (1965). Continuing importance of laboratory-acquired infections. *American Journal of Public Health* **55**, 190- 199,

PINCUS, S.H., MESER, K.G. NATA, P.L. *et al.* (1994). Temporal analysis of the antibody response to HIV envelope protein in HIV-infected laboratory workers. *Journal of Clinical Investigation* **53**, 2505–2513.

PIVNICK, H., WORTON, H., SMITH, D.L.T. *et al.* (1966). Infection of veterinarians in Ontario by *Brucella abortus* strain 19. *Canadian Journal of Public Health* **18**, 32–36.

PIZZI, T., NIEDMAN, G. & JARPA, A. (1963). Report of three cases of acute Chagas disease produced by accidental laboratory infections. *Bolitin Chileano de Parasitologia* **18**, 32–36.

POLAKOFF, S. (1986). Acute viral hepatitis B: laboratory report 1984. *British Medical Journal* **293**, 37–38.

POPOV, N.V. (1914). *Russ Vrach* 13, 848–849. Cited by Pike (1979).

POST OFFICE GUIDE (available at main UK post offices).

Pressure Systems and Transportable Gas Container Regulations 1989. London: The Stationery Office.

PRICE, J.E.L. & BENNETT, W.E.J. (1951). The erysipeloid of Rosenbach. *British Medical Journal* 2, 1061–1062.

PRICE, T.H. (1976). Isolation of salmonellas and shigellas from a laboratory bench. *Journal of Hygiene* **76**, 337–339.

PUBLIC HEALTH REPORTS (1944). Human case of pneumonic plague (laboratory infection) in San Francisco, California **59**, 962

RADACOVICI, R., ATANASIU, M. & COSTIN, C. (1962). Contribution to experimental studies on the treatment of toxoplasmosis. Infection following manipulation of virulent material. *Journal of Hygiene, Epidemiology, Microbiology and Immunology* (Prague) **6**, 89–99.

RAKE, B.W. (1978). Influence of cross drafts on the performance of a biological safety cabinet. *Applied Environmental Microbiology* **36**, 278–287.

RAMACHANDRA, R.T., SINGH, K.R.P. & PAVRI, K.M. (1964). Laboratory transmission of an Indian strain of Chikungunya virus. *Current Science* **33**, 235–236.

RAMSEY, R.K. & CARTER, G.R. (1952). Canine blastomycosis in the United States. *Journal of the American Medical Association* **120**, 93–98.

RAO, C.V. (1981) Laboratory infection with Ganjam virus. *Indian Journal of Medical Research* **74**, 315–324.

RAWAL, B.D. (1959). Laboratory infection with toxoplasma. *Journal of Clinical Pathology* **12**, 59–61.

RAYBURN, S.R. (1990). *The Foundations of Laboratory Safety.* New York: Springer Verlag.

READY, D. (1998). Microbial keratitis and contact lens wear. *Biomedical Scientist* **42**, 300–301.

REDFEARN, M.S. & PALLERONI, N.J. (1975). Glanders and melioidosis. In: *Diseases Transmitted from Animals to Man.* Springfield, IL: Thomas.

REID, D.D. (1957). The incidence of tuberculosis among workers in medical laboratories. *British Medical Journal* 2, 10–14.

REID, H.W., GIBBS, C.A., BURRELLS, C. *et al.* (1972). Laboratory infections with louping ill virus. *Lancet* i, 592–593.

REINICKE, J.J. (1894). Ein Fall von Todlicher Laboratoriums-cholera. *Deutsche Medizinische Wochenschrift* **20**, 795–797

REITMAN, M., ALG, R.L., MILLER, W.S. *et al.* (1954). Potential hazards of laboratory techniques. III. Virus techniques. *Journal of Bacteriology* **68**, 548–554.

REITMAN, M., FRANK, M.A., ALG, R. *et al.* (1953). Infectious hazards of the high speed blender and their elimination by a new design. *Applied Microbiology* **1**, 14–17.

REITMAN, M. & PHILLIPS, G. B. (1955). Biological hazards of some common laboratory techniques. I. The pipette. *American Journal of Medical Technology* **21**, 338–342.

REITMAN, M. & PHILLIPS, G.B. (1956). Biological hazards of common laboratory procedures. III. The centrifuge. *American Journal of Medical Technology* **22**, 14–16.

REITMAN, M., SUTTON, L.S., ALG, R.L. *et al.* (1955). Agglutinins in the serum of laboratory workers exposed to *Serratia marcescens. Proceedings of the Society for Experimental Biology and Medicine* **89**, 236–240.

REITMAN, M. & WEDUM, A. G. (1956). Microbiological safety. *Public Health Reports* **71**, 659–665.

REMINGTON, J. S. & GENTRY, L.O. (1970). Acquired toxoplasmosis: Infection versus disease. *Annals of the New York Academy of Science* **174**, 1006–1007.

REPORT (1958). Precautions against tuberculosis infections in the diagnostic laboratory. Monthly Bulletin of the Ministry of Health and the Public Health Laboratory Service **17**, *10–18.*

REPORT (1974) of the Committee of Inquiry into the Smallpox outbreak in London, March and April 1973. Cmnd 5626. London: The Stationery Office.

REPORT (1992) of the Committee appointed to enquire into the circumstances, including the production, which led to the contaminated infusion fluids in the Devonport Section of the Plymouth General Hospital. London: The Stationery Office

Reporting of Injuries, Diseases and Dangerous Occurrences Regulations 1992. London: The Stationery Office.

REUBEN, B., BAND, J.D., WONG, P. *et al.* (1991). Person to person transmission of *Brucella melitensis. Lancet* **337**, 14–15.

REVICH, S.J., WALKER, A.W. & PIVNICK, H. (1961). Human infection by *Brucella abortus* strain 15. *Canadian Journal of Public Health* **52**, 285–289.

REWELL, R.E. (1949). An outbreak of *Shigella schmitzii* infection in men and apes. *Lancet* i, 220–222.

RICHMOND, J.Y., KNUDSEN, R.C. & GOOD, R.C. (1996). Biosafety in the clinical mycobacteriology laboratory. *Clinical and Laboratory Medicine* **16**, 527–550.

RIDZON, R., KENYON, T., LUSKIN-HAWK, R. *et al.* (1997). Nosocomial transmission of human immunodeficiency virus and subsequent transmission of multidrug-resistant tuberculosis in as healthcare worker. *Infection Control and Hospital Epidemiology* **18**, 422–423.

RIESMAN, D. (1898). Two cases of diphtheria, one from laboratory infection and one in an infant eleven days old. *Philadelphia Medical Journal* **1**, 423–426.

RINGERTZ, O. & DAHLSTRAND, S. (1968). Culture of *P. tularensis* in the 1966 67 outbreaks of tularemia in Sweden. Laboratory methods and precautions against laboratory infections. *Acta Pathologia et Microbiologia Scandinavica* **72**, 464.

RIVERS, T.M. & SCHWENKER, F.F. (1934). Louping ill in man. *Proceedings of the Society for Experimental Biology and Medicine* **30**, 1302–1303.

ROBBINS, F. C. & RUSTIGIAN, R. (1946). Q fever in the Mediterranean area: report of its occurrence in Allied troops IV. A laboratory outbreak. *American Journal of Hygiene* **44**, 64–71.

ROBBINS, G.D. (1906). A study of chronic glanders in man with a report of a case. In: *Studies from the Royal Victoria Hosital*, Vol 2. Montreal: Guertin Print Co.

ROBERTS, F.J. (1971). Undiagnosed tuberculosis at autopsy. *Canadian Journal of Public Health* **662**, 496–502.

ROBERTSON, D.H.H., PICKENS, S., LAWSON, J.H. *et al.* (1980). An accidental laboratory infection with African trypanosomes of defined stock. *Journal of Infection* **2**, 105–112.

ROBINSON, R. (1944). Human infection with *Pasteurella septica. British Medical Journal* 2, 725.

ROSEBURY, T., ELLINGSON, H.V. & MEIKLEJOHN, G. (1947). A laboratory infection with psittacosis virus treated with penicillin and sulphadiazine and experimental data bearing on the mode of infection. *Journal of Infectious Disease* **80**, 64–77.

ROWSELL, H.C., KENNEDY, A.H. & FISCHER, J.B. (1954). A dermatophyte infection in chinchillas transmitted to man (abstr.). *Canadian Journal of Public Health* **45**, 31.

ROYAL COLLEGE OF NURSING (1987) *Introduction to Hepatitis B and Nursing Guidelines for Infection Control.* London: RCN.

RUBBO, S.D. & GARDNER, J.F. (1965). *A Review of Sterilization and Disinfection.* London: Lloyd-Lake.

RUDDY, S.L., MOSLEY, J.W. & HELD, J.R. (1967). Chimpanzee-associated hepatitis in the US in 1963. *American Journal of Epidemiology* **83**, 634.

RUGIERO, H.R., PARODI, A.S., GOTTA, H. *et al.* (1962). Epidemic haemorrhagic fever: laboratory infection and interhuman passage. *Revista de la Asociacion medica argentina* **76**, 413–417.

RUSSELL, A.D. (1981). Neutralization procedures in the evaluation of bactericidal activity. In: *Disinfectants, their Use and Evaluation of Effectiveness* (Eds C. H. Collins, M. C. Allwood, S. F. Bloomfield & A. Fox). pp. 45–60. London: Academic Press.

RUSSELL, A.D., HUGO, B. & AYLIFFE, G.R. (1992). *Principles and Practice of Disinfection, Sterilization and Preservation.* London: Blackwell.

RUTTER, D.A. & EVANS, C.G.T (1972). Aerosol hazards from some clinical laboratory apparatus. *British Medical Journal* **1**, 594–597.

RUTTY, G.N., HONOVAR, M. & DOSHI, B. (1991). Malignant glioma in laboratory workers. *Journal of Clinical Pathology* **44**, 868–869.

RYDER, R.W. & GANDSMAN, E.J. (1995) Laboratory-acquired Sabia virus infection. *New England Journal of Medicine* **333**, 1716-

SABIN, A.B. (1949). Fatal B virus encephalomyelitis in a physician working with monkeys. *Journal of Clinical Investigation* **28**, 808.

SABIN, A.B. & BLUMBERG, R.W. (1947). Human infection with Rift valley fever virus. *Proceedings of the Society for Experimental Biology and Medicine* **64**, 385–389.

SABIN, A.B. & WARD, R. (1941). Poliomyelitis in a laboratory worker, exposed to the virus. *Science* **94**, 113–114.

SABIN, A.B. & WRIGHT, A.M. (1934). Acute ascending myelitis following monkey bite with isolation of virus capable of reproducing disease. *Journal of Experimental Medicine* **59**, 115–136.

SADUSK, J.F., BROWNE, A.S. & BORN, J.L. (1957). Brucellosis in man resulting from *Brucella abortus* (strain 19) vaccine. *Journal of the American Medical Association* **164**, 1325–1328.

SAHN, S.A. & PIERSON, D.J. (1974). Primary cutaneous inoculation of drug-resistant tuberculosis. *American Journal of Medicine* **57**, 676–678.

SAINT-PAUL, M., DELPLACE, Y., TUFEL, C. *et al.* (1972). Tuberculoses professionelles dans les laboratoires de bacteriologie. *Archives des Maladies Professionelles de Medicin* **33**, 305–309.

SAKULA, A. (1977). Accidental self-inoculation of killed *Mycobacterium tuberculosis* in Freund's complete adjuvant. *Tubercle* **58** 221–223.

SALS (1980). Subcommittee on Arbovirus Laboratory Safety of the American Committee on Arthropod-borne Viruses. Laboratory safety for arboviruses and certain other viruses of vertebrates. *American Journal of Tropical Medicine and Hygiene* **29**, 1359–1381.

SALZMAN, B.R., MOTYL, M.R. FRIEDLAND, G.H. *et al.* (1986). *Mycobacterium tuberculosis* bacteramia in the acquired immunodefiency syndrome. *Journal of the American Medical Association* **256**, 390–391.

SAMPAIO, R.N., DE LIMA, L.M.P., VEXENAT, A. *et al.* (1983). A laboratory infection with *Leishmania braziliensis. Transactions of the Royal Society for Tropical Medicine* **77**, 274.

SANYAL, S.C., SIL, J. & SAKAZAKI, R. (1973). Laboratory infection by *Vibrio parahaemolyticus. Journal of Medical Microbiology* **6**, 121–122.

SARASIN, G., TUCKER, D.N. & AREAN, V.M. (1963). Accidental laboratory infection caused by *Leptospira icterohaemorrhagiae. American Journal of Clinical Pathology* **40**, 146–150.

SASAGAWA, A., KONO, R. & KONNO, R. (1976). Laboratory-acquired infection of the eye with AHC virus. *Japanese Journal of Medical Science and Biology* **29**, 96–97.

SASLOW, A.R. & IAMMARINO, R. (1974). Viral hepatitis in clinical chemistry workers. *Clinical Chemistry* **20**, 514–515.

SATTAR S.A. & SPRINGTHORPE, V.S. (1994). Survival and disinfectant activation of the human immunodeficiency virus: an update. *Reviews in Medical Micobiology* **5**, 139–150.

SAWYER, W. A., MEYER, K. F., EATON, M. D. *et al.* (1968). Human follicular conjunctivitis caused by the psittacosis agent. *Proceedings of the Society for Experimental Biology and Medicine* **127**, 292–294.

SCHACTER, J., ARNSTEIN, P., DAWSON, P. *et al.* (1968). Human follicular conjunctivitis caused by the psittacosis agent. *Proceedings of the Society for Experimental Biology and Medicine* **127**, 292–294.

SCHAEFER, W. (1950). Ueber Laboratoriumsinfektion, insbesondere mit Typhusbazillen. *Archiv für Hygiene und Bakteriologie* **132**, 15–32.

SCHAFER, T.W. (1976). biohazard potential: recovery of infectious virus from the liquid nitrogen of a virus repository. *Health Laboratory Science* **13**, 23–24.

SCHEID, W., JOCHEIM, K.A. & MOHR, W. (1956). Laboratoriumsinfektionen mit dem Virus der Lymphocytarem choriomeningitis. *Deutches Archiv fur Klinische Medizin* **203**, 88–109.

SCHEIDT, R. (1939). Tetanus-intoxikation bei fehlen Lebender Tetanus-bazillen. *Munchener medizinische Wochenschrift* **86**, 959–960.

SCHLECHT, W. F. (1981). Laboratory-acquired infection with *Pseudomonas pseudomallei* (melioidosis). *New England Journal of Medicine* **305**, 1135–1134.

SCHLECHT, W.F., TURCHIK, J.B., WESTLAKE, R.E. *et al.* (1981). Laboratory-acquired infection with *Pseudomonas pseudomallei* (melioidosis). *New England Journal of Medicine* **305**, 1133–1135.

SCHMID, H. J. (1931). Uber eine Psittackoseanliche epidemie in einen Tierspital. *Zeitschrift für Medicin* **117**, 563–593.

SCHMIDT, L.H., GREENLAND, R. & GENTHER, C.S. (1961). The transmission of *Plasmodium cynomolgi* to man. *American Journal of Tropical Medicine and Hygiene* **10**, 679–688.

SCHUBLAADZE, A.K., GAYDMAMOVITCH, S.Y. & GARILOV, V.I. (1959). Virological studies of laboratory infections with Venezuelan equine encephalomyelitis. *Problems of Virology* **4**, 305–310.

SCHUFFNER, W. & BOLHANDER (1942). Klinische und Bakteriologische Beobachtung einer Laboratoriumsinfektion mit Schlammfieber Leptospirurie. *Zentralblatt für Bakteriologie* Abt. 1. Orig. **149**, 193–202.

SCHWARZ, J.C. & BAUM, G.L. (1951). Blastomycosis. *American Journal of Clinical Pathology* **21**, 999–1029.

SCHWENTKER, F.F. & RIVERS, T.M. (1934). Rift Valley fever in man: Report of a fatal laboratory infection in man. *Journal of Experimental Medicine* **59**, 305–313.

SCIENCE JOURNAL (1966). Deliberate spreading of typhoid in Japan. **2**, 11–12.

SEAL, D.V. & HAY, J. (1993). The microbiologist as a contact lens wearer (Editorial). *Journal of Medical Microbiology* **39**, 1–2.

SEARS, H.J. (1947). Cutaneous infection with *Neisseria gonorrhaea* with development of lymphangitis resulting from a laboratory accident. *American Journal of Syphilis, Gonorrhea and Venereal Diseases* **31**, 63–64.

SEDER, R.H., DESAI, P.M. & KOFF, R.S. (1975). Laboratory-acquired hepatitis B. *Lancet* 2, 1316.

SEWELL, D.L (1995). Laboratory associated infections and biosafety. *Clinical Microbiology Reviews* **8**, 389–405.

SEXTON, R.C., EYLES, D.E. & DILLMAN, R.E. (1953). Adult toxoplasmosis. *American Journal of Medicine* **14**, 366–377.

SEXTON, D.J., GALLIS, H.A., McRAE, J.R. *et al.* (1975) Possible needle-associated Rocky Mountain spotted fever. *New England Journal of Medicine* **292**, 645 (letter).

SHAFER, T.W., EVERETT, J., SILVER, G.H. *et al.* (1976). Biohazard potential recovery of infectious virus from the liquid nitrogen of a virus repository. *Health Laboratory Science* **13**, 23–24.

SHANAHAN, R.H., GRIFFIN, J.R. & VON AUERSPERG, A.P. (1947). Anthrax meningitis. Reports of a case of internal anthrax with recovery. *American Journal of Clinical Pathology* **17**, 719–722.

SHANSON, D.C. (1989). *Microbiology in Clinical Practice.* 2nd edn. Chs. 6 and 21. Oxford: Butterworth-Heinemann.

SHARPE, A.N. (1963). Automation and instrumentation developments for the bacteriology laboratory. In: *Sampling Microbiological Monitoring of Environments* (Eds R. E. Board & D. W. Lovelock). pp. 197–232 London: Academic Press.

SHAW, E.W., MELNICK, J.L. & CURNEN, E.C. (1950). Infection of laboratory workers with coxsackie viruses. *Annals of Internal Medicine* **33**, 32–40.

SHAW, C. (1941). Accidental inoculation with *Spirochaete pallida. Archives of Dermatology and Syphilology* **44**, 868–882.

SHEEHAN, H.L. (1944). Epidemiology of infeetious hepatitis. *Lancet* **2**, 8.

SHIBATA, S. (1997). Towards prevention of biohazards. *Seizen Review* No. 5. pp. 126–127. (English).

SHIMKIN, N.I. (1946). Conjunctival haemorrhage due to an infection of Newcastle virus of fowls in man. *British Journal of Ophthalmology* **30**, 260–264.

SHIMOJO, H. (1975). Virus infections in laboratories in Japan. *Bibliotheca Haematologie* **40**, 771–773. Basel: Karger.

SHINTON, N.K., ENGLAND, J.M. & KENNEDY, D.A. (1982). Guidelines for the evaluation of instruments used in haematology laboratories. *Journal of Clinical Pathology* **35**, 1095–1102.

SHIRAISHI, H., SAZSAKI, T., NAKAMURA, M. *et al.* (1991). Laboratory infection with human parvovirus B19. *Journal of Infection* **22**, 308–310.

SHIREMAN, P.K. (1992) Endometrial tuberculosis acquired by a health care worker in a clinical laboratory. *Archives of Pathology and Laboratory Medicine* **116**, 521–523.

SHISH, K.V. & BARON, S. (1965). Laboratory infection with Chikungunya virus. A case report. *Indian Journal of Medical Research* **53**, 610–613.

SHUBLADZE, A.K., GAYDAMOVICH, S.Y. & GARILOV, V.I. (1959). Virologieal studies of laboratory infections with Venezuelan equine eneephalomyelitis. *Problems of Virology* **4**, 305–310.

SILVA, R. & KOPCIOWSKA, L. (1945). Contaminations de laboratoire chez les individus vaccines, dans le typhus exanthematique. *Bulletin de la Societe de Pathologie Exotique* **38**, 320–323.

SIMMONS, P., McORMISH, F., McCULLOUGH, P. *et al.* (1990). Contamination of immunoassay controls with hepatitis C virus. *Lancet* **338**, 1539–1542.

SIMPSON, D.H. & ZUCKERMAN, A.J. (1975). Lassa by letter. *Lancet* **2**, 701.

SIMPSON, D.G. (1965). Tuberculosis first registered at death. *American Review of Respiratory Disease* **92**, 863–869.

SIMPSON, W.M. (1929) *Tularaemia: History, Pathology, Diagnosis and Treatment.* New York: Hobner.

SKINHOJ, P. (1974). Occupational risk in Danish clinical chemistry laboratories. II. Infections. *Scandinavian Journal of Clinical and Laboratory Investigations* **33**, 27–29.

SKINHOJ, P. & SOEBY, M. (1981). Viral hepatitis in Danish health care personnel, 1974–78. *Journal of Clinical Pathology* **34**, 408–411.

SLEPUSHKIN, A.N. (1959). An epidemiological study of laboratory infections with Venezuelan equine encephalomyelitis. *Problems in Virology* **4**, 311–314.

SLOANE, R.A. (1942). Experiments on the airborne spread of tuberculosis. *New York State Journal of Medicine* **42**, 133–138.

SMADEL, J.E. (1951). The hazard of acquiring virus and rickettsial diseases in the laboratory. *American Journal of Public Health* **41**, 788–795.

SMADEL, J.E., GREEN, R.H., PALTAUF, R.M. *et al.* (1942). Lymphocytic choriomeningitis: two human fatalities following an unusual febrile illness. *Proceedings of the Society for Experimental Biology and Medicine* **49**, 683–686.

SMIRNOV, V.P. (1963). From the diary of a physician who sustained experimental plague. *Zhurnal mikrobiologii, epidemiologii i immunologii* **40**, 68–72.

SMITH, A.E. (1992). Formaldehyde. *Occupational Medicine* **42**, 83–88.

SMITH, C.E. (1943). Coccidioidomycosis. *Medical Clinics of North America* **27**, 790–807.

SMITH, C.E., PAPPAGIANIS, D., LEVINE, H.B. *et al.* (1961). Human coccidiomycosis, *Bacteriological Reviews* **25**. 310–320.

SMITH, C.E.G., SIMPSON, D.I.H., BOWEN, E.T.W. *et al.* (1967). Fatal human disease from vervet monkeys. *Lancet* **2**, 1119–1121.

SMITH, C.H. (1958). Accidental infection with trachoma. *British Journal of Ophthalmology* **42**, 721–722.

SMITH, D.J.W., BROWN, H.E. & DERRICK, E.H. (1939). A further series of laboratory infections with Q fever. *Medical Journal of Australia* **26**, 13–14.

SMITH, D.T. & HARRELL, E.R. (1948). Fatal coccidioidomycosis. Case of laboratory infection. *American Review of Tuberculosis* **57**, 368–374.

SMITH, G.S. (1953). Tuberculosis as a necropsy room hazard. *Journal of Clinical Pathology* **6**, 132–134.

SMITH, J.A., SKIDMORE, A.S. & ANDERSON, R.G. (1980). Brucellosis in a laboratory technologist. *Canadian Medical Association Journal* **122**, 1231–1232.

SMITH, J.G., HARRIS, J.S., CONANT, W.F. *et al.* (1955). An epidemic of North American blastomycosis. *Journal of the American Medical Association* **158**,641–646.

SMITH, W. & STUART-HARRIS, C.H. (1936). Influenza infection of man from the ferret. *Lancet* 2, 121–123.

SMITHBURN, K.C., MAHAFFY, A.F., HADDOW, A.J. *et al.* (1949). Rift Valley Fever: accidental infections among laboratory workers. *Journal of Immunology* **62**,213–227.

SNEATH, P.H.A., ABBOTT, J.R. & CUNLIFFE, A.C. (1961). The bacteriology of erysipeloid. *British Medical Journal* 2, 1063- 1066.

SOLTOROVSKY, M., ROBINSON, H.J. & KNIAZUK, H. (1953). Design and operation of a laboratory for experimental tuberculosis. *American Review of Tuberculosis* **68**, 212–219.

SOLTYS, M.A. (1948). Anthrax in a laboratory worker, with observations on the possible source of infection. *Journal of Pathology and Bacteriology* **60**, 253–257.

SONCK, C.E. (1961). Laboratory infections by skin pathogenic fungi in Finland. *Zhurnal Haut Ceschlechtskrift* **31**,117–122.

SONGER, J.F. (1993). Laboratory safety management: the assessment of risk. In: *Laboratory Safety. Principles and Practice.* (Eds D.O. Fleming, J.H. Richardson, J.I. Tulis & D. Vesley). 2nd edn. pp. 257–268. Washington: American Society for Microbiology.

SPICKNALL, C.E., HUEBNER, R.J., FINGER, J.A. *et al.* (1947). Report of an outbreak of Q fever at the National Institutes of Health. *Annals of Internal Medicine* **27**, 28–40.

SPICKNALL, G.G., RYAN, R.W. & CAIN, A. (1956). Laboratory-acquired histoplasmosis. *New England Journal of Medicine* **254**, 210–214.

SPINK, W.W. (1946). Human brucellosis. *Proceedings of the United States Livestock Sanitary Association* **50**, 274–286.

SPINK, W.W. (1956) *The Nature of Brucellosis.* Minnesota.

SPINK, W.W. (1957). The significance of bacterial hypersensitivity in human brucellosis. Studies in infection due to strain 19 *Brucella abortus*. *Annals of Internal Medicine* **47**, 861–874.

SPINK, W.W. & THOMPSON, H. (1953). Human brucellosis caused by *Brucella abortus strain* 19. *Journal of the American Medical Association* **153**, 1162–1165.

SPRAY, R.S. (1927). Diphtheria: a case of laboratory infection. *Journal of American Medical Association* **89**, 112.

STAAT, R.H. & BEAKLEY, J.W. (1968). Evaluation of laminar flow biological safety cabinets. *Applied Microbiology* **16**,1478–1482.

STASZKIEWICZ, C.J., LEWIS, C.M., COLVILLE, J. *et al.* (1991). Outbreak of *Brucella melitensis* among microbiology workers in a community hospital. *Journal of Clinical Microbiology* **29**,287–290.

STECKELBERG, J.M., TERRELL, C.L., EDSON, R.S. (1988). Laboratory-acquired *Salmonella typhimurium* enteritis: association with erythema nodosum and reactive arthritis. *American Journal of Medicine* **85**, 705–707.

STERN, E.L., JOHNSON, J.W., VESLEY, D. *et al.* (1974). Aerosol production associated with clinical laboratory procedures. *American Journal of Clinical Pathology* **62**, 591–600.

STERN, L. (1958). Rift Valley Fever in Rhodesia. Report of a case in a laboratory worker. *Central African Journal of Medicine* **4**, 281–284.

STEWART, J.C. (1904). Pyaemic glanders in a human subject. Report of a recent case of laboratory origin terminating in recovery. *Annals of Surgery* **40**, 109–113.

STILES, W.W. & SAWYER, W.A. (1942). Leptospiral infection (Weil's disease), as an occupational hazard. *Journal of the American Medical Association* **118**, 33–38.

STILLE, W., BOHLE, E., HELM, E. *et al.* (1968). Uber eine durch Cercopithecus aethiops ubertragene Infektionskrankheit ('Grune-Meerkatzen-Krankheit', 'Green Monkey Disease'). *Deutsche Medizinische Wochenschrift* **13**, 475–478.

STOENNER, H.C. & MACLEAN, D. (1958). Leptospirosis (ballum) contracted from Swiss albino mice. *Archives of Internal Medicine* **101**, 606–610.

STOKER, M.G.P. (19S7). Q fever down the drain. *British Medical Journal* 1, 425–426.

STOKES, J. (1953) Q fever in Southern Australia. *Medical Journal of Australia* 2, 779.

STOKES, J.H. (1925) Primary inoculation tuberculosis of the skin with metastasis to regional lymph nodes. *American Jounal of Medical Science* **169**, 722–736.

STROM, J. (1951–52). Toxoplasmosis due to laboratory infection in two adults. *Acta Medica Scandinavica* **139**, 244–252.

STUPPY, C.(1936). Laboratoriumsinfektion mit Malaria tertiene, *Munchener medizinische Wochenschrift* **83**, 932–933.

SUGITA, M, TSUTSUMI, Y., SUCHI, M. *et al.* (1989). High incidence of pulmonary tuberculosis in pathologists at Tokai University: an epidemiological study. *Tokai Journal of Experimental Medicine* **14**, 55–59.

SULKIN, S.E. (1964). Laboratory acquired infections. *Bacteriological Reviews* **25**, 303–211.

SULKIN, S.E. & PIKE, R.M. (1951). Laboratory-acquired infections. *Journal of the American Medical Association* **147**, 1740–1745.

SUTNICK, A.I., LINDON, W.T., MILLMAN, I. *et al.* (1971). Ergasteric endemic hepatitis associated with Australian antigen in a research laboratory. *Annals of Internal Medicine* **75**, 35–40.

SUTTON, L.S. & SHANAHAN, A.J. (1954). Laboratory infections with *Shigella flexneri* 3 and *Shigella sonnei. Journal of the American Medical Association* **154**, 1420–1421.

SYKES, G. (1969). Methods and equipment for sterilization of laboratory apparatus and media. In: *Methods in Microbiology I.* (Eds J. R. Norris & D. W. Ribbons), pp. 77–122. London: Academic Press.

TAYLOR, D.M. (1991). Inactivation of uncommon agents of scrapie, BSE and CJ disease. *Journal of Hospital Infection* **18**, SA 140–146.

TAYLOR, R.E. (1927). A case of diphtheria, probably acquired by laboratory inoculation. *Journal of the American Medical Association* **88**, 1967.

TAYLOR, L.A., BARBEITO, M.S. & GREMILLION, G.G. (1969). Paraformaldehyde for surface sterilization and detoxification. *Applied Microbiology* **17**, 614–618.

TEGESTROM, A. (1942). A case of accidental laboratory tuberculosis infection. *Acta Tuberculosea Scandinavica* **16**, 330–333.

TEJERSON, S. E. & CHERRY, G. B. (1978). The removal of micro-organisms from air by filtration. *Transactions of the Institute of Chemical Engineers* **25**, 89–96.

TEMPLETON, G.L., ILLING, L.A., YOUNG, L. *et al.* (1996). The risk of transmission of *Mycobacterium tuberculosis* at the bedside and during autopsy. *Annals of Internal Medicine* **122**, 922–925.

TERRY, L.L., LEWIS, J.L. & SESSOMS, S.M. (1950). Laboratory infection with *Leishmania donovani*: a case report. *American Journal of Tropical Medicine* **30**, 643–649.

TESH, R.B. & SCHNEIDAU, J.D. (1966). Primary cutaneous histoplasmosis. *New England Journal of Medicine* **275**, 597–599.

THOMPSON, D.W. & KAPLAN, W. (1977). Laboratory acquired sporotrichosis. *Sabouraudia* **15**, 167–170.

THOMSON, S. & INWOOD, M.J. (1976). Laboratory-acquired hepatitis B. *Lancet* 1, 489.

TIGGERT, W.D., BENESON, A.S. & GOCHENOUR, W.S. (1961). Airborne Q fever. *Bacteriological Reviews* **25**, 285–292.

TILLOTSON, J.R., AXELROD, D. & LYMAN, D.O. (1977). Rabies in a laboratory worker—New York. *Morbidity and Mortality Weekly Report* **26**, 183–184, 249–250.

TIMES (1977). Man got typhoid after container toppled over. 25 March.

TOKAREVICH, K.N. (1944). Laboratory infection with typhus exanthematicus. *Zhurnal mikrobiologii, epidemiologii i immunologii* No. 1–2, 26–29.

TOKARS,, J.I, MARCUS, R., CULVER, D.H. *et al.* (1993). Surveillance of HIV infection and zidovudine use among health care workers after occupational exposure to HIV-infected blood. *Annals of Internal Medicine* **118**, 913–919.

TOMLINSON, A.J.H. (1957). Infected air-borne particles liberated on opening screw-capped bottles. *British Medical Journal* 2, 15–17

TOMLINSON, C.C. & BANCROFT, P. (1928). Granuloma coccidioides. *Journal of the American Medical Association* **91**, 947–951.

TOMLINSON, C.C. & BANCROFT, P. (1934). Granuloma coccidioides. *Journal of the American Medical Association* **102**, 36–36.

TREES, D. (1992). Laboratory-acquired infection with *Haemophilus ducreyi* type strain CIP 542. *Medical Microbiology Letters* **1**, 330–331.

TREVER, R.W., CLUFF, L.E., PEELER, R.W. *et al.* (1959). Brucellosis—laboratory acquired acute infections. *Archives of Internal Medicine* **103**, 381.

TREXLER, P. C., EDMOND, R. T. & EVANS, B. (1979). Negative pressure plastic isolator for patients with dangerous infections. *British Medical Journal* 2, 559.

TREXLER, P.C. & GILMOUR, A.M. (1983). Use of flexible film isolators in performing potentially hazardous necropsies. *Journal of Clinical Pathology* **36**, 527–529.

TREXLER, P. C. & REYNOLDS, R. J. (1957). Flexible film apparatus for rearing and use of germ-free animals. *Applied Microbiology* **5**, 406–412

TRIMBLE, J.R. & DOUCETTE, J. (1956). Primary cutaneous coccidioidomycosis. Report of a case of laboratory infection. *Archives of Dermatology* **74**, 405–410.

TRUMBELL, M.L. & GREINER, D.J. (1951). Homologous serum jaundice - an occupational hazard. *Journal of the American Medical Association* **145**, 965.

TSAI, T.F. (1987). Hemorrhagic fever with renal syndrome; mode of transmission to humans. *Laboratory Animals* **37**, 428–430.

TULLIS, J.K., GERSH, I., JENNEY, E. *et al.* (1947). Tissue pathology of experimental tsutsugamushi disease and the report of human case acquired in the laboratory. *American Journal of Tropical Medicine* **27**, 245–269.

TUNG, T. & ZIA, S. H. (1936). Undulant fever among laboratory workers; report of three cases with bacteriological study. *Chinese Medical Journal* **50**, 1203–1210.

TURNER, A.G., WILKINS, J.R. & CRADDOCK, J.G. (1975). Bacterial aerosolisation from an ultrasonic cleaner. *Journal of Clinical Microbiology* **1**, 289–293.

UHLENHUTH, P. & GROSSMAN, H. (1926). Die Aetiologie und Epidemiologie der Ansteckden gelbsucht (Weilschen Krankheit) im Lichte Experimenteller Untersuchngen uber die Typenfrage ihreserrgers (*Spirochaeta icterogenses*). *Klinische Wochenschrift* **5**, 1113–1117.

UHLENHUTH, P. & ZIMMERMAN, E. (1933). Weisse (Zahme) Ratte els Ubertragerin des Erregers der Weilschen Krankheit (*Spirochaeta icterogenses*). *Deutsche medizinische Wochenschrift* **59**, 1393-1395.

UHLENHUTH, P. & ZIMMERMAN, E. (1934). Uber eine Laboratoriumsinfektion mit Weilscher Krankheit Sowie uber die Serumtherapie dieset Erkrankung. *Medizinische Klinik* **30**, 464–467.

UMENAI, T., LEE, H.W., LEE, P.W. *et al.* (1979). Korean haemorrhagic fever in staff in an animal laboratory. *Lancet* **1**, 1314–1316.

UNITED NATIONS COMMITTEE OF EXPERTS ON THE TRANSPORT OF DANGEROUS GOODS, Division 2 (1996). Infectious Substances 10th ed. revised. New York: UN.

US TREASURY (1950). Epidemiology. Laboratory infections. *Public Health Reports* **65**, 16.

VAN CLEVE, J. V. (1936). Coccidioidal granuloma. *Journal of the Kansas Medical Society* **37**, 54–55.

VAN DEN ENDE, M., LOCKET, S., HARGREAVES, W.H. *et al.* (1946). Accidental laboratory infection with tsutsugamushi rickettsia. *Lancet* **2**, 4–7.

VAN DEN ENDE, M., STUART-HARRIS, C.H., HARRIES, E.H.R. *et al.* (1943). Laboratory infection with murine typhus. *Lancet* **1**, 328–332.

VAN DER GROEN, G., TREXLER, P.C. & PATTYN, S.R. (1980). Negative pressure flexible film isolator for work with Class IV viruses in a maximum security laboratory. *Journal of Infection* **2**, 165–170.

VAN GOMPEL, A., VAN DEN ENDEN, E., VAN DEN ENDEN, J. *et al.* (1993) Laboratory infection with *Schistosoma mansonii*. *Transactions of the Royal Society for Tropical Medicine and Hygiene* **87**, 554.

VAN METRE, T.E. & KADULL, P.J. (1959). Laboratory-acquired tularemia in vaccinated individuals: a report of 62 cases. *Annals of Internal Medicine* **50**, 621 632

VAN SOESTBERGEN, A.A. (1957). Laboratory-acquired toxoplasmosis. *Nederlands Tijdschrift voor Geneeskunde* **101**, 1649.

VANSELOW, N.A., DAVEY, W.N. & BOCOBO, F.C. (1962). Acute pulmonary histoplasmosis in laboratory workers: report of two cases. *Journal of Laboratory and Clinical Medicine* **59**, 236–243.

VARELA-DIAZ, V.M., IMAS, B., SOTO, B. *et al.* (1974). Laboratory investigations on neuro-paralytic accidents associated with suckling mouse brain rabies vaccine. *Annals d'Immunologie* **125**, 925–938.

VARMA, A.J. (1982). Malaria acquired by accidental inoculation. *Canadian Medical Journal* **126**, 1419–1420.

VENJATRAMAN, J.T. & FERNANDEZ, G. (1997). Exercise, immunity and aging. *Aging (Milano)* **91**, 42–56.

VESLEY, A.K. & CHAGA. A.H. (1989). Laboratory acquired brucellosis. *Journal of Hygiene and Infection Control* **14**, 69–71.

VESLEY, D.L. (1995). Respiratory protection devices. *American Journal of Infection Control* **32**, 165–168.

VESLEY, D. & HARTMANN, H.M. (1988). Laboratory-acquired infections and injuries in clinical laboratories: a 1986 survey. *American Journal of Public Health* **78**, 1213–1215.

VETTER J.F. (1977). Microbial aerosols from a freezing microtome. *American Society of Clinical Microbiologists*. Summary report, January.

VON BRUNN, W. (1919). Uber die Uhrsachen die Haufigkeit des Vorkommens des Rotzes beim Menschen. Sowie über Massregeln zur Verhütung der Rotzubertragungen *Vierteljahrrschrift für gerichtliche Medizin und Offentliches Sanitätswesen (Berlin)* **58**, 134–161.

VON GARA, P. (1931). Eine Laboratoriumsinfektion mit Typhusbazillen. *Archiv für Hygiene und Bakteriologie* **107**, 105–107.

VON MAGNUS, H. (1950). Laboratory infection with St. Louis encephalitis virus. *Acta Pathologica and Microbiologica Scandinavica* **27**, 276–286.

WAKERLIN, G.E. (1932). Laboratory infection in man by the *Spirochaeta pallidum* of experimental rabbit syphilis. *Journal of the American Medical Association* **98**, 479.

WALDRON, H.A. (1997) Role of the occupational health department. In: *Occupational; Blood-borne Infections.* (Eds C H. Collins & D.A. Kennedy), pp. 219–232. Oxford: CAB International.

WALKER, J.E. (1928). Infection of laboratory worker with Bacillus influenza. *Journal of Infectious Disease* **43**, 300–305.

WARD, B.Q. (1948). The apparent involvement of *Vibrio fetus* in an infection of man. *Journal of Bacteriology* **55**, 113–114.

WEBB, H.E., CONOLLY, J.H., KANE, F.F. *et al.* (1968). Laboratory infections with louping ill with associate encephalitis. *Lancet* 2, 255–258.

WEBBER, W.J. (1956). Laboratory infection with *Mycobacterium tuberculosis. Journal of Medical Laboratory Technology* **13**, 489.

WEDUM, A.C. (1950). Nonautomatic pipetting devices for the microbiological laboratory. *Journal of Laboratory and Clinical Medicine* 35, 648–651.

WEDUM, A.G. (1953). Bacteriological safety. *American Journal of Public Health* **43**, 1428–1437.

WEDUM, A.G., BARKLEY, W.E. & HELLMAN, A. (1972). Handling infectious agents. *Journal of the American Veterinary Association* **161**, 1557–1567.

WEDUM, A.G. (1978). (Level 4 lab at Fort Detrick—423 cases of LAI in 25 years.) In: *Biorevolution* (Ed. R. Hutton). New American Library.

WEDUM, A.G. (1964). Laboratory safety in research with aerosols. *Public Health Reports* **79**, 619–633.

WEGMAN, P. & PLEMPEL, M. (1974). Das Krankheitsbild der Coccidiodomykose, dargesfellt an einer Laboratoriumsinfektion. *Deutsche Medizinische Wochenschrift* **99**, 1653–1656.

WEILBACHER, J.O. & MOSS, E. S. (1938), Tularaemia following injury while performing post-mortem examination on a human case. *Journal of Laboratory and Clinical Medicine* 24, 34–38.

WEISS, S.H., SAXINGER, W.C., RECHTMAN, D. *et al.* (1985). HTLV-III infection among health care workers. Association with needlestick injuries. *Journal of the American Medical Association* **254**, 2089–2093.

WEISSENBACHER, M.C., SAXINGER, W.C., RECHTMAN, D. *et al.* (1978). Inapparent infections with Junin virus among laboratory workers. *Journal of Infectious Disease* **137**, 309–313.

WELCKER, A. (1938). Laboratoriumsinfektionen mit Weilscher Krankheit, *Zentralblatt fur Bakteriologie*, Abt. 1. Orig. **141**, 400–410.

WELLS, W.F. (1934). Airborne infection II. Droplets and droplet nuclei, *American Journal of Hygiene* **20**, 611–618.

WELLS, W.F. (1955) *Airborne Contagion and Air Hygiene.* Cambridge, MA: Harvard University Press.

WELLS, W.F., RATCLIFFE, H.L. & CRUMB, C. (1948). on the mechanics of droplet nuclei infection. *American Journal of Hygiene* **47**, 11–28.

WENNER, H.A. & PAUL, J.R. (1974). Fatal infection with poliomyelitis virus in a laboratory technician. *American Journal of Medical Science* **213**, 9–18.

WESTWOOD, J.C.N., CHAUDHARY, R.K. & PERRY, E. (1973). Short term inapparent infection after accidental injection of hepatitis B-positive serum. *Lancet* 2, 1395.

WHALE, K. (1986). Is it time to rethink 'high risk' labelling? *Journal of Clinical Pathology* **39**, 41.

WHERRY, W.B. & LAMB, B.H. (1914). Infection of man with *Bacterium tularense. Journal of Infectious Disease* **15**, 331–340.

WHITWELL, F., TAYLOR, P.J. & OLIVER, A.J. (1957). Hazards to laboratory staff in centrifuging screw-capped containers. *Journal of Clinical Pathology* **10**, 88–91.

WHO (1979). Safety measures in microbiology. Minimum standards of laboratory safety. *World Health Organization Weekly Epidemiological Record* No. 44, 340 342

WHO (1980) Guidelines for the management of accidents involving microorganisms: a WHO memorandum. *Bulletin of the World Health Organization* **58**, 245–256.

WHO (1987) *Acceptability of Cell Substrates for the Production of Biologicals.* WHO Technical Series No. 74. Geneva: World Health Organization.

WHO (1993). *Laboratory Biosafety Manual*, 2nd edn, Geneva: World Health Organization.
WHO (1995) *Biosafety Guidelines for Personnel Engaged in the Production of Vaccines and Biological Products for Medical Use*. Geneva: World Health Organization.
WHO (1996) *Report on the Tuberculosis Epidemic*. Geneva: World Health Organization.
WHO (1997a) *Safety in Health-care Laboratories*. Geneva: World Health Organization.
WHO (1997b) *Guidelines for the Safe Transport of Infectious Substances and Diagnostic Specimens*. Geneva: World Health Organization.
WICHT, J.F. (1969). Unusual case of infection with *Corynebacterium diphtheria*. *British Medical Journal* 2, 1082–1083.
WIEBEL, H. (1937). Uber louping ill beim Menschen. *Klinische Wochenschrift* 16, 632–634.
WILDER, W.H. & McCULLoUGH, C.P. (1914). Sporotrichosis of the eye. *Journal of the American Medical Association* 63, 1156–1160.
WILKS, S. & POLAND, A. (1862). Disease of the skin caused by post-mortem examinations, or Verruca necrogenica. *Guy's Hospital Reports*, Series 3, 8, 263.
WILL, R.G., IRONSIDE, J.W., ZEIDLER, M. *et al.* 1996) A new variant of Creutzfeldt-Jacob disease in the UK. *Lancet* 347, 921–925.
WILLEKE, K., QIAN, Y., GRINSHPUN, S. *et al.* (1996). Penetration of air-borne microorganisms through a surgical mask and a dust-mite respirator. *American Industrial Hygiene Association Journal* 57, 348–355.
WILLET, F.M. & WEISS, A. (1945). Coccidioidomycosis in Southern California; report of a new endemic and with a review of 100 cases. *Annals of Internal Medicine* 23, 349–375.
WILLIAMS, J.L., INNIS, B.T., BURKOT, T.R. *et al.* (1983). Falciparum malaria: accidental transmission to man by mosquitoes after infection with culture-derived gametocytes. *American Journal of Tropical Medicine and Hygiene* 32, 657–659.
WILLIAMS, R.E.O. (1981). In pursuit of safety. *Journal of Clinical Pathology* 34, 232–239.
WILLIAMS, R.E.O. & LIDWELL, O.M. (1957). A protective cabinet for handling infective material in the laboratory. *Journal of Clinical Pathology* 10, 400–402.
WILLIS, M.J. & FURCOLOW, M. L. (1956). Laboratory infections with *Histoplasma capsulatum*. *Public Health Monographs* No. 39, 48–51.
WILSON, G.S. & MILES, A.A. (1975). *Topley and Wilson's Principles of Bacteriology, Virology and Immunity*, 3rd. edn. p.1571. London: Edward Arnold
WILSON, J.W., CAWLEY, E.P., WEIDMAN, F.D. *et al.* (1955) Primary cutaneous North American blastomycosis. *Archives of Dermatology* 71, 39–45.
WINKLER, W.G., FASHINELL, T.R., LEFFINGWELL, L. *et al.* (1973). Airborne rabies transmission in a laboratory worker. *Journal of the American Medical Association* 226, 1219–1221.
WOLBACH, S. B. (1919). Studies on Rocky Mountain Spotted Fever. *Journal of Medical Research* 41, 1–197, 263.
WONG, D. & NYE, K. (1991). Microbial flora on doctors' white coats. *British Medical Journal* 303, 1602.
WONG, T.W., CHAN, Y.C., YAP, E.H. *et al* (1988). Serological evidence of hantavirus infection in laboratory rats and personnel. *British Journal of Industrial Medicine* 43, 500–501.
WOO, J.H. (1991). A case of laboratory-acquired murine typhus. *Korean Journal of Internal Medicine* 5, 118–120.
WOOLPERT, O., MARSH, H.F. & YAW, O.F. (1939). Bacillary dysentery resulting from an accidental laboratory infection. *Journal of the American Medical Association* 113, 753–755.
WORK, T.H., TRAPIDO, H., MURPHY, D.P.N. *et al.* (1957). Kyasanur forest disease: a preliminary report on the nature of the infection and clinical manifestations in human beings. *Indian Journal of Medical Science* 11, 619–645.
WORMALD, P.J. (1950). Salmonella infection in a post-mortem room. *Monthly Bulletin of the Ministry of Health and Public Health Laboratory Service* 9, 28–30.
WRIGHT, A.E. (1985). Health care of laboratory personnel. In: *Handbook of Laboratory Health and Safety Measures* (Ed. S.B. Pal). pp. 61–78. Lancaster: MTP Press.
WRIGHT, A.E. (1987). Health care in the laboratory. In: *Safety in Clinical and Biomedical Laboratories* (Ed. C. H. Collins). London: pp. 118–132. Chapman & Hall.
WRIGHT, L.J., BARKER, L.F., MICKENBERG, I.D. *et al.* (1968). Laboratory-acquired typhus fevers. *Annals of Internal Medicine* 63, 731–738.
WRIGHT, W.H. (1985) Laboratory-acquired toxoplasmosis. *American Journal of Clinical Pathology* 28, 1.
WU, L.T., CHUN, J.W.H. & POLLITZER, R. (1923). Clinical observations upon the Manchurian plague epidemic, 1920–1921. *Journal of Hygiene* 21, 289–306.

WU, L.T. (1926). *A Treatise on Pneumonic Plague*. Geneva: League of Nations.

YATOM, J. (1946) An outbreak of conjunctivitis in man associated with the virus of Newcastle disease. *Refuah Veterinarith* **3**, 69–70.

ZERVOS, M.J. & BOSTIC, G. (1997). Exposure to brucella in the laboratory. *Lancet* **349**, 651.

ZIMMERMAN, W.J. (1976). Prevalence of *Toxoplasma gondii* antibodies among veterinary college staff and students. *Public Healh Reports* **91**, 526–532.

ZLATGOROFF, S. J. (1909). Ein Fall von Laboratoriumsinfektion mit einem aus dem Wasser Gewonnenen Choleravibrio. *Berliner Klinische Wochenschrift* **46**, 1972–1973.

Index